INEQUALITIES, YOUTH, DEMOCRACY AND THE PANDEMIC

This book brings together studies from various locations to examine the growing social problems that have been brought to the fore by the COVID-19 outbreak. Employing both qualitative, theoretical, and quantitative methods, it presents the impact of the pandemic in different settings, shedding light on political and cultural realities around the world. With attention to inequalities rooted in race and ethnicity, economic conditions, gender, disability, and age, it considers different forms of marginalization and examines the ongoing disjunctions that increasingly characterize contemporary democracies from a multilevel perspective.

The book addresses original analyses and approaches from a global perspective on the COVID-19 pandemic, its governance, and its effects in different geographies. These analyses are organized around three main axes: 1) how COVID-19 pandemic worsened social, racial/ethnic, and economic inequalities, including variables such as migration status, gender, and disability; 2) how the pandemic impacted youth and how younger generations cope with public health alarms, and containment measures; 3) how the pandemic posed a challenge to democracy, reshaped the political agenda, and the debate in the public sphere. Contributions from around the world show how local and national issues may overlap on a global scale, laying the foundation for connected sociologies. Based on qualitative as well as quantitative empirical analysis on various categories of individuals and groups, this edited volume reflects on the sociological aspects of current planetary crises which will continue to be at the core of our societies.

A wide-ranging, international volume that focuses on both unexpected social changes and new forms of agency in response to a period of crisis, *Inequalities, Youth, Democracy and the Pandemic* will appeal to scholars with interests in the sociology of health, social problems, and inequalities.

Simone Maddanu is Assistant Professor of Instruction at the University of South Florida, USA. His research explores social movements, immigration, Islam in Europe, common goods, and modernity. He is co-author of *Restless Cities on the Edge: Collective Actions, Immigration and Populism* (2021) and co-editor of *Global Modernity from Coloniality to Pandemic: A Cross-Disciplinary Perspective* (2022).

Emanuele Toscano is Associate Professor of Sociology at Marconi University of Rome, Italy. His research focuses on inequalities, subjectivation processes, and social movements. He is editor of *Researching Far-Right Movements: Ethics, Methodologies, and Qualitative Inquiries* (Routledge, 2019) and author of numerous journal articles and book chapters.

THE COVID-19 PANDEMIC SERIES

Series Editor: J. Michael Ryan

This series examines the impact of the COVID-19 pandemic on individuals, communities, countries, and the larger global society from a social scientific perspective. It represents a timely and critical advance in knowledge related to what many believe to be the greatest threat to global ways of being in more than a century. It is imperative that academics take their rightful place alongside medical professionals as the world attempts to figure out how to deal with the current global pandemic, and how society might move forward in the future. This series represents a response to that imperative.

Titles in this Series:

Women and COVID-19
A Clinical and Applied Sociological Focus on Family, Work and Community
Edited by Mariam Seedat-Khan and Johanna O. Zulueta

State-Society Relations around the World through the Lens of the COVID-19 Pandemic
Rapid-Test
Edited by Federica Duca and Sarah Meny-Gibert

Contagion Capitalism
Pandemics in the Corporate Age
Sean Creaven

Modernity and the Pandemic
Decivilization, Imperialism, and COVID-19
Sean Creaven

Inequalities, Youth, Democracy and the Pandemic
Edited by Simone Maddanu and Emanuele Toscano

INEQUALITIES, YOUTH, DEMOCRACY AND THE PANDEMIC

Edited by Simone Maddanu and Emanuele Toscano

Routledge
Taylor & Francis Group
LONDON AND NEW YORK

Designed cover image: © Marcelo Renda

First published 2024
by Routledge
4 Park Square, Milton Park, Abingdon, Oxon OX14 4RN

and by Routledge
605 Third Avenue, New York, NY 10158

Routledge is an imprint of the Taylor & Francis Group, an informa business

British Library Cataloguing-in-Publication Data
A catalogue record for this book is available from the British Library

ISBN: 978-1-032-60565-4 (hbk)
ISBN: 978-1-032-60570-8 (pbk)
ISBN: 978-1-003-45968-2 (ebk)

DOI: 10.4324/9781003459682

Typeset in Sabon
by Taylor & Francis Books

CONTENTS

ILLUSTRATIONS

Figures

Tables

PREFACE

On 5 May, 2023, the WHO declared the end of the COVID-19 pandemic: worldwide collected data at that time say that 7 million people died, while the virus is still killing and still changing. This book wants to provide a standstill understanding of an exceptional pandemic and its multi-geographical localized extents, its repercussions on individuals and groups, perceptions, imaginaries, and narratives.

Doing sociology in an age of crisis, and more specifically exploring the extent of the pandemic in our societies, has meant dealing constantly with different analysis on a planetary scale. Our work aimed to emphasize a multilevel and multi-approach view. The latter, more particularly, resulted in connecting different sociologies and their methods, frameworks, and lenses. We hope that the reader will benefit from this variety of contributions; we strongly encourage creative synthesis when necessary, allowing opposite perspectives to unfold.

As always, many colleagues and friends must be acknowledged for this work, particularly those who actively participated in fruitful discussions, in public or privately. Beside the contributors that took part in this edited book, we want to thank Ana Arán Sánchez, Breno Bringel, Aishwarya Bhuta, Smita Chakraborty, Vishal Chaudhari, Richard Cooper, Isabella De Vivo, Kalpana Dixit, Elisabeth Dobbins, Milena Gammaitoni, Debapriya Ganguly, Sara Green, Santosh Kumar, Carole Perrot, Geoffrey Pleyers, Shweta Rani, Vera Lucía Ríos Cepeda, Virginia Romano, Maria Livia Stefanescu, Magdalena Szaflarski, Sai Thakur, Magdalena Szaflarski, and Sabrina Zajak.

In memory of our fathers.

The editors

31 July 2023

CONTRIBUTORS

Antonio Álvarez-Benavides holds a Ph.D. in Sociology from the Complutense University of Madrid and the School for Advanced Studies in the Social Sciences in Paris. He is currently a María Zambrano Research Fellow at the Department of Sociology III (Social Trends), National University of Distance Education (UNED) and researcher at the Society and Politics Studies Group (GESP) and at the Contemporary Sociocultural Studies Group (GRESCO). He has been adjunct professor at John Jay College of Criminal Justice (CUNY), Carlos III University of Madrid and University of Valladolid. He has participated in more than twenty research and social intervention projects in both the public and private spheres and has more than thirty publications. His work deals with the sociology of social movements, sociological theory, research methodologies and social intervention.

Rosario Aparicio holds a Ph.D. in Demography from the University of Campinas and an MA in Economics from the National Autonomous University of Mexico. From 2018 to 2020, she was a postdoctoral fellow at the Seminar for Labor and Inequalities from El Colegio de México. She is a specialist in ethnic demography, and her main lines of research are gender violence, ethnicity, indigenous women, labor markets, and discrimination. She was the coordinator of the Latin American Population Association's Demographic Network of Indigenous and Afro-Descendent Peoples (PIAFAL) from 2020 to 2022 and a member of the Latin American Interdisciplinary Gender Network (LAIGN) based at Yale University.

Anil Yasin Ar, Tecnológico de Monterrey, MEXICO – earned his Ph.D. at Southern New Hampshire University. His research mainly revolves around corporate social responsibility (CSR), internationalization of emerging market multinationals, sustainability, and sustainability education in higher education institutions. He currently teaches at the International Business and Logistics Department at Tecnologico de Monterrey, Queretaro campus. He published several scholarly articles and book chapters.

Demetrio Gómez Ávila is a leading Rroma human rights activist who has worked for over three decades advocating for social justice and Romani rights through decolonial and intersectional perspectives. During his activist career, he became a founding member of the "Forum of European Roma Young People", the first International Romani young organization in Europe, and President of "Ververipen, Rroms for Diversity", a pioneering Spanish Romani LGTB+ organization. He has served as an expert and trainer for the Council of Europe, the European Commission, and other organizations and institutions connected to racial justice, antifascism and the fight against xenophobia and discrimination.

Erika Busse, Ph.D., is Associate Professor in the Department of Sociology at Macalester College. Busse studies the social construction of motherhood in the context of migration. Her research interests are connected by an underlying focus on the relationship between inequality regimes and social justice. Her scholarship examines the experiences of transnational mothers juggling gender, class, and racial hierarchies in both their home countries and the countries of reception, and the ways in which they engage in homemaking in the process. Her work has been published in journals such as Sociology of Race and Ethnicity; Ethnic and Racial Studies; and Diversities.

Maria Carmela Catone is Senior Lecturer in Sociology at the Department of Political and Social Studies, University of Salerno. Her area of expertise includes in particular the new epistemological and methodological frontiers of social research in the digital era, the sociological educational paths also in the light of the interconnections between technologies and ways of constructing knowledge, the analysis of integration and social inclusion processes.

Enzo Colombo is Professor of Sociology of Culture and Intercultural Relations at the Department of Social and Political Sciences, University of Milan, Italy. His research interests lie in everyday multiculturalism, active citizenship, cultural aspects of the globalisation process, young adults' identification and civic participation. He has published in top peer-reviewed journals. He is author of *Framing Social Theory, Reassembling the lexicon of Contemporary Social Sciences* (Routledge 2022, eds with P. Rebughini); *Youth and the Politics of the Present. Coping with Complexity and Ambivalence* (Routledge, 2019: eds. with P. Rebughini); *Children of Immigrants in a Globalized World: A Generational Experience* (Palgrave, 2012; with P. Rebughini), *Sociologia delle relazioni interculturali* (Carocci, 2020) and *Le società multiculturali* (Carocci, 2011).

Gabriella D'Ambrosio received her Ph.D. in Methodology of Social Sciences at Sapienza University of Rome in 2018 – Department of Communication and Social Research with a thesis on the study of marital instability in Italy using the social simulation approach. Her research interests span on family issues, immigration flows and higher education systems.

Rubén Díez García is Professor at the Department of Applied Sociology at the Complutense University of Madrid (Spain). He is a specialist in applied social research and data analysis by the Centro de Investigaciones Sociológicas (CIS). His main lines of research focus on the study of civil society and civic culture, risks and social reflexivity, emotions and youth activism. His publications include the book Democracy, dignity and social movements, together with E. Laraña, published by the CIS in 2017.

Kirstie Lynn Dobbs, Ph.D., is an assistant professor of practice in political science and public policy and in the Early College Program at Merrimack College. Her research analyzes various modes of youth political participation, such as voter behavior, involvement in political parties, and civic engagement through protests and civil society.

Laura Flamand is a research professor at El Colegio de México and a National System of Researchers member. She is also the founding director of the Network for the Study of Inequalities. She holds a Ph.D. in Political Science from the University of Rochester. Her research focuses on social and gender inequalities, intergovernmental public policies, especially in the health sector, and applied statistics. She has published six books, more than 40 peer-reviewed articles, and book chapters. She has received research fellowships from Oxford University, the Woodrow Wilson Center in Washington D.C., and the Maria Sibylla Merian Centre Conviviality-Inequality in Latin America.

Theodoros Fouskas is an Assistant Professor of Sociology with emphasis on Migration and Public Health at the Department of Public Health Policy, University of West Attica, Greece. He combines studies on migration, migrant health and access to healthcare, health disparities, precarious employment, domestic work and care, racial and ethnic inequalities, migrant community organizations, pro-/anti-migrant mobilizations, social integration and exclusion. Latest authored monograph: 2021 Precarious Lives of Maids, Nannies and Caregivers in Greece, Nova Science Publishers. Latest edited volume monograph: 2021 Immigrants, Asylum Seekers and Refugees in Times of Crises (Volume A & B), EPLO Publications. Latest research projects: 2020–2022 "Voices of Immigrant Women" (Erasmus+/EU); 2021–2022 "Migrant and Refugee integration into local societies during the COVID-19 pandemic in Spain and Greece" (GSRI/UNIWA); 2022–2023 "From reception, to gender empowerment and social integration of female refugees, asylum seekers and immigrants during the COVID-19 pandemic in Athens" (Ministry of Migration and Asylum/Panteion University).

Stephanie Garrone-Shufran, Ph.D., is an assistant professor of education in the Winston School of Education and Social Policy at Merrimack College. Her research is focused on English as a Second Language teachers' advocacy for emergent bilingual students in K-12 schools and the integration of language instruction across the curriculum.

Lotta Haikkola (Ph.D.) works as Academy Research Fellow at the Finnish Youth Research Network. Her current project explores young people working in the logistics sector. Her research focuses on young people, work, and activation policies and she also specializes on young migrants.

Konsta Happonen (Ph.D.) works as a Statistical Researcher at the Finnish Youth Research Network. Previously an ecologist, he has experience in applying advanced statistical methods.

Alix Helfer (M.Soc.Sci) works as a Researcher at the Finnish Youth Research Network. She has been studying the experiences of young persons during the COVID-19 pandemic. Previous research focuses on mental health and substance use treatment services in Finland.

Laura M. Hsu, Ed.D., is an associate professor of human development and human services in the Winston School of Education and Social Policy at Merrimack College. Her research focuses on how relationships influence identity development and in the role of identity in learning processes.

Francisco Jiménez Aguilar is Juan de la Cierva Postdoctoral Fellow at the Department of Contemporary History of the University of the Basque Country, Spain. He was Visiting researcher at The University of Sheffield and Complutense University of Madrid. He holds an International Ph.D. in history and arts from the University of Granada. That dissertation explored discourses and subjectivities on masculinities during the first decades of Franco regime. A Forthcoming book based on its conclusions will be published this year. His research interests Include women, gender, fascism, far right, and antifeminism in modern Spain.

Premalatha Karupiah is an associate professor of sociology at the School of Social Sciences, Universiti Sains Malaysia, Penang, Malaysia. She teaches research methodology and statistics. Her research interests are in the areas of beauty culture, femininity, Tamil movies, and issues related to the Indian diaspora. In 2022 she co-edited a book entitled *A Kaleidoscope of Malaysian Indian Women's Lived Experiences: Gender-Ethnic Intersectionality and Cultural Socialisation.*

Jenni Lahtinen (M. Soc.Sci) is a doctoral candidate at the University of Eastern Finland. Her dissertation deals with vocational students' well-being from the perspective of Capability-approach and ecological sustainability. Previously she has studied young people's experiences and well-being during the COVID-19 pandemic.

Simone Maddanu earned his Ph.D. in Sociology at the School for Advanced Studies in Social Sciences (EHESS) of Paris (France), and he is currently assistant professor of instruction at the University of South Florida, Department of Sociology and Interdisciplinary Social Sciences where he teaches Contemporary Social Problems, Sociology, and Classical Theory. He authored several books in three different languages. Recently, he edited the book (with H. N. Akil) *Global Modernity from Coloniality to Pandemic: A cross-disciplinary perspective*, Amsterdam University Press (2022); and authored the monograph (2021) *Restless Cities on the Edge: Collective Actions, Immigration and Populism*, Palgrave Macmillan (with AL Farro).

Antonio Montañés Jiménez is anthropologist and sociologist with an interested in the study of Rroma people, Christianity, and social movements. He is a Margarita Salas Postdoctoral Fellow affiliated with the School of Anthropology and Museum Ethnography at the University of Oxford and member of St. Antony's College (Oxford). Previously, he held a ESRC postdoctoral fellowship at the University of St. Andrews.

Veronica Montes is an Associate Professor in the Department of Sociology. Montes earned her doctorate from the University of California at Santa Barbara and was an Andrew W. Mellon Postdoctoral Teaching Fellow at the University of Southern California. Her research falls into two areas: immigration from Mexico and Central America to the United States and the intersection between gender, belonging, and migration. Her work has been published in journals such as Gender & Society; Gender, Place and Culture; Apuntes; Latino Studies Journal, and several chapters in edited volumes. Currently, Montes is working on a book examining the intersection between transnational motherhood, family separation due to deportation, and migration.

Beatriz Padilla holds a Ph.D. and a Master's in Sociology from the University of Illinois at Urbana-Champaign; a master in Public Affairs from the University of Texas at Austin, and a Licenciatura (BA) in Political Sciences and Public Administration from the National University of Cuyo, Argentina. She is Associate Professor in the Department of Sociology of the University of South Florida and the Director of the Institute for the Study of Latin America and the Caribbean. She is also affiliated to the Centro de Investigação e Estudos de Sociologia (CIES), Instituto Universitario de Lisboa (ISCTE-IUL), Portugal. She has coordinated many research projects, including The Venezuelan Humanitarian Crisis: Migration,

Trauma and Resilience, Trajectories of Refuge: gender, intersectionality and public policies in Portugal; "Multilevel governance of cultural diversity in a comparative perspective: EU-Latin America – GOVDIV"; Health and Citizenship: Gaps and needs in intercultural health care to immigrant mothers, Conviviality and Super-diversity in Lisbon and Granada, and "Understanding the practice and developing the concept of welfare bricolage». She has published in the Journal of Ethnic and Migration Studies, International Migrations, Ethnic and Racial Studies, Health Policy, among others. Her main research interests are migrations, public policies, health and diversity, gender, race, ethnicity and discrimination.

Fiorenzo Parziale is Senior Lecturer in Sociology of Culture in the Department of Communication and Social Research, Sapienza-University of Rome. His research program mainly focuses on the following topics: educational inequalities, social class subcultures and ideological conflict. These topics are developed through a perspective combining sociology of culture, sociology of knowledge and sociology of education. Some of his recent articles appear in Italian Journal Sociology of Education, Scuola Democratica and Athens Journal of Social Sciences.

Juan Ignacio Piovani is currently a Professor of Social Research Methods at the National University of La Plata and a Principal Researcher at the National Scientific and Technical Research Council (CONICET) and at Mecila (Maria Sibylla Merian Centre Conviviality-Inequality in Latin America). He holds a Ph. D. in Social Science Methodology from Sapienza Università di Roma and a MSc in Advanced Social Research Methods and Statistics from City University London. His research focuses on social inequalities and on the Social Science System in Argentina

Paola Rebughini is professor of Sociology of Culture and Social Theory at the Department of Social and Political Sciences, University of Milan, Italy. Her research interests lie in social theory, agency in everyday life, social movements, cultural aspects of globalization processes and youth civic participation. She has published widely in top peer-reviewed journals. Her latest books are *Children of Immigrants in a Globalized World: A Generational Experience* (Palgrave 2012, with E. Colombo); *In un mondo pluralista: grammatiche dell'interculturalità*, Utet, 2014); *Youth and the Politics of the Present: Coping with Complexity and Ambivalence* (Routledge 2019, eds. with E. Colombo); *Sociologia delle differenze: genere, cultura, natura*, (Carocci, 2022); *Framing Social Theory: Reassembling the Lexicon of Contemporary Social Sciences* (Routledge 2022, eds with E. Colombo).

Raquel Rojas is currently a visiting lecturer at the Institute for Latin American Studies at the Freie Universität (FU) Berlin. She holds a Ph.D. in Sociology from the FU Berlin and a MA in Social Sciences from the Humboldt University of

Berlin. Raquel is originally from Paraguay, where she earned a Specialist Degree in Social Development from the Facultad Latinoamericana de Ciencias Sociales (FLACSO) and a BA in Social Sciences from the Universidad Nacional de Asunción. Her research focuses on inequalities and intersectionality, labor relations and care work. She was a Mecila Junior Fellow in 2021.

Kenjiro Sakakibara is a senior researcher at Japan's National Institute of Population and Social Security Research. His research interests include the sociology of disability, disability theory, and disability statistics that investigate the social exclusion of disabled people. He has published a book, *Social Inclusion and the Body: Disability Definitions and Different Treatments Following Disability Antidiscrimination Legislation* (in Japanese), which won the Japanese Young Sociologist Award (Book Division). In addition, he has edited *The Sociology of Disability as a New Perspective: From the Social Model to the Sociological Reflection* (in Japanese).

Marianna Knothe Sanfelicio is a Graduate Research Student at the Department of Anthropology at the University of São Paulo. She is part of the Research Group on Cemeterial Studies at the Laboratório do Núcleo de Antropologia Urbana (LabNAU – USP); part of the Laboratório de Imagem e Som em Antropologia (LISA), and part of the study group on Memory, Grief and Testimony at Faculdade de Educação da Universidade de São Paulo (FEUSP). Her interests focus on the intersection between Urban and Visual Anthropology, working with themes of body, mourning, death, cemeterial spaces, photography and cinema.

Ariel Sribman Mittelman, Ph.D. in Political Science by the University of Salamanca (Spain). Has lectured at the University of Salamanca, University of Girona and Open University of Catalonia. Currently working at the Nordic Institute of Latin American Studies, Stockholm University (Sweden). Main lines of research: political institutions; political history; nations, nationalism and plurinationality; political sociology.

Barbara Sonzogni is Associate Professor of Sociology at Sapienza University of Rome, where she received also her Ph.D. in Methodology of Social Sciences. Her main scientific interests include sociological historiography, sociology of knowledge, sociology of culture, political sociology, digital social research and, within the methodology, the applications and developments of agent-based social simulation. Her fields of research are deviance, inter-ethnic coexistence, social policies, religiosity, network analysis, lifestyles.

Emanuele Toscano is associate professor of Sociology at Marconi University of Rome, Department of Human Sciences. He earned his Ph.D. in Sociology at the School for Advanced Studies in Social Sciences (EHESS) of Paris (France). His research focuses on inequalities, subjectivation processes, and social movements. Among his publications, (2019) *Researching Far-Right Movements: Ethics, Methodologies, and Qualitative Inquiries*. Routledge; with Consorti F., Ginsburg S., Ho M.J., Potasso L. (2018) "A Phenomenological Study of Italian Students' Responses to Professional Dilemmas: A Cross-Cultural Comparison", in *Teaching and Learning in Medicine*. (2013) "Towards a full integration of teaching/learning professionalism and clinical competence in medical students", in Giardino A.P., Giardino E.R., (eds), *Medical Education: Global Perspectives, Challenges and Future Directions*, pp. 27–60, Nova Science Publishers.

Yaprak Dalat Ward, Fort Hays State University, USA. earned her Ed.D. at Sam Houston State University in 2007. Her research topics include cultural diversity, digital divides, diversity, equity, and inclusion and online teaching and learning. She is an associate professor at Fort Hays State University College of Education, where she teaches graduate-level cultural diversity and educational research courses.

1

SOCIOLOGY OF THE PANDEMIC

Simone Maddanu and Emanuele Toscano

The most indisputable point of no return in sociology in the first decades of the 21st century was, and is, the global extent of economic, social, communication, and cultural processes and, consequently, social change. In the last few decades, it has been pointed out that global connectivities through communication technology (Castells 2009) – as well as through international migration (Appadurai 1996), compression of space and time (Beck 1992; 1996; 2000), globalization and transnationalism (Sassen 1998; 2006), global modernity as global capitalism (Dirlik 2002; 2007), and, in one word, glocalization (Robertson 1992) – have changed the methods and paradigms of social sciences. If, on the one hand, no one is pushing for a general theory – an omni-comprehensive sociological butterfly effect – then, on the other hand, structural approaches and actor–network theories are enlarging the level of analysis to a planetary interplay. Therefore, sociology can offer multiple angles of understanding about humans and their new dimensions – for instance, after a state of lockdown – in which we acknowledge a new reality that is more material and confined to limited spaces of life for ourselves and our dependants. Bruno Latour's (2021) Kafkian idea of metamorphosis seems to suggest the positive effects of prolonged lockdowns as being material, strictly terrestrial, and a realization of our finite dimension (92–98).

Classic sociology pointed out weakening bonds, alienation, instability, and shakiness that surfaced in the affluent society, and, more generally, in the post-industrial era. While this has been true for Western countries, the rest of the world is compromising with global capitalism, showing fast-growing development in major countries – first and foremost, China and India – in every sector of the economy and the military. However, with different speeds, outcomes, directions, purposes, and effects, globalization also means global awareness.

Considering the global extent of the COVID-19 pandemic, our sociological approach aims to reiterate the transformation capacity of modernity and society

DOI: 10.4324/9781003459682-1

itself, cognizant of Giddens' conceptualization of reflexivity: not only the inherent intertwined effects of remodeling and reinventing practices in light of new knowledge and accumulated experience but also the self-conscient willingness to generate historic change (Touraine 1969). The latter would assume societal repositioning in terms of living together and copying alternatives. To follow such "prophecies",[1] we should observe and retrace social actors' practices and creativity today in response to crises. Moreover, we also think that the classic view of social actors must be extended to all networks and fields of actions that, like never before, are, on a planetary level, profoundly connected and intertwined with human and non-human interactions – dependent and independent – institutions and technologies, artificial intelligences, bacteria, and viruses (Latour 2017).

Living in the midst of a prolonged narrative of crisis, from global warming to the economic crisis in 2008–9, the COVID-19 pandemic, and the Ukraine War and its impacts, may sound like an impossible time to cope with. While the Global North public sphere constantly reports on these uncertain and changing times, the Global South might have another temporal perspective and sense of upcoming challenges. Reflecting on pandemics and the importance of utopias, De Sousa Santos asserts that "the global South has become accustomed to living among ruins and to resisting and innovating on that basis. Perhaps this long experience will now prove more precious than ever, and not just for the global South" (De Sousa Santos 2023, 3). From this perspective, even considering the impact of pre-existing economic and financial inequalities affecting the Global South during the COVID-19 pandemic (McCann et al. 2022), societal expectations sedimented in collective imaginaries may be a source of resistance and resilience that opulent societies have forgotten. We do know that continuous crises nullify the idea of exceptionalism but introduce the possibility – and the risk – of a constant state of alarm and exception, during which we can activate rational discussions and practical measures that benefit the collective. However, we can also reinforce elitist control over massive majorities. This is true within a nation and, on a global scale, between the North and the South. Nevertheless, unequal material experiences between North and South (particularly wider for sub-Saharan countries, see Stein and Rowden 2022) in times of global crises do not change the common challenges: the spread of a highly contagious and deadly virus, global climate change, natural resource depletion, and wars. However, unequal conditions do change the ways in which we experience them and interpret the present and future. They change the perception of risk, but they do not change the global reality of the risks we all face.

Sociology in a Time of Pandemics

A global crisis like the COVID-19 pandemic seems to imply a global leveling of public health risk: who would have thought that a South European country like Italy would impose serious lockdowns and follow strict freedom limitations similar to what China did during the first wave? Unsurprisingly (at least for some), many mobility restrictions and confinement mandates, limited physical interactions, and public health logistics took place in almost all European countries within months, following disease-spread data and statistical projections. Surprisingly (for some), the first anti-COVID-19 measures and medical equipment (particularly masks) poured into Western countries like Italy (which was harshly hit by the first outbreak in Europe) and France. These came directly from China, which positioned itself as the leading country in fighting the early pandemic. From a geopolitical perspective of global public health, the severe outbreaks in China (January 2020) and then in Europe (February–March) [2] represented an example of a process of shrinking distances in a globalized world of human and non-human actors that call for planetary solutions. Human resource management and industrial capacities were tested: the extent of contemporary globalization unfolded in front of everyone's eyes.

Even more so today, the transition into an accelerated risk society being all-encompassing, precariousness and uncertainty fully characterize the generalized sense of lack of control over our personal, individual life. Moreover, during the COVID-19 pandemic, long periods of "state of exception" plunged individuals and communities into a resigned sense of distance between their everyday lives and the orientation of society. For these reasons, this volume aims to reflect on all crucial aspects that emerged during the COVID-19 pandemic to encompass many forms of inequalities with an original in-depth analysis of Youth, which we believe must be at the core of any new sociological understanding of a global crisis. With political institutions and democracy at stake (Fruscione 2021; Fung 2021), we see this pandemic (and potentially new ones) as one of the tipping points of a globalized society and, as such, a potential vector of transformation and recomposition. If, on the one hand, we see reflexivity as the capacity to use current and accumulated knowledge and historicized experience, then, on the other hand, the responses and adjustments do not produce a similar collective imaginary or a similar synthesis. In the midst of chaotic information and communication narratives (Qureshi et al. 2022), perceptions and collective sense are driven in different, even conflictual, directions (Bergmann 2018; Otto and Köhler 2018). Reality seems to appear and be digested in the most polarized way. Science, politics, culture, and ecology have become spheres of cognitive conflict in which the interlaced relation between individuals and the collective unfold. What made a theorization of a "generalized other" meaningful – in the original Durkheimian sense as "collective consciousness" – that would also make society real and alive, "as a result of the Mcluhanesque environment" (Collins and Makowsky 1993, 182), now fades out in the flux of communication between fakes and truth. It does so now in the midst of the complexity of what common knowledge is or should be. In the flux of compulsory information and multilevel communication, the comfort zone of taken-for-granted knowledge is accompanied by delusional beliefs and a lack of common cognitive sense (Mauer 2022; Ashwell 2023). As has been observed in the study of social media and its role in the rise of populism – between denial and generalized mistrust – cacophony and cognitive conflicts arise in the current public spheres (Morozov 2011; Moffitt 2016; Otto and Köhler 2018; Fitzi et al. 2019; Gerbaudo 2022). Even the information produced by experts and supported by their relative scientific communities is subject to harsh criticism; it can be miscommunicated, corrupted by misleading actors (with or without a political agenda), transformed, and challenged by a large public. Cacophony and cognitive conflictuality about scientific and technical knowledge and their sources – also when created in expert circles – are becoming more common within open societies. Open societies are where contrasting information is also produced and spread by ordinary individuals and groups that have extensive access to social media (Liu and Levenshus 2023). Potentially, cacophony and cognitive conflictuality remain at odds with the necessary public health measures. This is the case so long as the latter, to be successful, would require at least understanding, if not acceptance and complete trust.

The resistance against vaccination campaigns aimed at containing the disease's spread and, more generally, policy makers' mistrust of public health measures have both been interpreted through the "knowledge deficit model". Directly related to the 1985 Bodmer report (Collins and Bodmer 1986), the concept of the knowledge deficit correlates people's resistance to scientific innovation with persisting scientific illiteracy. Such illiteracy would find support for a "linear model" that would define the relation between science and politics (Pielke Jr. 2007). Therefore, according to this approach, we would see top-down scientific communication that includes scientific content, presented as indisputable, from the experts to the general public to fill the "knowledge gap" of ordinary people. However, such communication also aims to reinforce the level of public acceptance of science. Consequently, its aims to legitimize the "scientization" of policy – that is, the use of science, or its label – as unquestionable guarantees that political measures are following the "Truth" against which democratic conflict is neutralized. Encapsulating the defining field of pragmatic, theoretical, and rationalized knowledge in society, contemporary science takes on the character of a broadly understood social institution and, as such, enters a public space of conflict. Although it does not represent an entity per se, science symbolizes a set of practices and narratives that seem to assume control in the Age of Crises. Risk society theories point out the role of science and specialized knowledge in late modern society. On the one hand, the extent of a highly technically organized world must face a social world where different degrees of perceived risk reside. On the other hand, scientific divulgation goes through disputable communication channels that the free market offers. Through this process, both elements, when combined, may appear as a new instrument of power and control that is legitimized by 1) the *elitist* knowledge formed and reproduced within academic circles and the scientific community, and 2) the risk and alarms that only highly technical and scientific institutions can declare.

In a time of crisis, democracies face challenges that autocratic and authoritarian powers may dodge by implementing a high level of surveillance and control over the population and the public sphere (De Munck 2022). Controlling the main channels of information and stifling criticism may be associated with high levels of cohesion and loyalty/trust/fidelity that could make even the strictest lockdowns and preventive measures "successful" – meaning "doable" and without disruptions – as we saw in China during the first year of the pandemic. That being said, in the long term, handling unprecedented crises (or just unknown enemies, like the extent of COVID-19) requires the flexibility of an authority that can apologize, amend, and learn from its mistakes. The authority must not be afraid of acknowledging fallibility, inaccuracy of judgments and measures, and, finally, responsibility – all things that authoritarian systems are, at the very least, hesitant about. The challenge of a mature democracy, especially in a time of popular populism (Fitzi et al. 2019; Farro and Maddanu 2021; Fung 2021), is to find a balance between public health, cultural experience, cultural expectations, and the common good (Cooper 2022) to cope with uncertainty while rejecting authoritarianism.

Sometimes characterized by *faux pas,* ineffective, or valid practices, the handling of the COVID-19 pandemic has shown how open societies can use resourceful flexibility on the unstoppable reflexivity of modern societies. Although the consequences of this reflexivity could have led to a new stock of knowledge from the pandemic experience, they also left behind controversies, emotional conflicts, and polarized views. There is no denying that pre-existing privileges and capitalized resources (technological as well as financial) have aided positively in managing the pandemic crisis compared to countries that could not afford remote schooling or remote work. These countries could not afford to alleviate high unemployment rates, loan suspensions, or tax suspensions for low-income families in a time of exceptional economic stall or recession.

In the last few years (2020–23), the entanglement inequalities/COVID-19 pandemic has been at the core of the sociological debate, profiting from interdisciplinary and transnational approaches. First, the articulation of inequalities lies in individual potential exposure to the virus and its different responses. Contributing factors, such as age and pre-existing conditions, are intertwined with economic resources, socio-cultural status, working conditions, and spatial context (Bambra et al. 2021). Available living spaces with low density showed how privacy became an essential class privilege (DeParle 2020; Connolly 2022). Additionally, the ability and chance to work remotely, durably, and in well-covered working conditions and social benefits, along with education and professional expertise and skills, are all factors that have determined unequal substantial impacts on the population. Moreover, where data are collected, race and ethnicity, migration status, gender, and disability are evident variables of concrete disparity (Centers for Disease Control and Prevention 2023).

Second, the pandemic exacerbated pre-existing global inequalities related to systemic inequalities that lie in the global (lack of) distribution of wealth and material resources (Ferreira 2021) and that are differently reflected in each national and regional context (Milanovic 2005). These inequalities encounter different national healthcare structures, functionalities, and accessibility. Depending on how resourceful or poor, scarce, deficient, and inefficient the public health was, each country coped with the pandemic and its impact on the most vulnerable populations differently. Inequalities worsen when informal economies do not provide protection and rights for workers, including within the healthcare service. On an organizational level, inequalities worsen due to a lack of logistics and planning, when data trackers and surveillance fail to control the spread of the virus and when public health authorities struggle to obtain – and coordinate – testing systems and vaccination (Nanda 2021).

A Different Crisis

The emerging conflicts we are witnessing in this Age of Crises concern both the general orientation of a globalized society and its interconnections as well as the political and spiritual meaning of our living together. A general distrust of governments and institutions (including the economy, media, medicine, etc.) has been noted by national and international polling organizations. Following these trends, the climate crisis, health crisis, and the environment are not the only elements of concern that societies face. The extent of global migration and multilevel unsolved inequalities are bolded topics listed in the public agendas of the first decades of the 21st century. Following Bauman's (2000) previsions on the extent of a "liquid" society, institutions' roles face unique skepticism. Challenges of governance come from the inside of democracies, as populism and authoritarianism are gaining ground, ostensibly playing with people's sentiments of insecurity, instability, and disunity, but also exploiting a diffuse bewilderment about societal changes. Cultural and technological changes unfold quickly, much faster than ever before, while "resisting" cultural views and previous everyday practices (especially in the field of communication) are lagging behind.

Nevertheless, periods of crisis, such as the pandemic, have demonstrated government responses (Gunaratna and Aslam 2022), flexibility in the economy, and various degrees of social resilience within local and national communities (Esu and Dessì 2022; Mishra et al. 2022). Civil society resists and carries out renewed agencies, sometimes reimagining the social fabric, even when basic socialization is diminished by restrictive public health policies. The drama of isolation and the denial of open-space physical mobility aggravated individuals' mental health and constituted a lasting burden of stress, anxiety, and loneliness. Even when exceptional measures limit freedom and jeopardize financial and emotional stability, communities may reorganize social ties and cultural meanings (Ryan 2022a, 2022b). The idea of "utopian realism", as a potential social progressive characteristic of reflexive modernity (Beck, Giddens, Lash 1994), may be coupled with Charles Taylor's concept of "modern social imaginaries" (Taylor 2004). Imagining social justice that deals with reality in a post-ideological world means using the same practical knowledge produced by society itself, thus its capacity to act and change its own practices. Alain Touraine saw the potential of a "producing society" in social movements (1973) and the emergence of the Subject (1978). However, what we have learned in sociology about society in a classical way has always been related to the tendency of nurturing community within a moral and economic frame at the same time. By analyzing the turning points of modern societies, and all modernization processes, sociology has reiterated its concerns for the loss of community. Calling out the necessity of being community – or being engaged in its "quest" (Nisbet 1953) – also means reflecting on a reassembling project:

> Utopianism, after all, is social planning, and planning ... is indispensable in the kind of world that technology, democracy, and high population bring. Conservatives who aimlessly oppose planning whether national or local, are their own worst enemies.
>
> *(Nisbet 1962, xvii)*

If the pandemic has, in some ways, reconsidered the incontrovertibility of globalization (Ramsari 2021; Bringel and Pleyers 2022), the factual return of state-national governments, and borders' control (Gerbaudo 2021), it has also asserted the crucial importance of international institutions and global cooperation, planning, and knowledge sharing. However, apart from possible systemic and structural transformations, this pandemic has forced the world to reconsider our social interactions and the very way we live in our vital space, both physically and mentally. The grammar of interactions has been disrupted and artificially – medically, politically – redesigned for more than a year in a way that will leave traces for at least one generation. After the COVID-19 pandemic shook the world, we entered a different age of global crises, where institutions like public health, science and medicine, politics, and media became the most crucial and, at the same time, the most challenged and distrusted ones. Doing sociology in the age of crisis requires a multilevel, cross-disciplinary approach cognizant of all elements of social change and transformation that a major planetary event and its responses can trigger on a local and a global scale in the individual and institutional sphere. Avoiding the tempting national methodology, a sociology of the pandemic requires a reflection on the events, effects, and extents of the pandemic in its entirety – that is, through a constant comparison that seeks patterns and exceptions. We posit that there is a necessity for a cross-referenced analysis that is cognizant of phenomenological approaches, structural and systemic perspectives, and quantitative and qualitative approaches that include the intersubjectivity and commonality of emotions, images, and sensations. This book offers a variety of original research and in-depth analysis from multiple geographies and sociological approaches – quantitative and qualitative, technical, and humanitarian. The pandemic has certainly raised alarms about new contemporary social problems that are visible – and sometimes superposable – on a local and global scale, showing similar patterns and causal sources. Doing sociology in the Age of Crisis means questioning the current structuration of institutions (democratic or not), the transformation of technostructures and communications, and the unequal impact of biophysical events on and in society. The pandemic, climate change, resource depletion, and militarization are reshaping global narratives about the role of organized human societies on both an individual and collective scale. Expressions and the exercise of individuality must level with new global challenges that are not ascribable only to the local sphere or local management.

Pandemic and Inequalities, Gender, Migrants, and Disabilities

The first part of this volume offers a variety of topics related to multi-geographical inequalities regarding social class, race and ethnicity, gender, and disability all around the world, within and across nations. The effects of the pandemic and the extent of the countermeasures that have been enforced similarly, locally, and globally also caused suffering, fears, and incertitude, highlighting and exacerbating pre-existing inequalities. In a time of pandemic crisis, to all its extent, the global response cannot be measured only in terms of public health recommendations and disease control management. While global collaboration, scientific monitoring, and rational strategies are praised and advisable, local and global inequalities remain the major contributing factors to the aggravating outcomes we have observed.

By collecting qualitative and quantitative data in the metropolitan areas of Buenos Aires (Argentina), the Valley of Mexico (Mexico), and Asunción, the capital of Paraguay, Raquel Rojas, Lara Flamand, Juan Ignacio Piovani, and Rosario Aparicio (Chapter 2) analyze the "Exacerbation of Inequalities in the Aftermath of the COVID-19 Crisis and its Effects Within and Across Households". The study highlights the unequal distribution of responsibilities, chores, and schooling support that reflects gender inequality in low-income households during lockdowns and anti-COVID-19 restrictions. What emerges is a powerful hypothesis that connects the inequality faced by women (particularly in low-income classes) and "conviviality", which is defined within the sphere of social interactions and thus subject to the distribution of roles and tasks. The authors suggest that high inequality is closely linked to low or weak levels of conviviality due to an unequal distribution of arrangements and responsibility that correlates to pre-existing economic status and gender inequality.

Intersectionality is the lens through which Chapter 3 interprets worsening inequalities in Malaysia. Through qualitative interviews conducted when anti-COVID-19 confinement was reduced by the authorities, Premalatha Karupiah explores "Malaysian Indian Women Living in Poverty and the Challenges of the Pandemic". The valuable outcomes of this research reveal both the financial struggle that minority women in suburban areas face and the deterioration of essential services, especially for their children. In particular, we learn how the lack of access to education during the pandemic reshaped women's hopes to provide a better future for their children. As we saw in the case of conviviality in South American low-income households (Chapter 2), sedimented gender roles increase the burden (expected chores, caregiving work, and responsibility) on women during lockdowns.

Women are also at the core of Chapter 4 in "'*Rebuscarse la vida*": The Resourcefulness of Latinas Navigating COVID-19 in Philadelphia". Veronica Montes, Beatriz Padilla, and Erika Busse offer powerful observations and insights into the agency of Latinas living in a sanctuary for migrants. The authors' analysis encompasses poverty, lack of immigration status (undocumented migrants), and the health crisis. The exemplary stories collected in this study articulate the intersection of the statuses and material conditions of women who, while asserting their subjectivity, are experimenting with new coping strategies for the common good of their community. More than a resilient perspective, we see here a form of resistance that finds its source in migrant capital, "creative mobilization" (Phillimore et al. 2018, 6), "gendered enterprise", and "communitarian caring" (Chapter 4, p. 58).

Lockdowns, confinements, and movement restrictions have simplified and often halted travel across countries – in some cases, the domestic movement of people, even from town to town. The pandemic re-established strict border control as we have never seen it before. Such restrictions suggested the possibility of reversing globalization and migration as we knew it. Some formulated the hypothesis of a return to protectionism and an excuse to finally reinforce closed borders to migrants. Other global crises, such as climate change, the economy, or wars, accelerate migration phenomena. Although not all routes were closed, during the COVID-19 pandemic, international migration slowed (United Nations, n.d.). Racial and ethnic minorities holding immigrant status were more likely to experience the effects of ongoing inequalities and discrimination. The most affected by precarious conditions during the pandemic were certainly migrants who lived in the limbo of migrant reception centers as refugees or asylum seekers. The Greek coastline is one of the most utilized on entries into Europe for illegal immigration in the Mediterranean. In Chapter 5, "Sociology of Migration Amidst the COVID-19 Pandemic Precarity: Racial and Ethnic Discrimination in Greece", Theodoros Fouskas analyzes the outcomes of fieldwork research in Greece. Interviews and participant observation were implemented along with quantitative data about migrants' conditions before and during the COVID-19 pandemic. The chapter encompasses topics such as perceived racism, xenophobic narratives in the public sphere – including scapegoating – and material conditions experienced by already precarious, low-income, marginalized migrants. The framework that emerges points out unequal treatments in testing or treatment, mobility restrictions, segregation or quarantine in overcrowded and unhygienic conditions, delays in vaccinations, delays in the issue of residence permits, and access to services.

The pandemic had great impacts on people with disabilities who strongly depended on welfare and healthcare services. In Chapter 6, "The Impact of the COVID-19 Pandemic on Disability Services in Japan: Analysis of Administrative

Panel Data", Kenjiro Sakakibara explores, through a quantitative approach and statistical modelization, how COVID-19 affected the decline in short-term accommodation, day care, work activities, and home care services. Focusing on the Japanese context, this chapter analyzes anonymized monthly disability service data, which include all uses of nationwide services in middle-sized cities with a population of approximately 100,000. The statistical analysis uncovered the undermined living conditions of persons with disabilities experienced during COVID-19.

Inequalities can be observed in the materiality of people's everyday experiences as well as in media narratives and imaginaries. The first part of the volume ends with a visual anthropology of cemetery and burial images of COVID-19 victims in Brazil. In Chapter 7, "Images of Pandemic Inequality in Brazil", Marianna Knothe Sanfelicio reveals journalistic and mediated practices of ordinary inequalities. From a visual perspective, this research underlines how pictures of death taken in São Paulo's cemeteries during the pandemic reflect patterns of inequality and segregation in the city. The images reproduced by the press created a particular representation of death that expressed social inequalities in the urban environment. Inequalities become more subjective and individualized when pictures of corpses circulate in the press. Whether in life or in death, this visual and urban anthropology reflects on the inequality of disposable bodies.

Pandemic and the Youth

Given the societal importance of youth, as in the historic process of social change, global events such as global crises must be analyzed in their effects on young generations. Although sociology posits the central role of youth as a major and radical transformation agent in society, few collective works have focused on particular phenomena that may have reshaped new generations since 2020. The second part of the volume aims to highlight the various impacts of the pandemic on the education, everyday life, and civic engagement of young generations from different sociological traditions and theoretical perspectives. We might consider youth as a social category, keeping in mind that variables such as spatial and geographical context, economic inequalities, gender, race and ethnicity, or other statuses will always represent contributing factors that could worsen some of the negative effects of the pandemic. We can then consider how the anti-COVID-19 measures have affected younger people's vision of both the present and the future. Many existing scholarly works report mental health effects, learning difficulties, and, more generally, social behaviors that have changed due to lockdowns and confinements. By using different methodologies, the second part of this volume presents a variety of reflections, starting from the Finnish case, by Konsta Happonen, Alix Helfer, Lotta Haikkola, and Jenni Lahtinen. Through statistical multivariate analysis, Chapter 8, "COVID-19-Related Life Events and Life Satisfaction Among Young People in Finland", shows that even mild anti-COVID-19 policies implemented by the

Finnish government had long-lasting negative effects on the well-being of young people. However, the research also shows that the educational system softened the effects of the pandemic on young people's labor market status, especially among young women who worked in the service sector.

Chapters 9 and 10 both focus on the Italian context. "Generational Inequalities in Multiple Crises: Pandemic and the Italian Youth on the Edge", by Enzo Colombo and Paola Rebughini, analyzes how the pandemic had an impact on Italian youth – the generation between 18 and 30 years old. The chapter notes a growing sense of vulnerability that young people face in their everyday lives, their new perceptions about social mobility opportunities and, more generally, the future. According to the authors, the pandemic has increased the feeling of *presentification*, which has modified the perception of one's agency among the younger generation.

Living in a crisis has become a generational feature and a constant element of the biographical and existential horizons of contemporary Western young adults. Within this framework, Chapter 10, "The COVID-19 Emergency and University Students: An Analysis on Effects from Inequalities in Cultural and Socioeconomic Capital", by Gabriella d'Ambrosio and Barbara Sonzogni, presents the results of an internet-based survey conducted in 2021, targeting university students in Rome. Among the valuable results, the chapter demonstrates that students with lower cultural and socioeconomic capital are more likely to declare pessimistic cognitive views and negative feelings, such as anger, boredom, depression, nervousness, powerlessness, sadness, and uncertainty about the future.

Inequalities among the younger generation are also the main topic discussed in Chapter 11, "The Digital (In)Equity Crisis During the COVID-19 Pandemic: Narratives from the Field", by Yaprak Dalat Ward and Anil Yasin Ar. Through innovative qualitative research based on narrative design, the authors focus on the digital inequity crisis triggered by the COVID-19 pandemic in the education sector to understand further the concept of inequity, its root causes, and its interconnections with other forms of inequality.

The second part of the volume on pandemic and youth ends with a multilevel analysis of the role of education reform targeting skills building in civics education. In Chapter 12, "Generation Z and Civic Engagement in a Pre- and Post-Vaccine World", Stephanie Garrone-Shufran, Kirstie L. Dobbs, and Laura M. Hsu describe a new framework for building an out-of-school-time learning opportunity to motivate all members of Generation Z – particularly those who live in underserved communities – to become civically engaged. Based on 42 qualitative interviews conducted with members of Gen Z, aged 14–25, the research aims to explore the impact of the COVID-19 pandemic on Gen Z's political identity more deeply. This innovative collaborative research offers more than one opportunity to explore the creation of new social movements in a time of crisis. Furthermore, it provides new sociological approaches to observe practically and contribute to racial and ethnic minority agency at a high educational level.

Pandemic, Social Movements, and Democracy

While the second part highlights the impact of the pandemic on young generations as a social category – a new generational culture and lifeworld experience – the third and final part allows us to wrap up the macroanalysis, although empirical, that underlies political, cultural, and social changes that emerged during the pandemic in specific national contexts. These contributions offer five unique in-depth analyses of the new conflicting spheres of science, politics, culture, and ecology that complete the scope of this volume. Different theoretical approaches contribute to multilevel sociological perspectives in times of crisis. Starting with Chapter 13, "How Did the Pandemic Shape the Dynamics of Two Civic Communities? Unraveling Complementarities and Divergences Within Spain's Civic Culture", by Rubén Díez García and Ariel Sribman Mittelman, the reader will be introduced to civic engagement and collective actions during the COVID-19 pandemic in Spain. Based on a survey with a sample of 800 people, the authors' approach focuses on the behavioral patterns and political culture that individuals shared throughout the pandemic in 2020, suggesting the existence of two ideal dimensions of civic engagement: civic–normative and civic communitarian.

Chapter 14, "Moral Framing, Spanish Roma and Scapegoating in the Age of COVID-19", by Antonio Montañés Jiménez and Demetrio Gómez Ávila, completes the sociological analysis of civil society by introducing the topic of racism and public opinion during the pandemic. The chapter combines sociological insights with discourse analysis and highlights the role of mass and social media in reproducing negative views on social minorities during health crisis events. In particular, the authors focus on how Spanish Roma were blamed for the alleged dissemination of COVID-19 in Spain.

The next chapter, Chapter 15, explores the attitudes surrounding the criticism of science, vaccine refusal positions, and public opinion. "The Anti-vaxxer Attitude as a Socially Rooted Thought-style", by Fiorenzo Parziale and Maria Carmela Catone, aims to analyze the social roots behind COVID-19 vaccination aversion (refusal and hesitancy). By using data collected through a stratified sample of Italian upper secondary school students, the research shows a strong correlation between general distrust toward COVID-19 vaccines and low-income social class students.

Following the wave of populist ideas that arose during the pandemic in different societal spheres, the last chapter, Chapter 16, "'Feminism is the Real Plague': The Spanish Populist Radical Right Anti-feminism During the COVID-19 Pandemic", by Antonio Álvarez-Benavides and Francisco Jiménez Aguilar, analyzes the extent of anti-feminist rhetoric within far-right groups during the COVID-19 pandemic.

By presenting the impact of the pandemic in different settings and political and cultural realities around the world, this book covers fundamental subjects related to racial/ethnic and economic inequalities, gender, disabilities, marginality, and youth. In addition, both its theoretical and empirical chapters explore the ongoing disjunctions of contemporary democracies from a multilevel perspective, positing the emergence of planned or unexpected social changes and new agencies in the age of the pandemic and global crises. A sociology in the Age of Crisis must underscore the necessity of encompassing contemporary social problems, such as local and global inequalities, with a substantial focus on other elements of social change, such as youth, the public sphere, and the challenges of democracies. In the Age of Crisis, sociology must redirect its objects, methods, and epistemology to capture what successfully changes and what fails, what emerges, what collapses, or what simply disappears.

Notes

1 We refer here to the Tourainian classic envisioning of social movements and their historic role in society, as social and cultural forerunners and as the transformation capacity of social actors.
2 Following the first anti-COVID-19 measures in China (including lockdown and mask mandates), the February outbreak in northern Italy led to the first lockdown in March 2020 in the Lombardy region and then nationally (WHO, n.d.).

References

Ashwell, Doug. 2023. "Science communication and pandemics". In *Pandemic Communication*, edited by Stephen M. Croucher and Audra Diers-Lawson, 42–58. London and New York: Routledge.

Appadurai, Arjun. 1996. *Modernity at Large: Cultural Dimensions of Globalization*. Minneapolis: University of Minnesota Press.

Bambra, Clare, Julia Lynch, and Katherine E. Smith. 2021. *The Unequal Pandemic: COVID-19 and Health Inequalities*. Bristol: Policy Press.

Bauman, Zygmunt. 2000. *Liquid Modernity*. Cambridge: Polity.

Beck, Ulrich. 1992. *Risk Society: Towards a New Modernity*. London: Sage.

Beck, Ulrich. 1996. "World risk society as cosmopolitan society?" *Theory, Culture and Society* 13, 4: 1–32. https://doi.org/10.1177/026327649601300400l.

Beck, Ulrich. 2000. *What Is Globalization?*Cambridge: Polity.

Beck, Ulrich, Anthony Giddens, and Scott Lash. 1994. *Politics, Tradition and Aesthetics in the Modern Social Order*. Stanford: Stanford University Press.

Bergmann, Eirikur. 2018. *Conspiracy & Populism: The Politics of Misinformation*. Cham, Switzerland: Palgrave Macmillan.

Bhattacharyya, Rajib, Ananya Ghosh Dastidar, and Soumyen Sikdar. 2021. *COVID-19 Pandemic, India and the World: Economic and Social Policy Perspectives*. London and New York: Routledge.

Boyle, Mark, James Hickson, and Katalin Ujhelyi Gomez. 2022. *COVID-19 and the Case Against Neoliberalism: The United Kingdom's Political Pandemic*. Cham, Switzerland: Palgrave Macmillan.

Bradbury, Alice. 2021. *Ability, Inequality and Post-Pandemic Schools: Rethinking Contemporary Myths of Meritocracy*. Bristol: Policy Press.

Bringel, Breno, and Geoffrey Pleyers, eds. 2022. *Social Movement and Politics During COVID-19: Crisis, Solidarity and Change in a Global Pandemic*. Bristol: Bristol University Press.

Carey, Allison C., Sara E. Green, and Laura Mauldin, eds. *Disability in the Time of Pandemic*, Research in Social Science and Disability Series, Vol. 13. Bingley: Emerald Publishing Limited.

Castells, Manuel. 2009. *Communication Power*. Oxford and New York: Oxford University Press.

Centers for Disease and Control Prevention. 2023. "COVID-19 mortality overview: provisional death counts for COVID-19". *National Center for Health Statistics*, June 23. www.cdc.gov/nchs/covid19/mortality-overview.htm.

Collins, Peter, M.D., and Walter F. Bodmer. 1986. "The public understanding of science". *Studies in Science Education* 13, 1: 96–104. https://doi.org/10.1080/03057268608559932.

Collins, Randall, and Michael Makowsky. 1993 [1972]. *The Discovery of Society*. New York: McGraw-Hill.

Connolly, Creighton. 2022. "The urbanisation of spatial inequalities and a new model of urban development". In *Covid-19 in Southeast Asia: Insights for a Post-Pandemic World*, edited by Hyun Bang Shin, Murray Mckenzie, and Do Young Oh, 37–45. London: LSE Press.

Cooper, Richard. 2022. "Public health confronts modernity in the shadow of the pandemic". In *Global Modernity from Coloniality to Pandemic: A Cross-disciplinary Perspective*, edited by Hatem Akil and Simone Maddanu, 257–276. Amsterdam: Amsterdam University Press.

Cowan, Dave, and Ann Mumford. 2021. *Pandemic Legalities: Legal Responses to COVID-19: Justice and Social Responsibility*. Bristol: Bristol University Press.

Croucher, Stephen Michael, and Audra Diers-Lawson. 2023. *Pandemic Communication*. London and New York: Routledge.

De Munck, Jean. 2022. "Three political regimes, three responses to the COVID-19 crisis". In *Social Movements and Politics During COVID-19: Crisis, Solidarity and Change in a Global Pandemic*, edited by Breno Bringel and Geoffrey Pleyers, 26–33. Bristol: Bristol University Press.

DeParle, Jason. 2020. "The coronavirus class divide: space and privacy". *New York Times*, July 28. www.nytimes.com/2020/04/12/us/politics/coronavirus-poverty-privacy.html.

Della Porta, Donatella. 2022. *Contentious Politics in Emergency Critical Junctures: Progressive Social Movements During the Pandemic*. Cambridge and New York: Cambridge University Press.

De Sousa Santos, Boaventura. 2023. *From the Pandemic to Utopia: the Future Begins Now*. London and New York: Routledge.

Dirlik, Arif. 2002. "Modernity as history: post-revolutionary China, globalization and the question of modernity". *Social History* 27, 1: 16–39. https://doi.org/10.1080/03071020110094183.

Dirlik, Arif. 2007. *Global Modernity: Modernity in the Age of Global Capitalism*. London and New York: Routledge.

Esu, Aide, and Valeria Dessì. 2022. "Recasting solidarity during the COVID-19 pandemic: a case study". *Social Movement Studies*. https://doi.org/10.1080/14742837.2022.2134105.

Farro, Antimo L., and Simone Maddanu. 2020. "Popular populism". In *Understanding Social Conflict. The Relationship between Sociology and History*, edited by Liana M. Daher, 119–130. Milan: Mimesis International.

Ferreira, Francisco H.G., 2021. "Inequality in the time of COVID-19". *Finance and Development* 58, 2: 20–23.

Fisher, Thomas. 2022. *Space, Structures, and Design in a Post-Pandemic World*. Abingdon and New York: Routledge.

Fitzi, Gregor, Jürgen Mackert, and Bryan S. Turner, eds. 2019. *Populism and the Crisis of Democracy*. Vol. 2: *Politics, Social Movements and Extremism*. London and New York: Routledge.

Fruscione, Giorgio, ed. 2021. *The Pandemic in the Balkans: Geopolitics and Democracy at Stake*. Milan: Ledizioni.

Fung, Anchor. 2021. "Is democracy too much trouble in a pandemic?" In *Democracy in a Pandemic: Participation in Response to Crisis*, edited by Graham Smith, Tim Hughes, Lizzie Adams, and Charlotte Obijiaku, 169–181. London: University of Westminster Press.

Gadarian, Shana Kushner, Sara Wallace Goodman, and Thomas B. Pepinsky. 2022. *Pandemic Politics: The Deadly Toll of Partisanship in the Age of COVID*. Princeton: Princeton University Press.

Gerbaudo , Paolo. 2021. *The Great Recoil: Politics after Populism and Pandemic*. London: Verso.

Gerbaudo, Paolo. 2022. "Theorizing reactive democracy: the social media public sphere, online crowds and the plebiscitary logic of online reactions". *Democratic Theory*, 9, 2: 120–138. https://doi.org/10.3167/dt.2022.090207.

Giddens, Anthony. 1990. *The Consequences of Modernity*. Stanford: Stanford University Press.

Giddens, Anthony. 1991. *Modernity and Self-Identity: Self and Society in the Late Modern Age*. Stanford: Stanford University Press.

Giddens, Anthony. 1992. *The Transformation of Intimacy: Sexuality, Love and Eroticism in Modern Societies*. Stanford: Stanford University Press.

Gunaratna, RohanKumar, and Mohd Aslam. 2022. *COVID-19 Pandemic: The Threat and Response*. London and New York: Routledge.

Kettemann, Matthias C., and Konrad Lachmayerm, eds. 2022. *Pandemocracy in Europe: Power, Parliaments and People in Times of COVID-19*. Oxford: Hart Publishing.

Latour, Bruno. 2017. *Facing Gaia. Eight Lectures on the New Climatic Regime*, trans. Catherine Porter. Cambridge: Polity.

Latour, Bruno. 2021. *After Lockdown. Metamorphosis*, trans. Julie Rose. Cambridge: Polity.

Liu, Broke Fisher, and Abbey Blake Levenshus. 2023. "Interpreting the interpersonal: crisis communication insights for pandemics". In *Pandemic Communication*, edited by Stephen M.Croucher and Audra Diers-Lawson, 156–173. London and New York: Routledge.

Mauer, Barry. 2022. "The cognitive immune system: the mind's ability to dispel Pathological beliefs". In *Global Modernity from Coloniality to Pandemic. A Cross-disciplinary Perspective*, edited by Hatem N. Akil and Simone Maddanu, 221–248. Amsterdam: Amsterdam University Press.

McCann, Gerard, Nita Mishra, and Pádraig Carmody, eds. 2023. *COVID-19, the Global South and the Pandemic's Development Impact*. Bristol: Bristol University Press.

Mehta, Rimple, Sandali Thakur, and Debaroti Chakraborty, eds. 2023. *Pandemic of Perspectives: Creative Re-Imaginings*. London and New York: Routledge.

Milanovic, Branko. 2005. *Worlds Apart. Measuring International and Global Inequality*. Princeton: Princeton University Press.

Mishra, Nita, Sushree Sailani Suman, and Anuradha Mohanty. 2022. "NINE: Coping Mechanisms of Communities in Odisha: A Human Rights-Based Approach to the COVID-19 Pandemic". In *COVID-19, the Global South and the Pandemic's Development Impact*, edited by Gerard McCann, Nita Mishra, and Pádraig Carmody, 131–148. Bristol: Bristol University Press.

Moffitt, Benjamin. 2016. *The Global Rise of Populism: Performance, Political Style, and Representation*. Stanford: Stanford University Press.

Morozov, Evgeny. 2011. *The Net Delusion. How Not Liberate the World*. New York: Allen Lane.

Nanda, Serena. 2021. "Inequalities and COVID-19". In *COVID-19*. Vol. I*: Global Pandemic, Societal Responses, Ideological Solutions*, edited by J. Michael Ryan, 109–123. London and New York: Routledge.

Nisbet, Robert. [1953] 1962. *Community and Power*. New York: Oxford University Press.

Otto, Kim, and Andreas Köhler, eds. 2018. *Trust in Media and Journalism Empirical Perspectives on Ethics, Norms, Impacts and Populism in Europe*. Wiesbaden: Springer.

Pascale, Celine-Marie. 2021. *Living on the Edge: When Hard Times Become a Way of Life*. Cambridge: Polity.

Phillimore, Jenny, Hannah Bradby, Michi Knecht, Beatriz Padilla, and Simon Pemberton. 2019. "Bricolage as conceptual tool for understanding access to healthcare in superdiverse populations". *Social Theory & Health* 17: 231–252. https://doi.org/10.1057/s41285-018-0075-4.

Pielke, Roger A., Jr., 2007. *The Honest Broker. Making Sense of Science in Policy and Politics*. Cambridge: Cambridge University Press.

Qureshi, Israr, Babita Bhatt, Samrat Gupta, and Amit A. Tiwari. 2022. "Introduction to the role of information and communication technologies in polarization". In *Causes and Symptoms of Socio-Cultural Polarization. Role of Information and Communication Technologies* edited by Israr Qureshi, Babita Bhatt, Samrat Gupta, and Amit Anand Tiwari, 1–23. Singapore: Springer.

Ramsari, Atefeh. 2021. "The rise of the COVID-19 pandemic and the decline of global citizenship". In *Global Pandemic, Societal Responses, Ideological Solutions*, edited by J. Michael Ryan, 94–105. London and New York: Routledge.

Ringe, Nils, and Lucio Rennó, eds. 2023. *Populists and the Pandemic: How Populists Around the World Responded to COVID-19*. London and New York: Routledge.

Ritzer, George, and Jeffrey Stepnisky. 2017. *Sociological Theory*, 10th edition. Thousand Oaks: Sage.

Robertson, Roland. 1992. *Globalization: Social Theory and Global Culture*. Thousand Oaks: Sage.

Ryan, J. Michael, ed. 2021. *Global Pandemic, Societal Responses, Ideological Solutions*. London and New York: Routledge.

Ryan, J. Michael, ed. 2022a. *COVID-19: Surviving a Pandemic*. London and New York: Routledge.

Ryan, J. Michael, ed. 2022b. *COVID-19: Cultural Change and Institutional Adaptations*. London and New York: Routledge.

Sassen, Saskia. 1998. *Globalization and its Discontents. Essays on the New Mobility of People and Money*. New York: New Press.

Sassen, Saskia. 2006. *Territory, Authority, Rights: From Medieval to Global Assemblages*. Princeton: Princeton University Press.

Shin, Hyun Bang, Murray Mckenzie, and Do Young Oh, eds. 2022. *Covid-19 in Southeast Asia: Insights for a Post-Pandemic World*. London: LSE Press.

Smith, Graham, ed. 2021. *Democracy in a Pandemic: Participation in Response to Crisis*. London: University of Westminster Press.

Stein, Howard, and Rick Rowden. 2022. "Global finance and the COVID-19 pandemic in Africa". In *COVID-19, the Global South and the Pandemic's Development Impact*, edited by Gerard McCann, Nita Mishra, and Pádraig Carmody, 38–55. Bristol: Bristol University Press.

Tan, Sabine, and Marissa K. L. E. 2023. *Discourses, Modes, Media and Meaning in an Era of Pandemic: A Multimodal Discourse Analysis Approach*. London and New York: Routledge.

Taylor, Charles. 2004. *Modern Social Imaginaries*. Durham and London: Duke University Press.

Touraine, Alain. [1969] 1971. *The Post-Industrial Society: Tomorrow's Social History – Classes, Conflicts and Culture in the Programmed Society*, trans. Leonard F. X. Mayhew. New York: Random House.

Touraine, Alain. [1973] 1977. *The Self-Production of Society*, trans. Derek Coltman. Chicago: University of Chicago Press.

Touraine, Alain. 1978. *La Voix et le regard*. Paris: Seuil.

United Nations, n.d. "Growth of international migration slowed by 27%, or 2 million migrants due to COVID-19, says UN". Accessed June 30, 2023. www.un.org/en/desa/growth-international-migration-slowed-27-or-2-million-migrants-due-covid-19-says-un.

Völkl, Yvonne, Julia Obermayr, and Elisabeth Hobisch, eds. 2023. *Pandemic Protagonists: Viral (re)Actions in Pandemic and Corona Fictions*. New York: Columbia University Press.

Witzel, Morgen, ed. 2022. *Post-Pandemic Leadership Exploring Solutions to a Crisis*. London and New York: Routledge.

Woldegiorgis, Emnet Tadesse, and Petronella Jonck, eds. 2022. *Higher Education in the Face of a Global Pandemic*. Leiden: Brill.

Yamamoto, Nobuto, ed. 2023. *The COVID-19 Pandemic and Risks in East Asia: Media, Social Reactions, and Theories*. London and New York: Routledge.

PART I

Pandemic and Inequalities, Gender, Migrants and Disabilities

2

THE EXACERBATION OF INEQUALITIES IN THE AFTERMATH OF THE COVID-19 CRISIS AND ITS EFFECTS WITHIN AND ACROSS HOUSEHOLDS[1]

Raquel Rojas, Laura Flamand, Juan Ignacio Piovani and Rosario Aparicio

Introduction

The COVID-19 pandemic has generated a crisis of global dimensions and asymmetric effects. Stay-at-home mandates and mobility restrictions, both necessary measures to prevent the spread of the virus, have translated into significant socioeconomic costs that affect people who occupy disparate positions on the social scale differently. And while governments have intervened with various measures to mitigate the effects that the restrictions have brought with them, not all countries have the right tools or necessary budget to protect their economies and citizens from the backlash that closures – of borders, schools, industries, shops, among others – have generated.

In other words, while the crisis had the same *trigger* worldwide – the pathogen SARS CoV 2 – its effects varied greatly depending on the local conditions in terms of health-care access and social security coverage. Along this line, high levels of informality in the labor market, scarce social protection, poor housing conditions, as well as reduced connectivity levels and low access to technology, acted as *catalysts* for the crisis, making the pre-existing social inequalities much more visible and creating new ones that sedimented on the old ones. After more than two years of the declaration of the pandemic, we know that some groups of people were more affected in terms of mortality – the old, the sick, the poor, migrants, and ethno-racial minorities within countries – while the economic impacts were and are still felt more greatly by women, informal workers, and lower social classes. These developments have led some authors to favor the term "syndemic" (Horton 2020; Bambra et al. 2021), calling attention to the biological and social interactions that are to be considered when analyzing COVID-19 infection and death rates. All in all, the pandemic and its containment measures did not only produce and reproduce

DOI: 10.4324/9781003459682-3

inequalities, but inequalities have also undermined the response to the crisis, creating a vicious cycle.

While inequalities are by no means a novelty in current societies, their exacerbation produces a rupture in the daily course of convivial relations, affecting how we live and interact with each other. In fact, conviviality and inequality are reciprocally constituted, insofar as inequality is a relational concept that "assumes meaning and consequences in the realm of conviviality, that is, in the context of social interactions which, in turn, reflect existing inequalities" (Costa 2019, 28). The conviviality-inequality perspective focuses on the negotiations of differences and inequalities in everyday life. Drawing on this approach, this chapter discusses how the pandemic has rearranged the distribution of care responsibilities at the level of households and the effects this has had on pre-existing patterns of inequality.

To illustrate this discussion, we draw on qualitative and quantitative data collected between 2021 and 2022 in the Metropolitan Area of Buenos Aires (Argentina), the Metropolitan Area of the Valley of Mexico (Mexico), and Asunción, the capital of Paraguay.[2] A telephone survey was conducted in each city, where a probabilistic stratified sample of people aged 18 and older was selected (n=2,500 in Buenos Aires and Mexico City; n=1,200 in Asunción)[3] based on parameters such as gender, age, educational level, household size, and total population per district of the urban agglomerate. In addition, a series of focus groups with intentional samples based on gender, employment situation, social class, and family characteristics (for example, households with school-aged children) were carried out, to gather more detailed information about how particular segments of the population have been affected by containment measures and have adapted to them.

The analysis focuses on households and their material base, the home, understood as spaces of conviviality. The focus on Latin America provides evidence on how people in contexts with high levels of inequality, elevated degrees of informality, and lack of social security were affected by COVID-19 containment measures, and how the population organized to cope with these difficult circumstances. The collection of data around 1.5 years after the impositions of mobility restrictions allows assessing the changes in the mid- and longer term.

In this chapter, we discuss how the pandemic and its containment measures adopted by governments – such as mobility restrictions and confinement mandates – affected family arrangements regarding distribution of household chores, care work, and homeschooling support. We are interested in accounting for inequalities within households, with an emphasis on gender, and between households, considering the educational level of the main breadwinner as a proxy for social class. In so doing, the chapter explores if and how the new or exacerbated forms of inequality that have emerged during the pandemic have been negotiated and re-integrated into convivial arrangements at the level of the household.

The text is organized in five sections. Following this introduction, we elaborate on the nexus conviviality-inequality, arguing that this is a useful perspective to analyze the changes brought by the pandemic and its effects on social relations, particularly within households. The third section provides information about the cases under study, focusing on the socioeconomic effects of the containment measures implemented to reduce the spread of COVID-19 infections, as well as the pre-pandemic social organization of care, i.e., its distribution among different actors. The fourth section presents the quantitative and qualitative data we obtained between 2021 and 2022 concerning households' distribution of care work and allocation of new responsibilities, with a particular focus on homeschooling support. The last section discusses how these changes have reconfigured the nexus conviviality-inequality at the household level and have also rearranged the distribution of responsibilities between the State, the market, and families, exacerbating pre-existing inequalities.

The nexus conviviality-inequality as a lens to analyze the effects of the pandemic

Since the publication of Ivan Illich's *Tools for Conviviality* in 1973, discussions on this term have extended to different fields of knowledge. Reviewing various contributions that have engaged with this concept, Sérgio Costa (2019) argues that while most tend to focus on the cooperative dimension of convivial relations and disregard conflict, inequalities and conviviality are, in fact, reciprocally constituted. From this perspective, conviviality refers to everyday interactions in contexts characterized by inequalities and differences that highlight the "relational dimension of social life" (Costa 2019, 27; Mecila 2017). In this vein, we use conviviality as an analytical tool to address inequalities as "structuring elements of existing patterns of coexistence" (Nobre and Costa 2019, 10) that are produced and reproduced in everyday interactions. The organization of everyday life and the interactions between agents are shaped by social structures and negotiations between actors, resulting in different convivial configurations. This is in turn related to regimes of inequalities, as some forms of conviviality involve more or less equitable arrangements and allow for varying degrees of negotiation.

Care practices within households provide a paradigmatic context for observing the nexus between conviviality and inequality. Furthermore, households and family relations can be regarded as *primary* domains of conviviality that, while characterized by social cohesion, are also sites where inequalities are experienced and negotiated (Potthast 2021). Households are social organizations that not only share an interest in their maintenance but also rely on a structural base for conflict and struggle, as "each [member] has his or her own distinct and at times incompatible interests, based on individual positions within intra- and extra-domestic production and reproduction processes" (Jelin 1991, 33–4). The distribution of housework and care responsibilities is one potential element of conflict and change, as we will explore in this chapter, particularly since the declaration of the pandemic and the implementation of stay-at-home mandates. In fact, the context of global lockdowns has not only led to an unprecedented shift of the most various activities "from collective and public spaces to individualized and private ones", but has also positioned households "at the center of governments' response to the pandemic" (Strevano et al. 2021, 276–7), accelerating and exacerbating the privatization of care.

Certainly, analyses that highlight the privatization and commodification of care predate the COVID-19 pandemic. In Latin America, where welfare states were never a prominent institution, the provision of care is characterized by a strong family bias, which naturalizes the idea that the domestic group is the main – if not the only – actor responsible for providing care, disregarding the role of the State and the market. Consequently, the social organization of care is an intrinsically unfair one, and this can be observed at two levels: at the level of the distribution of responsibilities between institutions, since care is provided overwhelmingly by families; and at the level of families or households, since it is mostly women who assume care responsibilities (Esquivel 2011; Rodríguez Enríquez 2015, 2020; Soto et al. 2016). However, despite the feminization of care, not all women are affected by it to the same extent. Depending on their position in the social structure, some households have enough resources to pay for care services, commodifying care and transferring at least part of the burden to others, generally, other women. Class, ethnicity, and citizenship divides mark the separation between those who can outsource care and those who provide this service (Rollins 1985; Anderson 2000; Gutiérrez-Rodríguez 2010).

In other words, the high level of inequality in the region results in differentiated access to care (Esquivel et al. 2012). Analyzing the case of Argentina, but arriving to conclusions that apply to the region, Eleonor Faur (2011) has argued that households from different social classes and geographical areas have not only unequal access to care services, but also that the quality of the services available to them varies greatly. For example, while formally employed individuals can rely on employment-based care benefits such as protections during and after pregnancy, parental leave, or even access to child-care services at the workplace, these options remain completely out of reach for those working informally, who constitute half or more of the working population in the region. Since educational services for children under the age of 3 are particularly scarce, the main options to cover this demand are either family care or private centers, which translates into a high level of privatization for higher-income households and a high level of familiarization (and thus feminization) in the lower classes.

In this chapter, we focus on the distribution of care activities in the context of school closures and the transfer of responsibilities to households. We argue that decisions regarding which family member can prioritize wage work and who will reduce their participation in the labor market to provide care may appear to be a private matter, but they are inherently linked to social structures. Thus, care represents a point of intersection between micro- and macro-social levels of analysis, a relational concept that involves interpersonal interactions between actors marked by differences and inequalities, and a domain of conviviality (Rojas Scheffer 2022).

Addressing the effects of the COVID-19 crisis on households from this perspective reveals how social interactions at the micro level are inserted in broader structural dynamics and how systems of care characterized by an unequal distribution of responsibilities produce different family arrangements in which not only gender, but also socioeconomic differences, play a role in the allocation of responsibilities. This highlights, as will be further discussed, that negotiations occur within asymmetrical power relations and in a context of uneven access to resources.

Impacts of the pandemic and State responses

Since the beginning of the COVID-19 crisis, the structural weakness of the health-care system in Latin America has been a cause of great concern. Different actors have warned about the accentuated vulnerability of the region due to deficient infrastructure, underfunding of care services, and segmented access (Benza and Kessler 2022). These fears were materialized soon after: by the end of May 2020, the Pan American Health Organization (PAHO) declared that Latin America had become the epicenter of the pandemic (Boadle 2020), and, a year later, shortly before the application of our surveys, the region had already surpassed a million COVID-19-related deaths (PAHO 2021).

Now, as grim as the above-mentioned numbers are, it is widely assumed that they underreport the true extent of the pandemic's death toll. Many deaths attributable to COVID-19 have not been certified as such, because of the lack of testing capacities. In this regard, excess mortality – "the mortality above what would be expected based on the non-crisis mortality rate in the population of interest" (WHO 2022) – is considered a more accurate measure. According to the World Health Organization (WHO 2022), the average excess mortality rate per 100,000 people for 2020 and 2021 is 99 for Argentina, 138 for Paraguay, and 242 for Mexico, with cumulative estimates of 198, 275, and 483 respectively. Data at the national level show that the areas covered by our study (Buenos Aires, Mexico City, and Asunción) have been the most affected within each country. This is partly explained by the fact that these big urban conglomerates are the most densely populated areas, as well as the ones where COVID-19 tests have been more accessible.

Before vaccines were available, states resorted to lockdown measures and mobility restrictions to try to prevent the spread of the virus. By the end of March 2020, virtually all Latin American countries had containment measures in place. The extent of them, however, varied from case to case. In Argentina, the Government Stringency Index – a composite measure based on nine response indicators, such as school/workplace closures and travel bans, rescaled to a value from 0 to 100 – stayed at the maximum level (100) until the end of April 2020 and at around 80 until September 2021, fluctuating then between 40 and 50 up to the end of that year. In Paraguay, the index stayed above 90 until the end of May 2020, over 80 up to October 2020, slowly decreasing afterwards and staying between 40 and 50 throughout 2021, with occasional increases. Meanwhile, in Mexico this index never surpassed 82.5, falling to around 70 between June 2020 and February 2021 and staying around 40 for the rest of that year (Our World in Data 2022a). The relaxation of confinement measures was accompanied by an increase in vaccination rates, even though coverage was uneven. By the end of 2021, 74 percent of the population in Argentina, 57 percent in Mexico, and 44 percent in Paraguay had completed the initial vaccination protocol (Our World in Data 2022b).

As pointed out above, some measures were relaxed after a couple of months, yet schools remained closed for notably long periods. Between 2020 and 2021, UNESCO (2022) registered a total of 82 weeks of school closure in Argentina (22 weeks of total closure and 60 weeks of partial closure), 81 weeks in Mexico (53 total and 28 partial), and 74 in Paraguay (32 total and 42 partial). As we will see in the next section, homeschooling support was not only one of the most challenging tasks for parents during this period, but also a responsibility that was distributed in a markedly unequal manner.

Even if mobility restrictions and lockdown mandates were, without a doubt, necessary measures, they came at a high cost: according to the ILO, over 26 million people in Latin America and the Caribbean lost their jobs during 2020 (Maurizio 2021). In this region, where the coverage of the contributory social security system is limited and around 51 percent of the employed population was working in informality in 2019 (ILO 2020), non-contributory financial aid policies such as cash transfers programs (CTPs) were a crucial measure implemented by states to support those lacking economic security and a safety net. It is estimated that, during 2020, 18 percent of the Paraguayan population, 25 percent of the Argentinian, and 29 percent of the Mexican received a transfer from such programs (Stampini et al. 2021). Despite the centrality of these relief measures for securing some income in lower-class households, they also had important limitations, such as implementation flaws due to lack of logistical capabilities or of pre-existing information on population in need of the subsidies. Delays in payments and insufficient coverage have also been identified as major issues (see Benza and Kessler 2022).

It is also important to point out that the massive job losses resulting from restricting mobility did not affect all people equally. In this respect, between the first and second quarter of 2020, the reduction in female employment (18 percent) was greater than in male employment (14 percent) (Maurizio 2021), widening the already existing gap between men's and women's labor market participation. Several factors explain this. First, sectors that have been hit particularly hard by the crisis – such as tourism, commerce and services, and domestic work – are strongly feminized. There is also a greater rate of informality among women (Maurizio 2021). Moreover, women tend to assume most of the burden of unpaid care and domestic work, which creates significant barriers to their participation in the labor market.

Even before the pandemic, Latin American women were spending on average three times more time on unpaid care work than men (Stefanović et al. 2022). According to UN Women and ECLAC data, in Argentina men devote 9.3 percent of their time to unpaid domestic and care work; and women, 23.4 percent. In Mexico, the proportion is 7.5 percent for men and 23.7 percent for women and, in Paraguay, 4.4 percent and 15 percent respectively (UN Women and ECLAC 2020). It is therefore no surprise that around 60 percent of women in households with children under the age of 15 say that they do not participate in the labor market because they have family responsibilities. The figure drops to 18 percent in households without children (ECLAC and UN Women 2021).

In Mexico, care is still organized under a scheme where family provision and women's unpaid work dominate. In addition, social security systems that include care services only protect people who participate in the formal labor market, with minimal exceptions. As for State measures specifically oriented to care, they focus on vulnerable groups and, consequently, their results are assistance-based, not promoting any structural change (Villa-Ayala et al. 2021). Moreover, there are disjointed policies on health, education, food, and employment (Flamand 2018). During the government of President López Obrador (2018–24), several social plans providing care services have been discontinued, as was the case with the program *Escuelas de Tiempo Completo* [Full-Time Schools], an intervention that used to provide after-school programs in public facilities. In Mexico, as in many other countries in the region, significant advances have been made in legal matters and in making unpaid care visible, thanks to research and surveys on time use. However, the greatest challenge for building and operating an effective National Public System of Care is the allocation of the governmental budget.

Similarly, in Paraguay, care provision depends fundamentally on the family, where women play a preponderant role. Over the last years, there has been a slow transition from a totally family-based arrangement to one in which the State is starting to be recognized as an institution that should also participate in the provision of care through specific policies. That said, State programs that respond specifically to care demands have insufficient coverage and lack coordination among them. In addition, these programs tend to benefit only the population participating in the formal economy (Dobrée et al. 2021), even if most of the employment in the country is informal. The main advance in Paraguay in this area has been the creation of the Interinstitutional Group for the Promotion of Paraguay's Care Policy (GIPC), comprising a set of public institutions that elaborated a framework document for the design of the National Care Policy in 2020 (Batthtyány 2020).

In Argentina, previous analyses have shown that, the lower the socio-economic level, the higher the familiarization of care. Indeed, in the context of a public care provision system of variable quality and low coverage, households that do not have enough resources to access market solutions tend to transfer these responsibilities to members of their household – especially female members – or, if they commodify them, they do so to the detriment of their general wellbeing. In addition to the socioeconomic insertion of the household, the possibility of transferring part of the care is segmented according to age and region of residence. The gaps account for sharp differences in favor of households with higher socioeconomic status and those based in the Autonomous City of Buenos Aires (Faur and Pereyra 2018). Also, in this case, there is no unified care policy, effectively articulated and with broad coverage, and the care issue has not positioned itself as a priority on the public agenda (Faur and Pereyra 2018). However, in 2022, the inter-ministerial unit for policies of care was created within the national government, and a bill was sent to the Parliament for the creation of a National Comprehensive System of Care Policies (Presidencia Argentina et al. 2022).

To sum up, in Argentina, Mexico, and Paraguay, care needs are met primarily through high family participation, with the aid of some government programs that generally function only as support. In addition, only middle- and high-income urban sectors can purchase services in the market, revealing a fragile, fragmented, and narrowly focused institutional architecture, with services available mainly in the main urban centers.

New responsibilities and inequalities within and between households

The context of global lockdowns turned households into the locus of social life (Pérez Sáinz 2021), increasing the share of care work carried out at home. Now, as it has been discussed above, housework tends to be unevenly distributed, with women bearing the brunt of it. Along this line, we wanted to know how the intensified familiarization of care work during the COVID-19 crisis had been approached, and if it had caused an impact on the division of labor at the level of the household. To this end, we asked our respondents if there had been any changes in the distribution of housework during the period of lockdowns. We found that 75.5 percent of households in Buenos Aires, 75.4 percent in Asunción, and 65.8 percent in Mexico City do not report any changes.

Considering that most of them had previously declared an increase in domestic chores since the beginning of stay-at-home mandates, this suggests that the domestic workload of women increased significantly, especially in the case of households with members in need of greater care. For example, in Asunción, over 76 percent of respondents declared having to deal with more housework since the beginning of the pandemic, a percentage that surpasses 81 percent in the case of households with children up to 12 years. Now, even if most households in all educational groups maintained their previous arrangements regarding care work, the ones that reported a change towards a more equitable distribution tend to have higher levels of education, as can be seen in Figure 2.1.

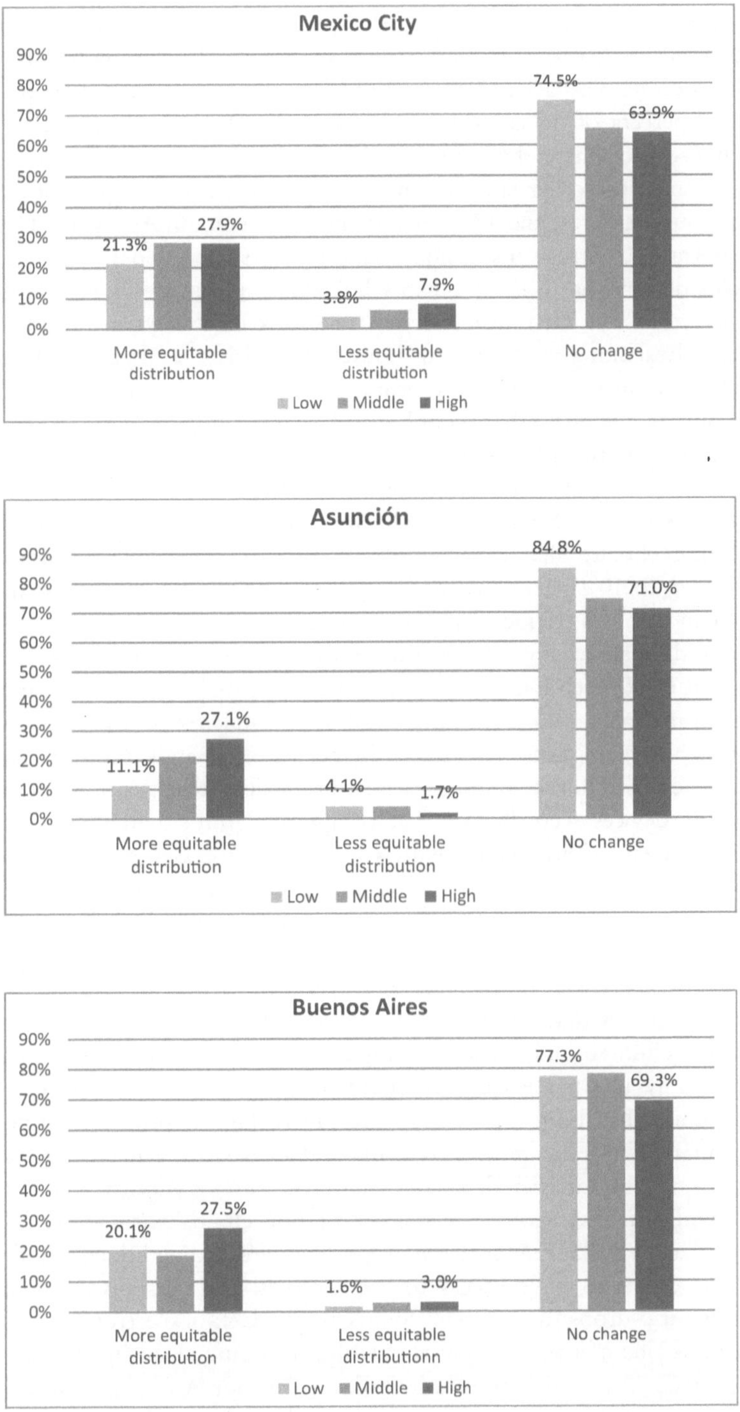

FIGURE 2.1 Changes in housework distribution during lockdown, by main breadwinner's level of education.[4]

The changes that took place during this period seem to reinforce a trend that has been registered before. In this respect, in Mexico City, respondents with a higher socioeconomic background declared an egalitarian distribution of housework in 32 percent of the cases, compared to only 19 percent of those stemming from a household where the main breadwinner has a lower level of education. The situation in the other cities is similar, with values of 27.3 percent and 21.6 percent in Buenos Aires, and 17.6 percent and 9.1 percent in Asunción. That said, it is important to stress once more that, in all socioeconomic groups, most households declare that it is a woman who primarily provides unpaid care.

In other words, women disproportionately took on the extra workload. This is particularly striking in the case of households with school-aged children that switched to homeschooling. Significantly more mothers than fathers were pointed out as the main household member providing help to children and adolescents during the almost two-year period of online classes. Again, our data suggests that there were some variations according to social class. For instance, in households with higher levels of education, there was an increase in responses declaring equally shared responsibility between mother and father, with differences up to 10.2 percentual points between households with low and high levels of education in Mexico City (see Figure 2.2).

Households that occupy a lower position in the social structure did not only see inequalities between family members get exacerbated, but also in comparison to other households, insofar as they had less resources to confront the new situation, while many times also facing higher care demands due to a more elevated presence of children. Along this line, insufficient access to the internet and to electronic devices were factors that complicated the situation. For instance, while 86.5 percent of households with a high level of education in Mexico City and 85.6 percent in Buenos Aires have at least one computer at home, these numbers drop to 46.2 percent and 59.5 percent respectively in households in which the main breadwinner has only up to primary level of education.

Concerning the usage of devices exclusively for virtual education, our data for Asunción shows that while in 52.9 percent of households with a higher level of education children had access to computers for their virtual classes, this was the case in only 11.7 percent of households in the lower level, in which the use of smartphones has been much more prevalent. This is problematic not only because smartphones are much less comfortable to work on, but also because their access to the internet depends heavily on having enough credit. Consequently, while in Asunción 27.9 percent of households with lower levels of education declared that one of the main problems regarding homeschooling was the lack of credit to have access to the internet, for the upper- and middle classes this ratio drops to 5 percent. Similarly, the lack of electronic devices was mentioned as one of the main barriers to be surmounted during this period in 20.6 percent of lower education households in Buenos Aires, in contrast to 9.5 percent of households with a higher level of education, and in 4.1 percent and 0.9 percent, respectively, in Mexico City.

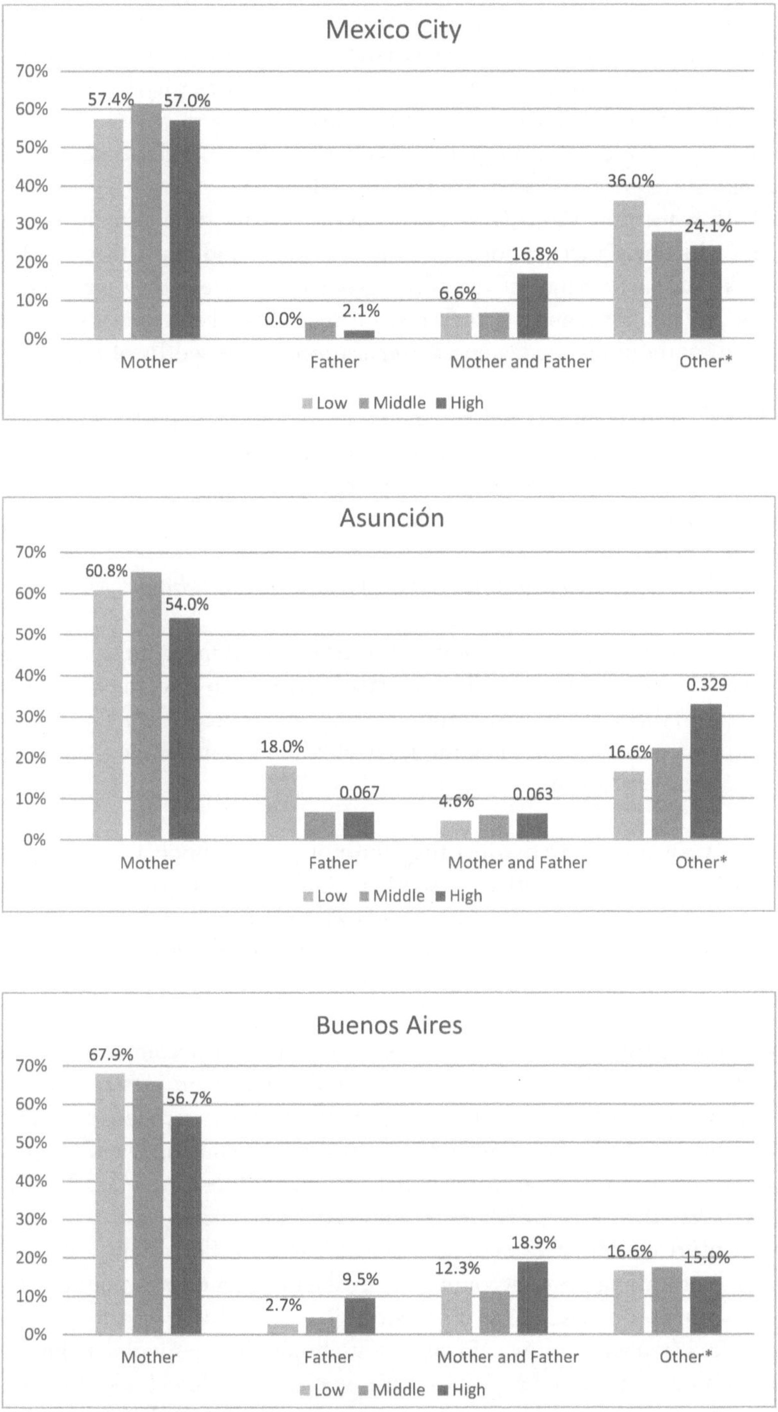

FIGURE 2.2 Household member responsible for assisting in homeschooling, by main breadwinner's level of education.

For sure, the access to quality education was already segmented before the pandemic. Yet this situation got exacerbated when a stable internet connection and availability of electronic devices became prerequisites for attending classes. This complicated matters even further in households with a larger number of children – as is the case in many low-income families –, where their members had to take turns to use the few devices available.

In addition to that, those with lower levels of education usually felt much less qualified to help their children with new content and assist them with their homework. As participants of the focus groups expressed, they were expected to be able to explain contents that many times they themselves did not fully understand, without any pedagogical preparation. In the words of a participant:

> When the pandemic started my daughter was in first grade; now she is in third grade, but she can't even read ... I asked the teacher to send her back to second grade and to teach her to read properly. Because my daughter doesn't understand me, and I don't understand her; I lack that pedagogy that teachers have.
>
> *(Meztli, 33 years old, works as a seller in the subway, Mexico City)*[5]

In addition to having to deal with insecure employment that many times translated into loss of income, these women also had to find the time to teach their kids and help them with schoolwork. Confronted with this situation, some of them resorted to completing their children's homework themselves, as another woman explained:

> It was very complicated when they did not go to school. I had to play the role of a teacher, a mother, a worker. And I would arrive home already stressed out, because there was no work, and they'd say, "I didn't do my homework". In the end, you had to do their homework for them.
>
> *(Anahí, 28 years old, domestic worker, Mexico City)*

Paradoxically, parents from lower classes also had to accompany their children's education more, insofar as virtual and synchronic classes (via zoom, meet, teams, etc.) with a direct interaction with teachers were less prevalent for children from this socioeconomic group. Data from Asunción shows that while in 87.1 percent of households with higher income children attended "real time" virtual classes, this was the case in only 60.9 percent of those with lower income. Unfortunately, the data does not allow to differentiate according to frequency but taking into account the problems mentioned above (lack of internet credit and of electronic devices), it is assumed that synchronic classes were also less frequent in lower-income households. It is no wonder then that a recurrent opinion in the focus groups with women from lower social strata was that the almost two years of homeschooling were nothing but "lost time" and that the children "did not learn anything", falling behind when they go back to school.

> It was very hard for me [teaching her kid] because I hardly remember anything. My son has just restarted in-person classes, and the teacher told me that he is "disoriented". Of course he is, if only I helped him, and I know almost nothing.
>
> *(Lucía, 30 years old, part-time salesperson, Asunción)*

All in all, our quantitative and qualitative data show an exacerbation of gender imbalances regarding care activities within households, which is in turn more pronounced in the lower social classes. Concurrently, it also calls attention to the greater difficulties that households with a lower socioeconomic background experienced regarding homeschooling and virtual education, which will probably further deepen the educational gap between those that come from households with higher and lower levels of education.

Concluding remarks

The COVID-19 pandemic has not only posed a global health emergency and taken a toll on the economy, but it has also disrupted people's intimate lives, changing the way in which we interact with each other. This was seen with remarkable clarity at the level of the household, as homes were forced to become overnight also the school, the workplace, the playground, and many other facilities that used to keep private and public life separate, forcing families to adapt to new scenarios. In this new context, the closure of schools and day centers did not only translate into an abrupt reduction of formal care options, but also into new responsibilities and roles for family members, particularly in households with school-aged children that switched to online learning. Yet while these changes occurred at a global level, it has affected people in disparate ways, since the extent and magnitude of the impacts have varied according to local characteristics and hierarchies based on gender, class, ethnicity, and citizenship.

Our results have shown that women were the most affected during the COVID-19 crisis, as they had to shoulder most of the burden that lockdown measures imposed on households. This was observed at all socioeconomic levels, including middle- and upper-middle class households that had made progress towards a more equitable distribution of domestic chores in the past decade. In this respect, data from the pandemic's early stages (when stricter mobility restrictions were imposed) revealed that households that had employed domestic workers before lockdown had widened the gender gap, implying that women were taking on the chores that were previously outsourced (Costoya et al. 2020). This underscores the persistence of the feminization of care across social classes. As Valeria Esquivel and colleagues contend, even when care responsibilities are outsourced, women are always responsible for managing and organizing everything related to them, also taking on responsibility in cases of emergencies (Esquivel et al. 2012).

That said, we also observed significant differences depending on socioeconomic standing, especially regarding virtual education. Higher-income households were better prepared for homeschooling (in terms of availability of devices and internet connection), while children in them could interact more often with their teachers, receiving thus more guidance and help with new content. For those in lower-income households, on the other hand, these options were many times not available, and the room for negotiating a more egalitarian distribution of chores seems to have been much smaller.

Certainly, the closure of schools was a major challenge for everyone, regardless of socioeconomic background. However, as discussed earlier, higher-income households have access to additional options beyond those provided by the state. For instance, many of them could still rely on paid domestic work, even during the strictest lockdowns, either because the domestic workers lived with them, or because their work was considered "essential", as was the case of nannies and those caring for the elderly. Working from home and being able to supervise the children during the workday, even if exhausting, was a measure that helped some families cope with the situation, yet again an option mostly available for middle- and upper-middle class professionals with a higher level of education.

For households that rely exclusively on public services, school closures meant higher familiarization – and thus, feminization – of care. With fewer options available, their ability to negotiate the allocation of the new responsibilities was restricted. This highlights a clear link between macro and micro levels of analysis: even if negotiations around the distribution of domestic and care work within households may seem like a private matter, they reflect the access that households have to services at the macro-social level. Thus, while gender inequalities in the allocation of care are seen in most households, regardless of their position in the social structure, they are exacerbated in the case of those with a lower socioeconomic background and fewer options.

Summarizing, the COVID-19 pandemic and its containment measures have amplified the central role of families in providing care, worsening the unequal distribution of responsibilities not only at an institutional level (between the state, market, families, and communities) but also within households. Through a conviviality-inequality perspective, we can see that the crisis has reorganized care within households and across society, exacerbating inequalities based on gender and class. Our data suggests that those in a less privileged position in society have had less ability to negotiate a fair distribution of chores within the family, leading to wider gender gaps. Thus, vertical inequalities resulting from unequal access to care services based on social status have a significant impact on household convivial configurations.

As previously mentioned, inequalities have undermined the response to the crisis, creating a vicious cycle. In this chapter we illustrated this dynamic through an analysis of households' responses to elevated care needs, highlighting how a segmented access to care services translates into deeper inequalities within and between households. Care, analyzed as a convivial realm, highlights how interpersonal negotiations at the microlevel are entrenched with broader dynamics at the macro level. The changes brought by the pandemic have made this relation even clearer.

Notes

1 The authors would like to express their gratitude to the funding agencies – the German Federal Ministry of Education and Research (BMBF) and the German Research Foundation (DFG) – for their crucial support in making this research possible. We would also like to thank the reviewers of our chapter for their valuable comments and suggestions, and the editors for organizing and coordinating the publication of this volume, which brings together a diverse collection of perspectives and ideas.
2 The data presented in this text stem from two broader projects on socioeconomic effects of the COVID-19 pandemic. The one covering the cases of the Metropolitan Areas of Buenos Aires and Mexico City was executed by Mecila and sponsored by the German Federal Ministry of Education and Research – BMBF (see https://mecila.net/en/homepage), while the one that focuses on Asunción was funded by the German Research Foundation – DFG (see https://gepris.dfg.de/gepris/projekt/468330077).
3 For further details regarding the survey carried out in Asunción and other Paraguayan cities, see Rojas Scheffer and Lachi (2022).
4 As previously mentioned, we use the education level of the primary earner as a proxy for social class. We believe that this variable is more suitable for cross-country comparisons as the measurement of income and the construction of the social class variable differ greatly between countries. In this text, "low level" comprises those whose highest level of education is primary school, "middle level" those who have attended or completed secondary school, and "high level" those who have attended or completed tertiary education.
5 All focus groups were carried out in Spanish. The translation, with minimal editing, was done by the authors.

References

Anderson, Bridget. 2000. *Doing the Dirty Work? The Global Politics of Domestic Labour*. London: Zed Books.

Bambra, Clare, Julia Lynch, and Katherine E. Smith. 2021. *The Unequal Pandemic: COVID-19 and Health Inequalities*. Bristol: Bristol University Press.

Batthyány, Karina. 2020. "Documento marco para el diseño de la política nacional de cuidados en el Paraguay". *EUROsociAL*. https://eurosocial.eu/wp-content/uploads/2020/01/Politica-Nacional-de-Cuidados-PY-DOCUMENTO-MARCO-1.pdf.

Benza, Gabriela, and Gabriel Kessler. 2022. "The impact of the pandemic on Latin America: social setbacks and rising inequalities." In *Persistence and Emergencies of Inequalities in Latin America. A Multidimensional Approach*, edited by Pablo Vommaro and Pablo Baisotti, 33–50. Cham, Switzerland: Springer.

Boadle, Anthony. 2020. "WHO says the Americas are new COVID-19 epicenter as deaths surge in Latin America". *Reuters*, 26 May. www.reuters.com/article/us-health-coronavirus-latam/who-says-the-americas-are-new-covid-19-epicenter-as-deaths-surge-in-latin-america-idUSKBN2322G6.

Costa, Sérgio. 2019. "The neglected nexus between conviviality and inequality". *Novos Estudos Cebrap* 38, 1: 15–32.

Costoya, Victoria, 2020. "Gender gaps within couples: evidence of time re-allocations during COVID-19 in Argentina". *Working Papers* 145.

ECLAC (Economic Commission for Latin America and the Caribbean) and UN Women. 2021. "Towards Construction of Comprehensive Care Systems in Latin America and the Caribbean: Elements for Their Implementation". ECLAC. Accessed 28 October 2022. https://lac.unwomen.org/sites/default/files/Field%20Office%20Americas/Documentos/Publicaciones/2021/11/TowardsConstructionCareSystems_Nov15-21%20v04.pdf.

Esquivel, Valeria. 2011. *La economía del cuidado en América Latina: Poniendo los cuidados en el centro de la agenda*: El Salvador: PNUD.

Esquivel, Valeria, Eleonor Faur, and Elizabeth Jelin. 2012. "Hacia la conceptualización del cuidado. Familia, mercado y Estado". In *Las lógicas del cuidado infantil: Entre las familias el Estado y el Mercado*, edited by Valeria Esquivel, Eleonor Faur, and Elizabeth Jelin. Buenos Aires: IDES.

Faur, Eleonor. 2011. "A widening gap? The political and social organization of childcare in Argentina". *Development and Change* 42, 4: 967–994.

Faur, Eleonor, and Francisca Pereyra. 2018. "Gramáticas del cuidado". In *La Argentina en el siglo XXI. Cómo somos, vivimos y convivimos en una sociedad Desigual – Encuesta nacional sobre la estructura social*, edited by Juan I. Piovani and Agustín Salvia, 497–534. Buenos Aires: Siglo Veintiuno Editores. www.jstor.org/stable/10.2307/j.ctvtxw2b7.

Flamand, Laura. 2018. "La reforma perdida. Tendencias de la política social en México (2012–2015)". In *Una agenda para la administración pública: reconocimiento a la trayectoria de María del Carmen Pardo*, edited by Fernando Nieto and Ernesto Velasco, 43–82. México: El Colegio de México.

Gutiérrez-Rodríguez, Encarnación. 2010. *Migration, Domestic Work and Affect: A Decolonial Approach on Value and the Feminization of Labor*. London: Routledge.

Horton, Richard. 2020. "Offline: COVID-19 is not a pandemic". *The Lancet* 396: 874.

ILO – International Labour Organization. 2020. "Impactos en el mercado de trabajo y los ingresos en América Latina y el Caribe". *Panorama Laboral en tiempos de la COVID-19*. Lima: ILO.

Jelin, Elizabeth. 1991. "Family and household: outside world and private life". In *Family, Household and Gender Relations in Latin America*, edited by Elizabeth Jelin, 12–39. London and Paris: Kegan Paul International and UNESCO.

Maurizio, Roxana. 2021. "Employment and informality in Latin America and the Caribbean: an insufficient and unequal recovery". Labour Overview Series for Latin America and the Caribbean 2021. Lima: ILO.

Mecila. 2017. "Conviviality in unequal societies: perspectives from Latin America – thematic scope and preliminary research programme". Mecila: Working Paper Series1, edited by Maria Sibylla Merian, International Centre for Advanced Studies in the Humanities and Social Sciences Conviviality-Inequality in Latin America. São Paulo: Mecila.

Nobre, Marcos, and Sérgio Costa. 2019. "Introduction: conviviality in unequal societies". *Novos Estudos CEBRAP* 38, 1: 9–13.

Our World in Data. 2022a. "COVID-19: Stringency Index". https://ourworldindata.org/covid-stringency-index.

Our World in Data. 2022b. "Coronavirus (COVID-19) vaccinations ". https://ourworldindata.org/covid-vaccinations.

PAHO – Pan American Health Organization. 2021."Latin America and the Caribbean surpass 1 million COVID deaths", 21 May. www.paho.org/en/news/21-5-2021-latin-america-and-caribbean-surpass-1-million-covid-deaths.

Pérez Sáinz, Juan Pablo. 2021. "Marginación social y nudos de desigualdad en tiempos de pandemia". *Nueva Sociedad* 293: 63–76.

Potthast, Barbara. 2021. "Mecila Merian Centre". www.youtube.com/watch?v=rZBXpI5HzSY.

Presidencia Argentina, Ministerio de las Mujeres, Género y Diversidad, and Ministerio de Trabajo, Empleo y Seguridad Social. 2022. "Proyecto de Ley "Cuidar en Igualdad" para la creación del Sistema Integral de Políticas de Cuidados de Argentina (SINCA)". www.argentina.gob.ar/sites/default/files/2022/06/cuidar_en_igualdad_-_sistema_integral_de_politicas_de_cuidados_de_argentina.pdf.

Rodríguez Enríquez, Corina. 2015. "Economía feminista y economía del cuidado. Aportes conceptuales para el estudio de la desigualdad". *Nueva Sociedad* 25: 30–44.

Rodríguez Enríquez, Corina. 2020. "Elementos para una agenda feminista de los cuidados". In *Miradas latinoamericanas a los cuidados*, edited by Karina Batthyány, 127–135. Ciudad de México and Buenos Aires: CLACSO and Siglo XXI.

Rojas Scheffer, Raquel. 2022. "Another turn of the screw: the COVID-19 crisis and the reinforced separation of capital and care". In Working Paper Series48, edited by Maria SibyllaMerian, International Centre for Advanced Studies in the Humanities and Social Sciences Conviviality-Inequality in Latin America. São Paulo: Mecila.

Rojas Scheffer, Raquel, and Marcello Lachi. 2022. "Socioeconomic impacts of the COVID-19 pandemic and its containment measures on Paraguayan border cities". https://doi.org/10.7802/2432.

Rollins, Judith. 1985. *Between Women: Domestics and Their Employers*. Philadelphia: Temple University Press.

Soto, Clyde, Lilian Soto, Myrian González, and Patricio Dobrée. 2016. *Panorama regional sobre trabajadoras domésticas migrantes en América Latina*. Asunción: OIT/ONU Mujeres.

Stampini, Marco, Pablo Ibarrarán, Carolina Rivas, and Marcos Robles. 2021. "Adaptive, but not by design: conditional cash transfers in Latin America and the Caribbean before, during and after the COVID-19 pandemic". Inter-American Development Bank. https://publications.iadb.org/publications/english/viewer/Adaptive-but-not-by-design-cash-transfers-in-Latin-America-and-the-Caribbean-before-during-and-after-the-COVID-19-Pandemic.pdf

Stefanović, Ana Ferigra, Lucía Scuro, and Iliana Vaca-Trigo. 2022. "The care economy and unpaid work: concepts and trends". In *Caring in Times of COVID-19: A Global Study on the Impact of the Pandemic on Care Work and Gender Equality*, edited by A. Ferigra Stefanović, 17–32. Santiago: ECLAC.

Strevano, Sara, Alessandra Mezzadri, Lorena Lombardozzi, and Hannah Bargawi. 2021. "Hidden abodes in plain sight: the social reproduction of households and labor in the COVID-19 pandemic". *Feminist Economics* 27, 1–2: 271–287.

UN Women and ECLAC. 2020. "Care in Latin America and the Caribbean during the Covid-19. Towards comprehensive systems to strengthen response and recovery". 19 August. https://repositorio.cepal.org/server/api/core/bitstreams/48f01d52-bbd3-486e-86e4-25dd93f65047/content.

UNESCO. 2022. "Global monitoring of school closures caused by COVID-19". Last modified March 2022. https://covid19.uis.unesco.org/global-monitoring-school-closures-covid19/regional-dashboard.

Villa-Ayala, Karina, Diana Lilia Trevilla Espinal, and Laura Ríos Quiroz. 2021. "México". In *Los cuidados del centro de la vida al centro de la política*, edited by Ailynn Torres, 100–147. Santiago de Chile: Friedrich-Ebert-Stiftung. http://library.fes.de/pdf-files/bueros/chile/18037.pdf.

WHO – World Health Organization. 2022. "Estimates of excess mortality associated with COVID-19 pandemic". Last modified 25 March 2022. www.who.int/data/sets/global-excess-deaths-associated-with-covid-19-modelled-estimates.

3

MALAYSIAN INDIAN WOMEN LIVING IN POVERTY AND THE CHALLENGES OF THE PANDEMIC IN MALAYSIA

Premalatha Karupiah

Introduction

The COVID-19 pandemic has changed our lives drastically. It has affected every aspect of our everyday life. As a measure to prevent the spread of the disease and loss of lives, many countries went into lockdown around the world. Malaysia had various levels of lockdowns from 18 March 2020 to October 2021 (see Boo (2021b) for a detailed discussion on lockdowns in Malaysia). During the various levels of lockdown, many restrictions were imposed on people, which include aspects such as the distance traveled, number of persons in a car, business/government agency operations, and public transportation. All educational, religious, and cultural institutions were closed to break the chain of infections. All types of social gatherings were also not allowed. Many people worked at home or were unable to work during these lockdowns. Schools were also closed for a long period. This meant that people were spending more time together at home during the COVID-19 pandemic.

Studies around the world have documented many challenges faced by women during the pandemic and the subsequent lockdowns. Some studies focused on the burden of unpaid work shouldered by women during the pandemic while others explored issues such as domestic violence, work-life balance, and access to health care (Borah Hazarika and Das 2020; McLaren et al. 2020; Boo 2021b; Chauhan 2021;Uddin 2021). In Malaysia, scholars also studied the challenges faced by specific groups such as entrepreneurs and single mothers. However, none of these studies looked at the experiences of minority women. This study focuses on challenges experienced by minority women living in poverty in an urban area in Malaysia, focusing on Malaysian Indian women. This is important, because ethnic minority women often face discrimination that is very different from other groups, including minority men. Taking this into consideration, this study uses

DOI: 10.4324/9781003459682-4

the intersectionality approach in understanding the challenges faced by minority women who are living in poverty during the pandemic.

Malaysian Indians

Malaysian Indians are a minority ethnic community in Malaysia. They are about 7 percent of the population. In terms of gender, 50.4 percent of Malaysian Indians are women. Malaysian Indians are not a homogenous group. They have diverse linguistic and religious affiliations. The majority of Malaysian Indians identify with Tamil as their mother tongue, but there are also Malaysian Indians who identify Telegu, Malayalam, Punjabi, or Gujarati as their mother tongue. Based on religious background, Malaysian Indians may be Hindus, Muslims, Christians, Sikhs, Bahai, etc. Hindus make up the largest group of Malaysian Indians (Karupiah and Fernandez 2022).

Malaysian Indians are mostly descendants of indentured laborers who migrated to Malaysia (then Malaya) during the British Colonial period in the late 19th and early 20th century. At the time, many migrants originated from Tamil Nadu (then Madras Presidency). Other than indentured laborers, there was also a small number of traders and professionals who migrated during this period. Most indentured laborers came to Malaya to escape class and caste oppression in India but suffered many kinds of discrimination and challenges in Malaya. The number of migrant female Indian workers was smaller than male workers, because traditionally women were not allowed to go for paid work or migrate for work. However, the hardship experienced in their homeland and the changes in the policies of the colonial government led to an increase in the number of female workers in Malaya. Female migrants during this period were oppressed both in their homeland and in the host country by colonial masters and other male workers. The female Indian migrants were marginalized in education, and healthcare, and were left behind in their personal and professional development, making them extremely vulnerable to poverty (Gopal and Musa 2022). During this time, most Indians lived in plantations and continued to suffer from impoverishment and oppression in the plantations (Sandhu 1993; Gopal and Karupiah 2013).

Malaya gained independence in 1957 and Malaysia was formed in 1963. After this, there was much growth in the industrial sector, leading to the rural to urban migration of Indians. Many left the plantations and settled in urban and suburban areas in Peninsular Malaysia. When they were living in the plantations, many were not able to acquire skills or education; therefore, when they relocated to urban and suburban areas, many ended up working in jobs with low wages and settled in squatter areas, particularly in the Klang Valley (Dass et al. 2014). While there has been progress in terms of socioeconomic development in Malaysia, Malaysian Indians still struggle with the issue of poverty, particularly urban poverty. Poverty eradication programs by the Malaysian government were not able to support the socioeconomic development of

Malaysian Indians (Gopal and Karupiah 2013). Taking this scenario into consideration, Indian women may be more vulnerable to poverty, because they are deprived of developing their capabilities due to traditional gender socialization and gender inequality in the household (Gopal and Sathyanarayanan 2021). Some Indian women remain poor and experience intergenerational poverty, because they lack the skills and capability to escape the cycle of poverty (Guna Saigaran, Karupiah, and Gopal 2018). Furthermore, statistics on mean household income also show that women in Malaysia are more vulnerable to poverty. This is because, among female-headed households, families headed by Indian women have lower mean monthly income than households headed by Bumiputera and Chinese women (Ministry of Women Family and Community Development Malaysia 2016). Intergenerational mobility among Malaysian Indians has been identified as being lower than other ethnic groups such as Malay and Chinese (Khalid 2018), which means that children born in lower-income families are less likely to move to higher-income groups among Malaysian Indians. All these indicators suggest that Malaysian Indian women are more vulnerable to poverty compared to men.

Intersectionality Approach

This study uses an intersectionality approach. The term was coined by Kimberle Crenshaw in 1989 (Bilge and Denis 2010). Intersectionality is a way of "conceptualizing the relation between systems of oppression which construct our multiple identities and our social locations in hierarchies of power and privilege" (Carastathis 2014, 304). An individual's social identity influences the multiple forms of oppression a person experiences. In other words, the influence of power on an individual experience is very much related to one's social identity, so one's experience of gender and other experiences in everyday life is influenced by their social identity. Therefore, the exploration of gender and related experiences must be done by taking into account individual social locations. (Shields 2008). A person with multiple subordinate identities may experience various forms of discrimination when compared to a person with a single subordinate identity. The overlapping nature of various forms of discrimination creates additional barriers for people with multiple subordinate identities. Ethnic minority women's experience of discrimination may be very different from that of ethnic minority men or other women. The intersection between gender and ethnicity could aggravate problems faced by ethnic minority women, because they may experience biases and stereotypes related to their gender, ethnicity, or even skin color (colorism). An intersectional approach enables us to understand these multiple types and levels of discrimination experienced by minority women. The women who participated in this study are minority women living in poverty; hence the intersection of ethnicity, class, and gender is pertinent in understanding their challenges during the pandemic.

Methods

This study is part of a bigger study focusing on the health and well-being of Malaysian Indian women living in poverty. The data were collected from ten Malaysian Indian women living in Penang using the in-depth interview technique. The participants of the study were selected using a purposive sampling technique. The criteria used for this selection is that they identify as Malaysian Indians and were living in poverty. Data collection was done during a time when movement restrictions were relaxed in Malaysia. It was conducted with adherence to the standard operating procedure given by the Malaysian government. Participants spoke in Tamil, with a mix of Malay and English.

All participants identified Tamil as their mother tongue. The average age of the participants was 31 years old. Eight of them were married, while two were single mothers. Four participants were homemakers, while six were working as security personnel, running a small business, and janitors. Most participants had some level of secondary education, while two participants only attended primary school. One participant did not attend school at all.

After the interviews were transcribed and translated, the researcher went through the transcripts in order to be familiar with the data before coding them. After three rounds of manifest coding, the researcher identified themes related to challenges faced by women during the pandemic. These themes are discussed in the next section. All names used in this chapter are pseudonyms.

Findings

Two themes were identified in the data analysis, i.e., financial burden and the burden of unpaid work. These themes show the various challenges that Malaysian Indian women living in poverty were experiencing during the pandemic.

Financial Burden

The most important challenge identified by all participants in this study is the financial burden brought by the pandemic. Women living in poverty were already struggling financially before the pandemic, and during the pandemic and the subsequent lockdown many businesses and workplaces were closed. Therefore, many people were unable to go to work or lost their job. Some women in this study were unable to work or lost their job, and this contributed to the worsening of their financial situations. Women who were homemakers also experienced a similar problem when their spouse lost their job or was unable to go to work.

Only participants who were janitors were able to continue working during the lockdown period because it was considered an essential service. However, they experienced many challenges to continue work. During the various levels of lockdown in Malaysia, there were different levels of restrictions imposed on everyday life, such as the number of persons in a vehicle, the distance one could travel, the number of passengers in e-hailing services, etc. There was a period when only limited service of public transportation was available to people, which made it very difficult for them to get to work on time or even to get to work at all. This contributed to the loss of pay, which made their financial burden even worse. One participant, Kanchana, shared her experience.

> During the first phase of MCO [lockdown which started in March 2020], there was limited bus service, and I was not able to get to work on time. Many days I was late to work, and I had problems at my workplace because of this. It also took me longer to get home after work. I got a salary that was lower than what I usually get. This made it very difficult for me to run the household. My husband lost his job, which made it worse.

Another participant shared her experience.

> We both lost our jobs and took us a long time to find a job after the restrictions were relaxed. We were unemployed for more than a year. I started doing odd jobs to earn as much money as possible, but it was extremely difficult. We depended on his mother's [mother-in-law] pension, which is not much. It was not enough to support everyone in the family. I am very grateful that she was willing to support us during that difficult time. Otherwise, I cannot imagine what I would have done.

The financial burden of the pandemic and lockdowns is something that is expected and documented by scholars (Gani 2021). Furthermore, the pandemic had disproportionate adverse financial and employment impacts on women who were more vulnerable to poverty even before the pandemic (Ou et al. 2022), particularly for those working in informal sectors. This was also made worse due to the new financial demands during the pandemic, such as the additional cost of masks, sanitizer, internet services, and devices. Kanchana went on to explain,

> Before the pandemic, we buy one bottle of soap [handwash] but during the pandemic, I had to budget for sanitizer and masks. These were not cheap. When my children started online classes, I struggled to buy a new device for my daughter. Otherwise, she would use my handphone [cellphone] for her class. I don't use data much, so it was not enough for my daughter to do her online class. It was better when we got free data from the government but that was still not enough … I wanted to install a wii connection at home, but I couldn't do it during the first lockdown. Also, I realized I could not afford it.

The participants' experiences show the extent of financial challenges women faced in their households. During this period, not only their income was lower than in pre-pandemic times, but the pandemic brought many new demands (in terms of products and services) that were not required before the pandemic and made their financial situations extremely strained.

The Burden of Unpaid Work

The theme "burden of unpaid work" is divided into two sub-themes: household chores, and care work and care work related to education. Both types of unpaid work were shared by most of the participants. This theme is important beyond the understanding of women's challenges during the pandemic. This is because women's experiences during the pandemic made them understand the magnitude of gender inequality that operates in a household. The participants of this study explained that the lockdown gave them a new perspective regarding the division of household chores. Before the pandemic, men in the household used to go out for paid work or other activities (such as games, meeting friends, and volunteering work). Women were not aware of the kinds of activities men participated in outside the house. Only some men would share what they were doing outside the house. Many participants explained that men would just tell them that "I am going out" without giving details regarding what they were doing when they were out. Regardless of the type of activities they participated in, it is often seen and emphasized as something important. Therefore, when they returned, they expected or demanded to be served or given time and space to relax. Women did not enjoy this freedom. Most participants shared that they would inform other members of the household about going out, but when they returned they would continue with household chores. They never had the "luxury" of being able to relax after returning from outside, even if whatever they were doing may be of great importance to the well-being of the family. However, many women tolerated this because they felt that men were coming back from working hard outside the house and they deserved time to rest and relax without thinking much about the inequality of this practice. Many explained that "that is how it has always been" or "that is what women do or my mom does". This shows that they have been socialized to follow gendered roles in the household and have internalized these values. Before the pandemic, they were more accepting and did not challenge these gendered norms.

However, the pandemic changed this scenario. When men were not able to go out for work or leisure, the participants realized that men were just sitting in the living room and not contributing to the running of the household. In addition to this, some men also expected to be served or had higher expectations regarding how they should be served while staying at home during the lockdown. Women also identified the lack of acknowledgment and appreciation for the work they do at home. One participant shared,

> When he was home, he expected me not only to prepare lunch and dinner but also something for tea because he kept saying that he usually would

> have something during teatime [while at work before the pandemic]. When I told him that I had too many things to do and could not prepare something for teatime, he was upset and we had a big argument. I never saw a problem with this until then. This is when I began to realize that this is not right. You cannot expect me to work all the time, while you are just sitting, watching TV, or playing with your phone.

Another participant shared that she was really upset and hurt when her husband was sitting in the living room and ordering her around. She admitted that she never realized the problem with the way housework was done before the pandemic. She started questioning herself and the situation: "Why am I the one running around, nonstop?" "How can he sit there and do nothing the whole day?" These are some questions that came to her mind and she could not answer. She also added that this situation made her think about her daughter. "Would she suffer the same fate? Would she be doing all the work at home? When would she rest?" she asked. That was when she realized that she did not want her daughter to experience the same level of inequality. While they begin to realize the level of gender inequality in their household, participants also admitted that they still see themselves as responsible for household chores and caregiving work. This is because they found it hard to change the situation in a short period. One participant, Meena, explained,

> As a mother and a wife, it is my duty to serve the family. I must ensure that everything in the house is well taken care of, even though I used to work. That is what I have been told and what my mother did. But now I begin to question myself. I am still unsure how to do this differently, but I want to be a good mother.

Meena's conundrum highlights the complexity of understanding gender inequality in a household, because household chores and caregiving work is often associated with being a good woman or a good mother. While it has given much meaning to her role as a mother, the pandemic has made question the level of inequality in her household. At the same time, she also wonders if her frustration or the "newfound" notion of sharing housework would make her a "bad" mother, one that does not play the role of the self-sacrificing mother which is cherished in Tamil society. This is closely related to the cherished form of femininity in Tamil society and how these women have performed their roles based on traditional feminine roles in society (Karupiah 2019; Karupiah and Fernandez 2022). The values related to the traditional notion of femininity are transmitted via the gender socialization process and are largely evident in cultural products such as songs, literature, films, and mythology. Therefore, they feel caught between the traditional expectation of femininity that they have internalized and their awareness of the extent of gender inequality they experience at home.

Based on their experience, the burden of unpaid work experienced by women during the lockdown enabled them to actually "see" the problem of gender inequality in the household which they accepted as the norm before the pandemic. The following sections discuss the two sub-themes related to unpaid work.

Household Chores and Caregiving Work

Studies in Malaysia and many countries highlight that women shoulder most of the household chores, even before the pandemic. However, during lockdowns, particularly in the initial stage of the pandemic, household chores became multifold (Borah Hazarika and Das 2020; Boo 2021a, 2001b; Chauhan 2021). This is mainly because, when all the members of the household were at home most of the time, they had more cleaning, cooking, and organizing work to do. All participants highlighted that they had to cook more meals per day during the lockdown when compared to pre-pandemic times. Before the pandemic, they would eat out or buy food regularly, which reduced the work in meal preparation. Even though restaurants were open for takeaways in the initial stage of the lockdown (strict lockdown), some were not able to afford to buy food for a few meals a day. Others were concerned about eating outside food for the fear of infection, and wanted to reduce going out. Also, they were worried about the cost involved in buying food, because many lost their income during this period. Furthermore, some explained that they had to save money to buy new tablets/phones/computers or spend more for internet services for their children, who were doing online classes.

One participant explained,

> I used to cook only two meals a day, but during the lockdown I was making four meals. When you cook four times, imagine all the preparation and cleaning up that I have to do before and after cooking. It felt like I was in the kitchen the whole day. Other than that, I also had to do other chores like washing clothes and cleaning the house, and the most difficult was to figure out what to do with the children [since schools were closed and children were not allowed to go out to play or go to school].

Other than household chores, women also had more caregiving work, because more members of the household were at home. Many participants felt responsible to plan what the children should be doing when they were not following their classes online. Other than this, they also had to spend time taking care of unwell household members. In the initial stage of the pandemic, anyone who was COVID-19 positive would be quarantined in hospitals and family members would be quarantined at home. But, in later stages of the pandemic, COVID-19-positive individuals could be quarantined at home. Therefore, two participants explained how difficult it was to ensure that the positive person was properly quarantined and other members were not infected. Another participant who was COVID-19-positive explained that the quarantine was almost like a "holiday" for her, because she has never had spent so much time by herself without doing anything. Even though she admitted at the time she was very worried about her health and her family's health, but on retrospection it made her realize the amount of work she was doing in the household.

The burden of household chores and caregiving work was made worse during the lockdown, because they were not able to get support from their social networks. Some women depended on their family or friends for food preparation or mobility. During the lockdown, particularly when they had restrictions on going to other households, they had to shoulder everything alone. Some did not visit their parents, because of the risk faced by older people.

> Usually, my mom would prepare lunch for my son because I am working. My son would go to her house after school, and I will pick him up after I finish work. Even though my mom's house is not far away, we did not visit her during the lockdown, because I was worried about her health, and I started cooking all the meals at home. Even when I bought groceries for her, I just left them outside the house, but I did not go inside.

Another participant shared:

> My neighbor usually accompanies me to the hospital, but during the first part of the lockdown we were not able to do that. There were restrictions on the number of people in a car and how far we could travel. Therefore, it was difficult to go to the hospital. Also, the hospital postponed my appointments because they were overwhelmed with dealing with COVID-19 patients.

All participants depended mainly on government clinics and hospitals for health services. They sometimes went to private clinics in case of emergency or minor health issues. During the pandemic, whenever the number of cases was high or increasing, government hospitals postponed their appointments or requested them to go to government clinics for health services, because the hospitals were focused on dealing with patients with COVID-19. This was also done to reduce the number of patients handled by the hospitals and also to protect outpatients from unnecessary risk of infection at the hospitals. When this happened, the participants had to plan how to go to the clinic that was suggested by the hospitals. Some participants were able to go to the hospital using public transportation, which was not available for the suggested clinic. With unexpected changes, mobility became a big problem for them. Even though taxi or e-hailing services were available, they would need to spend more for these services.

The unequal division of household chores and caregiving work shows the unequal power relations in society. While unpaid work is very important for the well-being of the family and society, it is seen as trivial and less valued;

hence it is performed mostly by women, while men are expected to focus on paid work. These values are reinforced by gender socialization in society and experiences when one is growing up (Boo 2021a). In addition to this, in a patriarchal society, women are expected to perform the role of nurturing and caregiving, which is closely associated with motherhood (Chauhan 2021). In Tamil society, women's service to the family and their caregiving role are seen as elements of a good/ideal woman (Karupiah 2019), which would explain why many participants felt that caregiving work was mainly theirs to perform and felt conflicted when they were unable to handle the burden of household chores or caregiving working during the pandemic.

Care Work Related to Education

During the pandemic, most schools and institutions of higher education shifted to online classes. There was a short period when students went to school, and there were also instances when only students who had public examinations attended school. Some participants with young children were directly involved with their children's education. They took time to teach the children and revise the lesson taught via online class. They spent more time with their children in educational-related activities compared to their spouses, even when they were at home during lockdowns.

Some participants were not directly involved in the teaching and learning process, because they felt that they did not know how to teach their children, particularly when the children were in secondary school or higher education. Some participants were not able to teach their children in primary school, because they studied in a school with a different medium of instruction from their children. Rathi explained,

> I went to Tamil[1] school, so I studied everything in Tamil, but my son goes to a Malay school, so I am not able to help him with his work.

Before the pandemic, a few participants sent their children to tuition, but this option was not available to them due to the financial burden they were experiencing. In poor households, the availability of devices such as tablets or laptops was a problem. Most students used their parents' cellphones. The cost of new devices and additional internet services added to their already-strained financial status.

Regardless of women's direct participation in education, many participants with older children took the bulk of chores at home to enable their children to spend as much time focusing on education. Meena admitted that before the pandemic, her children (particularly her daughter) would help her to do household chores like washing dishes and drying clothes. Meena explained,

> My daughter used to do more housework last time. But now I have asked her to reduce doing housework and focus on her studies. Sometimes, she

> struggles with online classes and I worry about her results ... After the lockdown, I realize how unfair the world is to women. I do not want my daughter to suffer like me. Now that I realize what is happening in my own house, I fear this when they go outside the house. Even though I might not be able to change my life, I want my daughter to have a better life. For us Indians, education is our only hope. Only if she has a degree, she will be able to have a better life ... As a mother, I will do anything possible to ensure that she has a bright future.

A few other participants shared the importance of their children's education and how much they contributed to supporting their children's education, such as taking over the chores that were previously done by the children, spending as much money as possible for their children's education while reducing the amount spent on their well-being (such as for leisure, health, and clothes). Some participants explained that, since their house was not very big and they did not have enough rooms for their children to follow online classes, they had to be extremely cautious while doing household chores (for example, they could not talk or use the blender).

Care work related to education is something that has not got much attention in the literature. O'Brien (2007) explains that when parents' involvement in education is discussed, it may refer to the mother's involvement in education, but the gendered nature of this type of care work is not widely discussed. The experiences of the participants in this study show that they spent much time and effort supporting the learning process of their children, even when their spouse was at home and was not doing other household chores.

Most participants gave much importance to the care work related to education, because they realized the importance of education for their children and did not differentiate between the importance of education for their sons or daughters. However, they admitted that, whenever they needed someone to support them with household chores, they often asked their daughters first, particularly if their daughter was playing or resting. This shows some level of disadvantage that young women experience in the household in terms of their right to leisure. Gender inequality in leisure activities, particularly in the household, is not uncommon in many countries (Beck and Arnold 2009; Craig and Mullan 2013), but this study shows gender inequality in leisure among children in low-income families. This is an aspect of gender inequality that needs to be explored further in future studies.

Care work related to education was often emphasized by the participants, because they associated it with the social mobility of their children. Women living in poverty realize that, as a member of a minority group, their children would face immense challenges to improve their socioeconomic status. As a result of this, they felt that higher education would be their only opportunity to escape poverty and improve their socioeconomic status.

Intergenerational educational mobility for Malaysian Indians is lower compared to other ethnic groups, such as Bumiputera[2] and Chinese. In a large study on social mobility, an Indian child born to parents in the bottom 40 percent income group is 0.4 times less likely to complete tertiary education compared to Bumiputera children. This is due to the lack of financial assistance that Indian students receive from the government, and the main focus of affirmative action programs in Malaysia is aimed at the Bumiputera group. The lower level of upward educational mobility among Indian children born to parents with low education also results in lower occupational mobility for Indian children with low-skilled parents. The study shows that only 19 percent of Indian children with low-skilled parents would get high-skilled jobs. This is much lower than other ethnic groups – 25 percent and 39 percent for Bumiputera and Chinese, respectively. This is related to lower income mobility among Indian children (Khalid 2018).

Participants show much understanding and acceptance of this reality. Their experiences during the pandemic also made them more aware of gender inequality. They acknowledged that they may not be able to change their present situation, but would put effort and sacrifice their comfort and well-being for intergenerational changes, particularly for the betterment of their daughters' (if they had daughters) lives. Even though the agency of the participants is not very clear when it comes to changing their present situation, this cannot be seen as being docile or passive. Davis (2009), in her study on cosmetic surgery, explains that women rarely make choices free from societal influence, but make them based on their understanding of their context and society, and this is also a form of agency. The women in this study show a great understanding of their context and society and were making important choices to make changes. However, their expectation is for intergenerational changes and not direct changes in their life. In many instances, their sharing regarding their role and expectations shows their acceptance and internalization of traditional expectations of femininity, but have rather different aspirations for their children. In addition, some participants shared their inner conflicts. Anitha shared:

> When I got married, my mom advised me to always serve my husband and his family. That is what she did and that was what I believed a good woman should do. But now I wonder if this is right. I don't think I want this for my daughter. I don't think she should suffer like me or my mother. It is just not fair, especially when women are also contributing to the finances at home. I don't know if I am capable of changing this, and I don't even know how to do things differently, but I hope my daughter will have a better life and I will do anything for that. I think I need to talk to my sons and perhaps make them see the challenges that women face and hope that they would act differently when they get married.

The burden of unpaid work, particularly during the pandemic, often affects the participants' well-being. Women spend many hours doing housework and caregiving work and neglect their well-being. They have very limited time for leisure, recuperation, and resting, which is again associated with the traditional notion of femininity (Guna Saigaran and Karupiah 2020).

Conclusion and Limitations

Women's experiences during the pandemic have amplified the extent of the inequalities they experienced. This chapter shows the challenges experienced by Malaysian Indian women living in poverty in an urban area in Malaysia. Two major challenges they experienced were the financial burden and the burden of unpaid work. Participants highlighted their important role in caregiving associated with education. The gendered nature of care work related to education performed by women is not widely discussed, in both popular and academic literature. This study gives some insights into the extent of care work related to education performed by women. Their efforts and sacrifices to support their children's education have escalated during the period of the pandemic, and this has given them the necessity to think deeply about the future of their children and their chances of escaping the cycle of poverty. This also contributes to the wider discourse on women's work. This is an important contribution of this chapter.

The pandemic, and particularly lockdowns, has amplified the level of inequality in the household, and this made the participants more aware of the inequality experienced by women. They identified the lockdown as the first time they were able to "see" inequality in their household. Prior to this, women accepted that work in the household (chores and caregiving) were their sole responsibility, because they expected men to be working outside the home. They have experienced the gendered nature of household chores and caregiving work throughout their lives, and this is something they have internalized as part of their meaning of being a woman. These values are also emphasized through gender socialization, making them seem like the natural order of how work should be divided. The pandemic, particularly the lockdown, brought a drastic change to this order and revealed the types and levels of gender inequality in a household. Men's lack of contribution toward housework when they were not doing any work during the lockdown periods was a revelation. It made women reflect on their experiences and revealed the level of gender inequality in the division of household chores and caregiving work in their household.

Women's experiences show a great understanding of their position as a minority and as a woman. Therefore, in a context where social mobility is very low, much importance was given to education as the only glimmer of hope for their children (particularly for their daughters) to escape poverty and negotiate the sharing of unpaid work with their spouse.

One of the limitations of this study is that it focused only on women living in an urban area. Future studies should explore the experiences of women in both urban and rural areas. Also, the experiences of women of various socioeconomic statuses will enrich our understanding of gender inequality. It will give some insights into the role of education and career in women's negotiation process in terms of the division of labor in the household.

Furthermore, this study did not explore men's experiences during the pandemic and their understanding of women's roles and work. A previous study in India showed how men and women had contrasting experiences during lockdown (Borah Hazarika and Das 2020). It is important to explore whether similar patterns are seen elsewhere.

Acknowledgment

This study was funded by the Ministry of Higher Education Malaysia Fundamental Research Grant Scheme with Project Code FRGS/1/2020/SS0/USM/02/7.

Notes

1 In Malaysia there are National School and National Type schools (for primary education). National schools use Malay as the medium of instruction, while National Type schools use Tamil or Mandarin as their medium of instruction. English and Malay are taught in all schools and a similar curriculum is used.
2 "Bumiputera" means "sons of the soil". It does not refer to a single ethnic group, but it encompasses ethnic groups such as the Malays (the largest ethnic group), Orang Asli, and natives from Sabah and Sarawak (Mason and Omar 2003).

References

Beck, Margaret E., and Jeanne E. Arnold. 2009. "Gendered time use at home: an ethnographic examination of leisure time in middle-class families". *Leisure Studies* 28, 2: 121–142. doi:10.1080/02614360902773888.

Bilge, Sirma, and Ann Denis. 2010. "Introduction: women, intersectionality and diasporas". *Journal of Intercultural Studies* 31, 1: 1–8. doi:10.1080/07256860903487653.

Boo, Harn Shian. 2021a. "Gender norms and gender inequality in unpaid domestic work among Malay couples in Malaysia". *Pertanika Journal of Social Sciences and Humanities* 29, 4: 2353–2369. doi:10.47836/pjssh.29.4.14.

Boo, Harn Shian. 2021b. "Unpaid domestic work and gender inequality in the time of COVID-19 in Malaysia". *Pertanika Journal of Social Sciences and Humanities* 29, 3: 1765–1781. doi:10.47836/pjssh.29.3.16.

Borah Hazarika, Obja, and Sarmistha Das. 2020. "Paid and unpaid work during the Covid-19 pandemic: a study of the gendered division of domestic responsibilities during lockdown". *Journal of Gender Studies* 30, 4: 429–439. doi:10.1080/09589236.2020.1863202..

Carastathis, Anna. 2014. "The concept of intersectionality in feminist theory". *Philosophy compass* 9, 5: 304–314.

Chauhan, P. 2021. "Gendering COVID-19: impact of the pandemic on women's burden of unpaid work in India". *Gender Issues* 38, 4: 395–419. doi:10.1007/s12147-020-09269-w.

Craig, Lyn, and Killian Mullan. 2013. "Parental leisure time: a gender comparison in five countries". *Social Politics* 20, 3: 329–357.

Dass, Mahaganapathy, Sarjit S. Gill, Ma'rof Redzuan, and Nobaya Ahmad. 2014. "Urban poverty among Indians in Malaysia: a naturalistic inquiry". *Life Science Journal* 11, 7: 21–26.

Davis, Kathy. 2009. "Revisiting feminist debates on cosmetic surgery: Some reflections on suffering, agency, and embodied difference". In *Cosmetic Surgery: A Feminist Primer*, edited by Cressida J. Heyes and Meredith Jones, 35–48. Surrey: Ashgate.

Gani, Irwan. 2021. "Poverty of women and the Covid-19 pandemic in Indonesia". *Budapest International Research and Critics Institute (BIRCI-Journal): Humanities and Social Sciences* 4, 1: 1034–1041. doi:10.33258/birci.v4i1.1710.

Gopal, Parthiban S., and Premalatha Karupiah. 2013. "Indian diaspora and urban poverty: a Malaysian perspective". *Diaspora Studies* 6, 2: 103–122. doi:10.1080/09739572.2013.853441.

Gopal, Parthiban S., and Gayathri Sathyanarayanan. 2021. "Gender socialization – an inhibitor of potential in capable poor urban women: a review on capability perspective in Malaysia". *International Journal of Development Issues* 21, 1: 54–71. doi:10.1108/ijdi-03-2021-0063.

Gopal, Syamala Nair, and Mahani Musa. 2022. "Migration of Indian women to Malaya: socio-economic status and sense of nationalism, 1900–1957". In *A Kaleidoscope of Malaysian Indian Women's Lived Experiences*, edited by Premalatha Karupiah and Jacqueline L. Fernandez, 21–42. Singapore: Springer.

Guna Saigaran, Nithiya, and Premalatha Karupiah. 2020. "The nexus of time poverty and well-being of women from poor households: a Malaysian Indian case scenario". *Malaysian Journal of Society and Space* 16, 4: 260–272. doi:10.17576/geo-2020-1604-19.

Guna Saigaran, Nithiya, Premalatha Karupiah, and Parthiban S. Gopal. 2018. "Gender socialization and capability deprivation on child urban poverty: experiences of Malaysian Indian women". *Geografia-Malaysian Journal of Society and Space* 14, 4: 346–356. http://ejournal.ukm.my/gmjss/article/view/29103.

Karupiah, Premalatha. 2019. "Femininity in everyday life: experiences of Malay and Indian women in Malaysia". In *Youth, Inequality and Social Change in the Global South*, edited by Hernan Cuervo and Ana Miranda, 113–128. Singapore: Springer.

Karupiah, Premalatha, and Jacqueline Liza Fernandez. 2022. "Negotiating femininity and empowerment: experiences of professional Malaysian Tamil women". In *A Kaleidoscope of Malaysian Indian Women's Lived Experiences*, edited by Premalatha Karupiah and Jacqueline Liza Fernandez, 127–141. Singapore: Springer.

Khalid, Muhammed Abdul. 2018. "Climbing the ladder: socioeconomic mobility in Malaysia". *Asian Economic Papers* 17, 3: 1–23. doi:10.1162/asep_a_00624.

Mason, Richard, and Ariffin S. M. Omar. 2003. "The '*Bumiputera* Policy': dynamics and dilemmas". *Kajian Malaysia* 21, 1&2: 1–12.

McLaren, Helen Jaqueline, Karen Rosalind Wong, Kieu Nga Nguyen, and Komalee Nadeeka Damayanthi Mahamadachchi. 2020. "Covid-19 and women's triple burden: vignettes from Sri Lanka, Malaysia, Vietnam and Australia". *Social Sciences* 9, 5: 87. doi:10.3390/socsci9050087.

Ministry of Women Family and Community Development Malaysia. 2016. "Statistics on women, family and community, Malaysia". www.kpwkm.gov.my/kpwkm/uploads/files/Penerbitan/Buku%20Perangkaan/Perangkaan%202016.pdf.

O'Brien, Maeve. 2007. "Mothers' emotional care work in education and its moral imperative". *Gender and Education* 19, 2: 159–177. doi:10.1080/09540250601165938.

Ou, J. Y., A. R. Waters, H. K. Kaddas, E. L. Warner, P. L. V. Lopez, K. Mann, J. S., et al. 2022. "Financial burdens during the COVID-19 pandemic are related to disrupted healthcare utilization among survivors of adolescent and young adult cancers". *Journal of Cancer Survivorship* 17, 6: 1571–1582. doi:10.1007/s11764-022-01214-y.

Sandhu, Kernial Singh. 1993. "The coming of Indians to Malaysia". In *Indian Communities in Southeast Asia*, edited by K. S. Sandhu and A. Mani, 151–189. Singapore: Institute of Southeast Asian Studies.

Shields, Stephanie A. 2008. "Gender: an intersectionality perspective". *Sex Roles* 59, 5–6: 301–311. doi:10.1007/s11199-008-9501-8.

Uddin, M. 2021. "Addressing work-life balance challenges of working women during COVID-19 in Bangladesh". *International Social Science Journal* 71, 239–240: 7–20. doi:10.1111/issj.12267.

4

"REBUSCARSE LA VIDA"

The Resourcefulness of Latinas Navigating COVID-19 in Philadelphia

Veronica Montes, Beatriz Padilla and Erika Busse

Introduction

On Friday 13 March 2020, the City of Philadelphia announced the shutdown of all non-life-sustaining businesses due to the COVID-19 pandemic. In a matter of days, thousands of people saw their livelihoods seriously impacted. The socioeconomic consequences quickly arose. By mid-April, the unemployment in the City of Brotherly Love increased from 5.8 percent, reported in February (Cohen and Babaseun 2020), to 16.1 percent (Keith 2021). As in the rest of the country, restaurants and bars were among the hardest-hit industries impacted by the pandemic. In Philadelphia, between March and April of 2020, about 42,000 people working in the food/drinking services lost their jobs (Cohen and Babaseun 2020). This dire situation was particularly challenging for the Latino immigrant community in Philadelphia, not only because 75 percent of them work in this sector (Henninger 2017), but more importantly because a considerable number are unauthorized workers, which prevented them from receiving federal emergency aid.

In times of crisis, such as this outbreak, state services retreat, leaving vulnerable populations, for example, those who already lack state protection – unauthorized immigrants and mixed-status families (e.g., Gavazzo and Nejamkis 2021) – to fend for themselves. These populations have developed coping strategies to manage these hardships. To cope with their unique challenges, marginalized communities work with both grassroots and NGOs (Lubbens et al. 2020). In so doing, such organizations become part of what Flores-Yeffal (2013) calls Migration-Trust Networks, as they earn the trust of the community. This collaboration becomes crucial in times of an unprecedented crisis such as the pandemic. Under these circumstances, many NGOs lost communication with their base, and only a few reacted, adjusted, and reorganized to respond in a timely fashion to the new needs

DOI: 10.4324/9781003459682-5

of the communities they normally assist; this was the case for the New Sanctuary Movement of Philadelphia (NSMP) during this pandemic. NSMP is an interfaith, multicultural, immigrant justice movement whose mission is to build a community that transcends faith, ethnicity, race, and class lines and ends injustices against immigrants regardless of their immigration status.

Its longstanding work with the Latino immigrant community allowed NSMP not only to continue its work during the pandemic but, more importantly, to quickly launch crisis-response programs such as *Oficinas Virtuales* (Virtual Offices, henceforth OV). OV was a volunteer-run project that emerged from the Philadelphia Area Immigrant Collective Action (PAICA) network of 20 immigrant advocacy and service organizations. This city-wide network shared a concern regarding Spanish speakers' accessibility to the Philadelphia Emergency Rental Assistance Program (ERAP) and thus set up this project to provide one-on-one support to assist the Latino immigrant community in completing applications.

ERAP aimed to provide emergency rental assistance to tenants and landlords affected by the COVID-19 pandemic. Since August 2020, OV has met with over 200 residents to submit applications to the different phases of the ERAP. Most people who NSMP has accompanied are Latino immigrants, many of them unauthorized, who work mainly in the service industry – restaurants, construction, cleaning, and so forth – in the informal economy. These socioeconomic characteristics led them to face additional layers of economic loss and uncertainty throughout the pandemic, not to mention the fact that many of these families are not only digitally challenged but also have limited levels of literacy both in Spanish and English, and thus would not be able to access the ERAP without support.

In this chapter, we argue that unauthorized Latino immigrants, due to their experience of precarity in their country of origin, have developed a set of practices to face the different crises they have to endure, including COVID-19. Moreover, our work in OV reveals that most of the people who used them were women, so OV was a gendered space where women developed specific strategies to deal with crises by rearticulating a series of life lessons that they accumulated overtime. We refer to these lessons as *rebusque*, and they include surviving and coping strategies learned and deployed in the country of origin, during the migration process and in their insertion in the country of destination. In this context, we argue that the concept of *rebusque* allows us to examine how marginalized communities, such as the unauthorized Latino immigrants in the US, tap on all resources they were able to find to support their families in times of crisis.

Thus, drawing on a mix of qualitative methods that complement each other – such as semi-structured virtual interviews, virtual participant, and non-participant observation as volunteers of OV, alongside virtual weekly self-reflection meetings among the three researchers – our work with the NSMP and Latino immigrants during and after the outbreak of COVID-19 contributes to the literature on women's agency, migrant capital, and Latino immigrants' structural precarity in the US context. First, we introduce the reader to the local context where the OV program was created. We then discuss the theoretical foundations of this study by exploring the intersection between women's agency, migrant capital, and precarity to describe next the virtual participatory research methodology used to underline the nuances from which we developed this project. In the empirical section, we present three paradigmatic cases that illustrate the collective *rebusque* that unauthorized Latina immigrants displayed, and we conclude with the implications of our findings.

Research Context: *Oficinas Virtuales*

While many studies focus on factors that contributed to the higher rates of COVID-19 cases among Latino populations (Figueroa et al. 2020), the impact of this pandemic on the Latino family economy and how it jeopardized their access, not only to a physical space to call "home" but also to maintain the sense of security that a home brings, is an issue that has not been studied yet. The Philadelphia Renters Report showed that, even before the COVID-19 outbreak, both Black and Latino families faced a lack of affordable housing, as about 141,000 (half of Philadelphia's) renters spend more than 30 percent of their income on rent. Furthermore, this report highlights that low-income renters are much more likely to be cost-burdened, as 88 percent of them cannot afford rent (Philadelphia Renters Report). Thus, the COVID-19 crisis further deepened housing insecurity for thousands of Black and Latino families.

In May 2020, in response to this dire housing plight, the City of Philadelphia began providing the ERAP to tenants and landlords affected by the pandemic. By February 2021, Philadelphia had spent over $65.5 million supporting more than 14,000 households (according to a City of Philadelphia Flyer). In the first three phases (May 2020–February 2021), only 45.3 percent of the 35,298 received applications were approved and, according to the city, 78 percent of the recipients were BIPOC[1] and 70 percent were women (City of Philadelphia Flyer).

Most people who used OV were women, on behalf of their families who had migrated from a handful of countries: Mexico, Honduras, El Salvador, and Guatemala. Most did not speak English, and all had children of different ages, with younger children born in the US, and thus were mixed-status families. Some women with young children stayed home, while others used to work until they lost their jobs due to the pandemic. Since most worked informally in cleaning services or restaurants, they lacked documents to prove employment, which rendered them ineligible for unemployment benefits. As our data show, immigrant women's wages are much lower than men's, some making $400 per month, while men make between $1,000 and $2,500. Only those with young US-born children receive some governmental assistance (e.g., WIC, SNAP, or Medicare). Regarding housing in Philadelphia, monthly rent ranged from $340 for a room to $1,300 for an apartment or house. The rental properties available to unauthorized immigrants tend to have pests, leaks, and/or improper electric wires, among other issues. Additionally, many landlords were reluctant to participate in ERAP.

Through OV, most women learned to use information and communication technologies (ICT), such as Zoom, to join sessions, while simultaneously using other platforms such as WhatsApp, the cellphone's camera and scanner, etc. They became acquainted with requesting letters from their present and/or former employers and contacting their landlords. Many times, these communications were difficult to establish, because most do not speak English. On many occasions, OV volunteers would make calls on their behalf to their landlords, provide them with template letters for their employers, or receive copies of English emails or correspondences to translate the content. These exchanges between women and volunteers in OV built the trust that enabled immigrant women to draw on volunteers' advice and support to make informed decisions on issues beyond their ERAP application.

Theoretical Framework

Emerging diseases are sources of instability, uncertainty, and even crises that can bring visibility to features of the social order ordinarily opaque to investigation (Dingwall et al. 2013). This was the case during the COVID-19 pandemic. Considering the nexus between NGOs and the unauthorized Latino immigrant community in Philadelphia during COVID-19, we ask why women were more active in OV. To address this question, we turn to the literature on several related issues: crisis, catastrophic events or pandemic, immigrant women's agency, precarity, and migrant capital.

A catastrophe such as the pandemic is an opportunity to analyze how people face a moment of calamity. On this, Zinn points out that these moments "[illustrate] how uncertain scientific knowledge and everyday life experience combine and change over time in political decision making as well as people's everyday life engagement with the virus and related regulations" (Zinn 2021, 435), allowing one to uncover unjust and unequal social conditions and power relations while also looking at solutions found by grassroots organizations and people. Drawing on Beck's notions of risk society and world at risk (1993, 2009), we focus on how unauthorized immigrants experienced the crisis, taking into account the multiple layers of precarity (migration status, job informality and insecurity, lack of access to health services and other governmental programs) that put them at greater risk. Moreover, the COVID-19 crisis highlighted the importance of extending the nation-state perspective to a cross-national approach, or as Beck (2009) suggests, shifting from *methodological nationalism* to *methodological cosmopolitanism* (Zinn 2021). We follow the methodological cosmopolitanism perspective, as we include experiences of *rebusque* to tackle crises that immigrant women have been facing even before leaving their country of origin, instead of assuming that women's knowledge is solely acquired in the country of destination.

The literature on Latina immigrants' agency and their political participation shows that mothers mobilize as political actors differently than their male counterparts (Jones-Correa 1998). First, immigrant mothers are more likely to be in contact with public institutions due to their responsibilities of taking their children to school, health appointments, etc. This close contact make them more aware of social programs. Second, women tend to develop collective alternative strategies to provide practical support to other immigrants, such as sharing childcare. Through these common activities, Latina immigrants in the US share information about services available to them, thereby creating a sense of community and cooperation (Hardy-Fanta 1993).

Women are active in their local communities, in both their countries of origin and destination, but for different reasons. As Andrews (2014) shows, women are even more active during periods of socioeconomic crisis in contexts of precarity. Marginalized communities and those living in perilous conditions in the US and other regions partner with both grassroots organizations and NGOs to get by (e.g., Lubbens, et al. 2020; Padilla et al. 2022). In the context of COVID-19, Gavazzo and Nejamkis (2021) showed how the networks immigrant women developed over the years in Greater Buenos Aires were crucial to care for the community, compensating for the State's absence during the pandemic. These "communitarian caring" strategies include soup kitchens and counseling for women affected by domestic violence.

Since precarity means different things depending on the context, we use it to refer to several situations of insecurity deriving from lack of immigration status, job loss, informal employment, etc. In this context, the concept of precarity is central. The study of precariousness tends to focus on the analysis of the vulnerabilities immigrants face regarding labor conditions (e.g., Ramirez et al. 2021), resistance to precarity (Paret and Gleeson 2016), and illegality (Dudley 2019). Building on these views, we focus on the unsteadiness of their livelihood, which during the pandemic translated into an increased risk of eviction. While COVID-19 exacerbated the already precarious conditions marginalized communities live in, in this chapter, we acknowledge that, for unauthorized immigrants, this represents another layer of crises.

To better understand the practices displayed by Latina immigrants during this time of exhaustion, we turn to the concept of migrant capital, which refers to the "knowledge gained about the state that allows them to successfully navigate migration control mechanisms" (Busse and Vásquez Luque 2016, 206). This conceptualization builds on Auyero's (2012) description of how immigrants learn about the State through interactions with state institutions in their country of origin and transit, mastering "the local legal logics" (Fonseca and Jardim 2010, 46). Likewise, Ramos (2018) indicates that migrant capital better positions them to know what to expect, focusing on the legal knowledge acquired while migrating and when arriving to a new place. Thus far, the research on the capital that immigrants accumulate refers to the knowledge learned on the move and when settling in their new country.

To enrich the conceptualization of migrant capital, we include the "lifelong human capital" that women learn in their home country. This is understood as the "learning and skill development as lifelong processes that begin at early ages in households and home communities and may include formal schooling and training but also informal learning experiences" (Hagan, Hernandez-León, and Demonsant 2015, 10). This connects what women learned about participation in their hometowns before migrating (e.g., Goldring 2001) with what they grasped throughout the migration experience by having to manage a series of precarious situations. Once in the country of reception, individuals draw on a bricolage of practices to overcome challenges to survive, turning challenges into opportunities (Phillimore et al. 2019). Due to the bonds of cooperation, they embrace, women tend to develop practices of collaboration that create a sense of belonging, which Montes (2020) calls *haciendo familia* (doing family). In this sense, women become competent to collectively work to provide for their families in their home country (Goldring 2001; Padilla 2004; Andrews 2014), when and while migrating (Busse and Vásquez Luque 2016) and once they settle (Phillimore et al. 2019). Thus, we see three big moments through which women develop and accumulate capital over time.

We combine this knowledge with what Flores-Yeffal calls migration trust networks (MTN), where immigrants, particularly unauthorized ones, assist others without expecting anything in return or, what she says, "a form of 'risk-pooling' … in which immigrants 'return' favors by helping others in the future" (Flores-Yefall 2013, 36). By combining MTN (Flores-Yeffal 2013) and communitarian caring (Gavazzo and Nejamkis 2021), we presume that experiencing increasing precarity more vividly activates these types of networks.

Weaving this literature together allows us to expand the concept of migrant capital in two ways. First, we identify that this capital is organized along gender lines. Second, by building on "lifelong human capital", we problematize the traditional concept of human capital by looking at how such capital, in the context of migration, is acquired in the three moments – before, during, and after migration – rather than one. Thus, we put forth what we call *rebuscarse la vida*, defined as the accumulation of formal and informal knowledge that immigrant women accrue along the way, from their community of origin, their migratory journey, and resettling in their new community. Our conceptualization centers around the action of *rebuscarse* (or "rummaging through") as a way to make ends meet. This disposition allows immigrants to overcome the different types of precariousness facing immigrants in general and unauthorized immigrants in particular.

Methodology

The empirical data for this chapter come from a larger project. which the three authors located in different cities across the US (Philadelphia, Minneapolis, and Tampa), embarked on since April 2020. To discover what was happening in the lives of Latino immigrants during the pandemic, we entered the field through the connections established by the author, who lives in Philadelphia. Thus, we approached the NSMP to offer our research capacity. To collect data, we opted for multiple complementary methods that aligned with action research: semi-structured virtual interviews, virtual participant and non-participant observations, and virtual weekly self-reflection team meetings. Along with data collection, we wrote emails/letters (to employers and landlords) and held meetings with city officials and representatives to red-flag the barriers Latino immigrants faced to access ERAP.

Although face-to-face interviews have been one of the traditional paths to data collection in qualitative studies (Creswell 2013), interviews conducted through other means were also available; however, they have occupied a secondary role (Holt 2010). Previous studies identified alternative methodologies, such as video conferencing including Zoom, suited for when meeting participants in person is not feasible due to being "geographically dispersed, unable or unwilling to travel, or research funding does not allow" (Gray et al. 2020, 1292). Here, we incorporate Zoom, Skype, and WhatsApp in different ways – first, by making the virtual world our fieldsite. In that sense, virtuality enabled us to see beyond the circumscribed physical space. People connected to the Zoom meeting from the intimacy – bedrooms, living rooms, kitchens – of their homes, inviting us in, sometimes surrounded by family members. Second, virtual fieldwork allows for ongoing accompaniment. Beyond ethnography, the time spent with these applicants was a way to accompany them throughout their application process, while witnessing both the main challenges Latino families faced during COVID-19 and the coping strategies developed to overcome them. Hence, these online platforms were instrumental in accompanying, assisting, and collecting data. Overall, we spent over 200 hours as OV volunteers in dialogue with community members, mainly women.

Along with the methodology, our positionality is relevant. The three researchers are women of immigrant background (from Mexico, Argentina, and Peru), Spanish native speakers, and feminist, who embraced and incorporated action research as a way to cope with the desperation brought by the pandemic and empathetically felt the level of distress this crisis brought to Latino immigrant families in the US. As the literature has highlighted, individuals categorized as vulnerable tend to collaborate in studies because they welcome the opportunity to talk about their experiences with an empathetic listener (Wolf 2021). Because of the role played by NSMP and the OV volunteers, and indirectly by the access to immigrants through OV, this dialogue was also welcomed, especially due to the implications this action research could directly bring to improving policies and services.

Empirical Findings: Stories of *rebuscarse la vida*

This section focuses on the practices carried out by unauthorized Latina immigrant women to cope with the challenges brought by the pandemic. We introduce three cases, which are paradigmatic, to illustrate the concept of *rebuscarse la vida*. First, we start with the case of Milagros,[2] whose story resembles her narrative shared in an interview along with our many participant observation sessions. While her case illustrates how past experiences navigating multiple crises throughout her life accumulated over time, the second and third cases describe the practices/strategies and knowledge used by two Latina immigrant women to navigate the COVID-19 crisis. By showing the strategies deployed by these women, we shed light on how the practice of *rebuscarse la vida* did not emerge now but, rather, is part of a series of practices that these women have used when facing a crisis.

Milagros

We met Milagros on 20 August 2020, in her capacity as a community liaison between NSMP and the Latino community in North Philadelphia. (She has been with NSMP since 2013.) Due to COVID-19, we met her at her house via Zoom in a staff meeting, when we presented NSMP with the work we were interested in conducting through OV. Since then, Milagros has played a vital role in the implementation and success of OV. She took her responsibilities so seriously that she would not stop even when she got infected with COVID and ended up in the hospital. From her hospital bed, she continued to reach out to the community to use OV to apply for ERAP.

Through volunteering, we saw how she contacted people in the community in two different, but complementary roles: as part of her job in NSMP, as well as an active member at her church in North Philadelphia. We learned that Milagros is well-known in the community, but, more importantly, people trust her. This trust is crucial for members of the community, who otherwise would be reluctant to participate in city programs. Milagros's work goes beyond OV and ERAP. We observed her guiding residents to apply to other support programs, such as a cash program or the distribution of food during the pandemic. NSMP staff and volunteers recognize that Milagros strengthens the work of NSMP; she even expands the trust that residents have in her toward the organization. Further, one characteristic that we observed is that Milagros carefully and emphatically listens to every person that contacts her.

Milagros is from a small community of about 2,000 individuals in the department of Olancho, Honduras (Honduras Instituto Nacional de Estadistica 2013). With a sixth-grade education, she ran a small grocery store in her village. As a married woman, she never thought of migrating to the US; on the contrary, she believed those migrating to the US were bad mothers for leaving their children behind. As a mother of six children ranging between 14 and two years of age, she eventually faced the very experience she criticized. Yet, it was not Milagros who decided to migrate, at least not in the same sense that other women spend time thinking and planning to embark on such a journey. Facing economic hardships in the early 1990s, she got a mortgage on her father-in-law's plot. The money was initially thought to be for stocking her grocery store. With the money at hand, women among her friends and family recommended that Milagros use the money to migrate to the US instead. While a bit hesitant at first, three months later Milagros followed their advice. From the very beginning, she discussed this possibility with her husband. With his support, she headed to the US, arriving in Philadelphia in 1994. A couple of years later, her husband reunited with her and, six years later, most of their children and their partners.

Milagros's way of *rebuscarse la vida* in her community of origin took different forms. Besides running a small grocery store (or bodega), she also participated in short-term jobs as a seamstress, which turned out to be handy later on when finding a job in a factory. As a devout Catholic, Milagros also participated as a catechesis leader. Further, living in a small rural town, many of the social services the community needed – like a health center, a primary school, and even drinking water – required community members to organize themselves to pressure the state. In the process of organizing, particularly women, they learn community-building skills. Milagros has been employing all these skills in her current job with NSMP.

The community organizing skills Milagros developed in her hometown, her creativity to find ways to make ends meet, along with the immigrant trust networks Milagros has established since she moved to the US, are still very present in her life. In Philadelphia, she has never stopped. Managing a tight budget and meager salary has required Milagros to find ways to save and make money. Upon arrival, she saved every penny by eating rice and chicken or just bread for long periods. She picked up every penny and nickel she found on the streets, adding them to her savings. Because her first job in a factory did not pay much, she learned to make tamales and bread, for sale during weekends, and took extra sewing jobs at home. All the bits of money she made combined to help her pay rent, eat, send, and save money to bring her family to the US.

In sum, Milagros's case illustrates how past experiences navigating multiple crises throughout her life accumulated over time – from the difficulties experienced in Honduras, on her way to the US, and once she settled down. It is this accumulation of knowledge that allows women like Milagros to cope with the precarious conditions they face throughout their lives. However, it was during the pandemic that practices of *rebuscarse la vida* became more evident, as the following cases illustrate.

Amparo

The first time I[3] spoke with Amparo was an afternoon in August 2020. She was the first person I accompanied to fill out her ERAP application. From the beginning, her confident and decisive personality was evident. Having hailed from Mexico, Amparo, in her early thirties, was married and a mother of two, the younger of the two requiring special education. From the beginning, I noticed Amparo's familiarity with filling out forms for social programs. Unlike other immigrants I accompanied that required time to explain in more detail each question, Amparo quickly and assertively answered all questions. For instance, for many applicants, convincing their landlords to participate in the program was challenging, not only because of the lack of English skills to communicate with them but also because some were intimidated by them. Not only did Amparo speak enough English to communicate with the management company, but also she was not afraid of directly contacting the landlord when the administration was not willing to support her application.

Rather than waiting for me to contact her to finish her application, as was the case with many applicants, it was Amparo who followed up each step by providing all the missing information to ensure a quick and complete submission. Her initiative made me acknowledge her lead on ensuring that her application was submitted; it was then when she mentioned that she had learned to navigate the bureaucracy of the social institutions to ensure her younger child received the care he required. Unless she were on top of the social worker to get what her child needed, nobody else would advocate for them. In this context, it becomes clear that Amparo knows that it was not enough to learn how to seek resources for her family, but more importantly it was also crucial to follow up closely until one gets the resources or services needed. That ability to get what one needs, regardless of the hurdles one must face, becomes the difference between life and death in times of crisis, as in the COVID-19 outbreak. However, Amparo used the skills she learned in solving her family problems to help others in the community. For instance, she provided assistance to neighbors to apply for ERAP and other city programs.

In early September 2020, we submitted Amparo's ERAP. Since then, we have stayed in contact, as we needed to closely follow the status of her application. In mid-October, Amparo contacted me to let me know she was selling tamales and asked me to help promote them among my networks. That weekend I contacted my friends and acquaintances, and together we bought 40 tamales and *atole* (traditional Mexican hot drink) from her. For several weeks Amparo continued selling tamales to her expanded social networks. For many Latino families, the support received from members of the community was what made the difference in grappling with the economic uncertainties brought about by the pandemic, particularly when they got infected with the virus.

In early November 2020, through her husband, I learned that Amparo contracted COVID-19. It had been almost three months since we had submitted Amparo's ERAP. Both Amparo and her husband had lost their jobs and, after having been economically supported by their church to pay their rent for three months, that assistance ended. They were already two months behind on rent. On 12 November 2020, Amparo entered the ICU. Their situation was so desperate that their only hope was to rely on collective solidarity. On 15 November, Amparo was released from the ICU, although she still stayed in the hospital. As soon as she could reach the phone, she called me to let me know that her husband had contracted the virus too. She asked for help to get her sister a humanitarian visa to come to Philadelphia to care for their children, in case her husband ended up in the hospital. In a matter of hours, I contacted several people in Philadelphia who could help her to figure out what could be done in such a case.

Although her husband did not need hospitalization at that time, several members of the community came to support Amparo's family. As her husband could not leave their house because he was sick and the only caregiver of their children, I put him in contact with several community programs to receive financial assistance. Through other community members, her family also got food delivered and toiletries while she stayed in the hospital, as the closest family members of her husband were in New Jersey and, therefore, support from his family was not possible.

On the evening of Thanksgiving, Amparo's husband entered the hospital. My family and I had prepared a Thanksgiving dinner for Amparo's family, and when my husband delivered it to Amparo, we learned about the situation. Knowing that my husband had gone to drop off the dinner, Amparo asked him to please take some clothes to her husband at the hospital. Fortunately, Amparo's husband was released the following day.

Before the end of 2020, Amparo's ERAP was approved. She recovered quicker than her husband, who unfortunately experienced some heart issues. Amparo began working at the beginning of 2021, but the economic repercussions of the long months of sheltering at home during COVID-19 hit Amparo's family hard. Since then, she did apply to the ERAP when Phase Four opened, but, as of the time of writing (July 2021), she has not heard back from the city, like most applicants. When I think of Amparo, not giving up and her determination are the two features that shape the way she embraces life and, more importantly, how her style of practicing *rebuscarse la vida* is defined.

Esperanza

I[4] met Esperanza in early November 2020 in OV when assisting her with her application to ERAP. Because of her involvement in church, she was familiar with NSMP and had heard about OV. Before I met her, Esperanza had made her case to receive an emergency assistance fund from NSMP, which helped her and her family survive early in the fall of 2020. At that time, she did everything possible to apply to Phase One of ERAP but was not able to. Later, when I met her at OV, we worked hard together to apply for Phase Two, finding alternative ways to get proof of residency and finally submitting all the documentation. Unfortunately, the application was denied, due to the landlord's inability to provide banking information.

Esperanza, aged 55, came from Honduras with her 16-year-old daughter. They were running away from violence and persecution. Even though she got temporary protected status (TPS), as did many other Hondurans, she was not sure what that meant, nor was she able to get any papers in hand because they were retained by the lawyer handling her case. Esperanza still owes some fees, so she has only seen pictures of her TPS permit in a WhatsApp message.

The COVID-19 pandemic drastically changed the living conditions of many immigrants, including Esperanza. She lost the steady job she had in cleaning services, and since then she has juggled to get short-term and even daily jobs: doing some house cleaning, removing trash from construction sites, harvesting, working in factories, and whatever comes up. Like many other immigrants, she thinks she does not have rights, and trusts that God will provide. Thus, she is not fully aware that, little by little, and with her tireless efforts, she is the one providing for herself and her daughter.

Persistence, an incredible capacity to keep trying in different ways, and never losing hope are what keeps her going. These features and her positive attitude define her. In addition to work, not having a place to live is what troubles her the most. Esperanza's home, located upstairs in a small house in a low-income neighborhood in North Philadelphia, is owned by her former boss from when she was working in cleaning services. When the pandemic was declared, her boss, an older guy from Central America, had to dismiss his employees, including Esperanza, because everyone canceled their contracts. Thus, he also lost his source of income. He was supportive of Esperanza applying to ERAP but, due to a complex situation, his bank accounts were frozen, making him ineligible to receive public funding. Thus, it was then when (creatively) Esperanza offered to open a bank account so her former boss and current landlord, along with her, could apply and eventually received rental support, which for both was a way to survive. On 28 December 2020, we completed the application for Phase Three. Then, Esperanza, the landlord, and I waited for news.

To apply, Esperanza, assisted by her teenage daughter and me, learned some skills. First, she became familiar with Zoom, to join OV, where we first met. Then, most of our communication was done by WhatsApp, involving video calls and document exchange. She would send information and news; I would send her final forms and confirmations. In addition to learning more about these platforms, she also had to open an email account, which she did with the endless assistance of her daughter, who, in addition to being a "good student" in high school, helped her with translations and checked her email. Both Esperanza and her daughter helped the former boss and current landlord, who is not ICT-savvy, to open an email account and monitor the -mails related to the application process. Furthermore, Esperanza, who has a caritative soul and is always willing to help others, took care of the landlord when he got COVID-19, as he was hospitalized, and was instrumental during his recovery.

After waiting for a few months, in mid-March, Esperanza (and her landlord) got the good news about the approval of their process, and the following week she got the payment in her bank account. As soon as she heard, she transferred the money to him, to pay for the late rent. To show his appreciation, her landlord gave her a small portion of the funds, and right after that she immediately called me with joy to share the good news. Overall, Esperanza's *rebusque* is not selfish (besides looking after herself and her daughter), caring for others as well.

Discussion

By examining these emblematic cases, we show what the concept of *rebuscarse la vida* entails and, more importantly, how its practice manifested during this pandemic.

Research on migration shows that unauthorized immigrants learn what to do to achieve their goals (Busse and Vásquez Luque 2016). One important lesson is taking care of and supporting others. Most of the times immigrants do this with people they just met on the way. Thus, Migration-Trust Networks (Flores-Yeffal 2013) are constructed on the go. In Milagros's case, her arrival in Philadelphia was a decision made on the go, as the initial plan was to relocate to Miami. However, because Milagros and the group of women with whom she initiated the migration journey took on the responsibility of bringing along a 14-year-old girl, at the special request of her family, Milagros had to bring the girl to Philadelphia, where her parents live. In return for bringing the girl, Milagros and her cousin had a place to stay for the first six months in the US, where she stayed for good.

Over the years, Milagros exemplifies what Flores-Yeffal (2013) calls Migration-Trust Networks, where immigrants, particularly unauthorized, assist others without expecting anything in return. It is this sense of uprooting that immigrants experience upon leaving their countries of origin, and resettling elsewhere, that makes them more easily trusting of others to ensure their physical and emotional survival. Perhaps more out of necessity than out of choice. For Milagros and her community, MTNs have been crucial because the support given by these networks became the core of tacit community reciprocity among those involved. In the end, the fact that NSMP developed MTNs with the Latino immigrant community in Philadelphia was what allowed a project such as OV to be accepted and successful.

In the case of Amparo, *rebuscarse la vida* included an independent and proactive attitude to seeking out public resources for her family's needs, engaging in income-generating activities, and reaching out to people in search of help, thus sharing with the community the migrant capital (skills and knowledge in dealing with public and private institutions) that she has accumulated throughout her life, both in Mexico and the US. Her determination to seek social services to satisfy her family's needs is what defines her way of *rebuscarse la vida*. Studies have shown (Jones-Correa 1998) that it is through their children that Latina immigrants come into broader contact with a range of public institutions if compared to their male counterparts. This exposure leads them not only to better navigate the bureaucracy of these institutions but, more importantly, it is through these experiences that many of these women enhance their practices of *rebuscarse la vida* to cope with the precarity their families and themselves endured in the new society

In the case of Esperanza, it was during the application process to ERAP that she discovered she could simultaneously help others, and thus she became instrumental in assisting her former boss and current landlord. Her determination led her to come up with the idea of opening a bank account, so they both could benefit from the assistance. But, later, she showed her solidarity when she took responsibility in caring for the well-being of the landlord while hospitalized and during his recovery.

Individual determination, however, is not enough to guarantee survival during times of crisis. Thus, the practice of *cuidados comunitarios* (Gavazzo and Nejamkis 2021) becomes pivotal for the survival of vulnerable communities. For Gavazzo and Nejamkis, *cuidados comunitarios* are "activities aimed at sustaining the common world" (Wlosko and Ros 2012), such as food, health, childcare, within the framework of the strategies deployed by families, in pursuit of the reproduction of life" (Gavazzo and Nejamkis 2021,105). Furthermore, Padilla (2004) and others have shown how impoverished communities organized themselves to access social services when the State fails to provide them. The concept of healthcare bricolage, defined as the "a creative mobilization, use and re-use, of wide-ranging resources, including multiple knowledges, ideas, materials, and networks to address particular health concerns" (Phillimore et al. 2018, 6), has been used to illustrate how both social service users and/or providers in superdiverse neighborhoods developed strategies to address everyday concerns. Moreover, research shows how social care is a gendered enterprise, as women take on more responsibilities in engaging with social services; thus the concept of bricolage allows also "to make visible the work which has been unseen, over-looked and naturalized, as part of a gendered caring role" (Bradby et al. 2019, 33). The example of these three women evidenced how *cuidados comunitarios* and bricolage are organized along gender lines and how the protagonists are women. While *rebuscarse la vida* could be a selfish strategy as a survival strategy, among these women *rebuscarse la vida* implies solidarity and community care.

Final Remarks

Our chapter contributes to the immigration literature in a couple of ways. First, we connect the literature on grassroots organizing in South America (e.g., Padilla 2004), the literature on what immigrants learned on the move and how they deploy their immigrant capital (Busse and Vásquez Luque 2016), and what they learned upon arrival to the new country (Jones-Correa 1998; Flores-Yeffal 2013; Gavazzo and Nejamkis 2021; Montes 2022). The backdrop of this research is the precarity people face in their hometowns, while migrating and in the country of arrival. We call the combination of knowledge, practices, and strategies women accumulate over time *rebuscarse la vida,* which is a form of migrant capital specifically developed by women. In doing so, we dispel the presumption that women learned how to organize themselves in the country of destination, but this is a skill they have been honing way before they migrated to the US. Women bring the experience of working together for the betterment of their community from their hometowns. Also, we shed light on the fact that

COVID-19, while strenuous and devastating, is not the only big crisis for unauthorized immigrants, but rather one more crisis they endured.

To conclude, we put forth the concept of women's migrant capital, or what we call *rebuscarse la vida*, which is the accumulation of knowledge, practices, and strategies immigrant women living in precarity develop when dealing with crises. This accumulation comes from their experiences in their hometown, when migrating, and when settling in a new city. While there are many topics that we would like to go into in more depth, at this point, we would like to conclude with a few questions that have emerged in our conversations and presentations of this research. If it is about the people, are there other unauthorized immigrant groups deploying what we call *rebuscarse la vida*? If it is about the place, what does the City of Philadelphia offer those women to deploy *rebuscarse la vida*? If it is about the grassroots organizations working with immigrant communities, what do they do to foster *rebuscarse la vida*?

Notes

1 The acronym "BIPOC" stands for "Black, Indigenous and People of Color" and is utilized as a political stand regarding the specific injustices affecting Black, Indigenous, and other People of Color in the context of the American socioeconomic, legal, political, and cultural systems.
2 The actual names were changed to protect participants′ confidentiality.
3 Here, the "I" refers to one of the authors who participated as a volunteer for the OV.
4 This "I" refers to the second author, who participated as a volunteer as well.

References

Aiken, Claudia, Vincent Reina, *et al.*2021. "Learning from emergency rental assistance programs". https://furmancenter.org/files/ERA_Programs_Case_Study_-_Final.pdf.

Allen, Taylor. 2021. "Philly courts just extended eviction protections again. Here's what that means", 1 July. https://whyy.org/articles/philly-courts-just-extended-eviction-protections-again-heres-what-that-means/.

Andrews, Abigail. 2014. "Women's political engagement in a Mexican sending community: migration as crisis and the struggle to sustain an alternative". *Gender & Society* 18, 4: 583–608.

Auyero, Javier. 2012. *Patients of the State: The Politics of Waiting in Argentina*. Durham, NC: Duke University Press.

Beck, Ulrich. 1993. *Risk Society*. London: Sage.

Beck, Ulrich. 2009. *World at Risk*. Cambridge: Polity.

Bradby, Hannah, Kristen Liabo, *et al.*2019. "Visibility, resilience, vulnerability in young immigrants". *Health: An Interdisciplinary Journal for the Social Study of Health, Illness and Medicine* 23, 5: 533–550.

Busse, Erika, and Tania Vásquez Luque. 2016. "The legal-illegal nexus: Haitians in transit migration deploying migrant capital". *International Journal of Sociology* 46, 3: 205–222.

Creswell, John W. 2013. *Qualitative Inquiry and Research Design: Choosing Among Five Approaches*, 3rd edition. Sage: Los Angeles: Sage.

Cohen, Julia, and Ige Babaseun. 2020. "*Restaurants in the Age of COVID-19: How Does Philadelphia Stack Up?*", 7 October. https://econsultsolutions.com/restaurants-covid-philadelphia-stack-up/.

De Genova, Nicholas. 2002. "Migrant 'illegality' and deportability in everyday life". *Annual Review of Anthropology* 31: 419–447.

Dingwall, Robert, Lily M. Hoffman, and Karen Staniland. 2013. *Pandemics and Emerging Infectious Diseases: The Sociological Agenda*. Malden, MA: Wiley-Blackwell.

Dudley, Mary Jo. 2019. "These U.S. industries can't work without illegal immigrants", January 10. www.cbsnews.com/news/illegal-immigrants-us-jobs-economy-farm-workers-taxes/.

Figueroa, Jose F., Rishi K. Wadhera, *et al.*2020. "Community-level factors associated with racial and ethnic disparities in COVID-19 rates In Massachusetts: study examines community-level factors associated with racial and ethnic disparities in COVID-19 rates in Massachusetts". *Health Affairs*, 39, 11:1984–1992.

Flores-Yeffal, Nadia. 2013. *Migration-Trust-Networks: Social Cohesion in Mexican-US Bound Emigration*. College Station: Texas A&M University Press.

Fonseca, Claudia, and Denise F. Jardim. 2010. "Kinship, migrations and the state". *Suomen Antropologi: Journal of the Finnish Anthropological Society* 35, 4: 45–49.

Gammage, Jeff. 2020. "With undocumented families excluded from coronavirus aid, immigrant organizations step in to help keep food on the table", 11 June. www.inquirer.com/news/immigrant-migrant-aid-unemployment-coronavirus-stimulus-20200611.html.

Gavazzo, Natalia, and Lucila Nejamkis. 2021. "'If we share, it is more than enough': networks of communitarian caring among women migrants in the Great Buenos Aires against COVID19". *REMHU Revista Interdisciplinaria Mobilidad Humana*. 29 (61):97–120.

Goldring, Luin. 2001. "The gender and geography of citizenship in Mexico-US transnational spaces". *Identities Global Studies in Culture and Power* 7 (4): 501–537.

Goodman, Laurie, Kathryn Reynolds, *et al.* 2021. "Many people are behind on rent: how much do they own", 24 February. www.urban.org/urban-wire/many-people-are-behind-rent-how-much-do-they-owe.

Gray, Lisa M., Gina Wong-Wylie, *et al.* 2020. "Expanding qualitative research interviewing strategies: Zoom video communication". *The Qualitative Report 2020*, 25, 5: 1292–1301.

Hagan, Jacqueline, Ruben Hernandez-León, and Jean-Luc Demonsant. 2015. *Skills of the "Unskilled": Labor and Social Mobility across the US-Migratory Circuit*. Berkeley, CA: University of California Press.

Hardy-Fanta, Carol. 1993. *Latina Politics, Latinos Politics: Gender, Culture, and Political Participation in Boston*. Philadelphia, PA: Temple University Press.

Henninger, Danya. 2017. "Immigrants plan to walk off their Philly restaurant jobs on Feb. 16". *BillPenn*, 14 February. https://billypenn.com/2017/02/14/immigrants-plan-to-walk-off-their-philly-restaurant-jobs-on-feb-16/.

Holt, A. 2010. "Using the telephone for narrative interviewing: a research note". *Qualitative Research*, 10, 1: 113–121. https://doi.org/10.1177/1468794109348686

Honduras Instituto Nacional de Estadística. 2013. *XVII Censo de Población y VI de Vivienda*, Vol. 228. Tegucigalpa: Instituto Nacional de Estadística.

Jones-Correa, Michael. 1998. "Different paths: gender, immigration and political participation". *International Migration Review* 32, 2: 326–349.

Keith, Charlotte. 2021. "The inside story of how Pennsylvania failed to deliver millions in coronavirus rent relief". *Philadelphia Inquirer*, 15 February. www.inquirer.com/news/pennsylvania/spl/pa-rent-relief-application-deadline-pennsylvania-failure-tenants-landlords-20210215.html?utm_medium=email&utm_campaign=Morning%20email%202-15-21&utm_content=Morning%20email%202-15-21+CID_c9b32e6dd5b8ec4af85579a5e70e760c&utm_source=newsletter_edit&utm_term=deliver%20millions%20in%20coronavirus%20rent%20relief#loaded.,

Lubbens, Miranda J., et al. 2020. "Do networks help people to manage poverty? Perspectives from the field". *ANNALS, AAPSS* 689: 7–25.

Montes, Veronica. 2022. "*Mujeres luchadoras*: Latino immigrant women's homemaking practices to assert their belonging in a Philadelphia suburb". In *Beyond Deportability: Latinx Belonging, Community-Building, and Resilience in the United States*, edited by Natalia Deeb-Sossa and Jennifer Bickham Mendez. Tucson, AZ: University of Arizona Press.

Padilla, Beatriz. 2004. "Grassroots participation and feminist gender identities: a case study of women from the popular sector in metropolitan Lima, Peru". *Journal of International Women's Studies* 6, 1: 93–113.

Padilla, Beatriz, Simone Castellani, Vera Rodrigues. 2022. "Who cares? Civil society organizations as healthcare life vest for migrants in post troika Portugal". *Journal of Ethnic and Migration Studies*. DOI:doi:10.1080/1369183X.2022.2157802.

Paret, Marcel, and Shannon Gleeson. 2016. "Precarity and agency through a migration lens". *Citizenship Studies* 20, 3–4: 277–294.

Philadelphia Renters Report. 2021. "COVID-19's impact on race and housing security across Philadelphia". *Philly Tenant*, 17 February. https://clsphila.org/wp-content/uploads/2021/02/20210222-Philadelphia-Renters-Report.pdf.

Phillimore, Jennifer, Hannah Bradby, *et al.*2019. "Bricolage as conceptual tool for understanding access to healthcare in superdiverse populations". *Social Theory & Health* 17: 231–252.

Ramirez, Catherine, *et al.*2021. *Precarity and Belonging. Labor, Migration, and Noncitizenship*. New Brunswick, NJ: Rutgers University Press.

Ramos, Cristina. 2018. "Onward migration from Spain to London in times of crisis: the importance of life-course junctures in secondary migrations". *Journal of Ethnic and Migration Studies* 44, 11: 1841–1857.

Wlosko, Miriam, and CeciliaRos. 2012. "Violencia Laboral en el sector salud: abordajes conceptuales y resultados de investigación en personal de enfermería en la Argentina". In *Personas Cuidando Personas: Dimensión Humana y Trabajo en salud*, edited by Elisa Ansoleaga Moreno, Osvaldo Artaza, and Julio Manuel Suarez Jiménez. Santiago de Chile: Representación.

Wolf, Sonja. 2021. "Talking to migrants: invisibility, vulnerability, and protection". *Geopolitics* 26, 1: 193–214.

Zinn, Jens O. 2021. "Introduction: towards a sociology of pandemics". *Current Sociology* 69, 4: 435–452.

5

THE SOCIOLOGY OF MIGRATION IN THE COVID-19 PANDEMIC

Racial and Ethnic Discrimination and Barriers to Integration in Greece

Theodoros Fouskas

Introduction: Unhealthy Conditions in the Reception and Identification Centers (RICs) and Accommodation Facilities

As the World Health Organization (WHO) (2020) states, asylum seekers, refugees, and migrants are at an increased risk of contracting diseases, such as COVID-19, as they live mostly in overcrowded facilities with deplorable and unhygienic living conditions, including lack of running water and sanitation, and an inappropriate sewage system without essential public health amenities (Veizis 2020; WHO 2020) and health services (including medical doctors, social workers, and psychologists). The daily routine of asylum seekers, refugees, and migrants includes two to three hours of waiting in queues to receive meals, often described as being of a low quality, which leads some to abandon the queue or not to eat (Jalbout 2020). Shortages of medicines and lack of healthcare facilities characterize the access to healthcare of asylum seekers, refugees, and migrants in humanitarian settings (WHO 2020). In Greece, thousands of asylum seekers, refugees, and migrants live under inhumane, unsafe, and degrading conditions at camps on the Aegean islands and several others in mainland Greece (Kathimerini 2019, Oxfam 2019). Camps are severely overcrowded, and a lack of medical doctors is marked, resulting in numerous health issues in general, but also compounded by lack of heating and insulation in the winter months. Many third country nationals (TCNs) feel insecure under these conditions, while many have suffered sexual abuse or mental traumas. In the RICs, there are frequent outbreaks of violence and fires – for example, in Lesvos (March 2020) (Kathimerini 2020a) and Samos (April 2020) (Kathimerini 2020b), where the fire spread quickly due to the flammable materials in the camp used for cooking inside the tents. These violent clashes were the result of differences between migrant groups (for example, African and Afghan migrants residing in the camp), poor living conditions, lack of healthcare and overcrowding,

DOI: 10.4324/9781003459682-6

as multiple different nationalities live in the same area and there exists psychological stress and tension intensified by the ongoing immobility and uncertainty. The RICs have been operating inappropriately. They are mostly set up in old facilities, such as abandoned army camps and factories, which have been extended beyond their intended capacity. Newcomers set up tents wherever they can find available space in the surrounding area, taking no safety measures and being exposed to the elements. TCNs inside the RICs are crammed into small individual tents or separate makeshift spaces made by wooden walls under a larger umbrella tent. These spaces offer little or no privacy, blankets are used for doors and mats for flooring, while they provide insufficient insulation from the elements and temperature changes (summer heat/winter cold). There is no segregation between men, women, and children (including unaccompanied minors), while containers are used as living spaces. The RICs, in general, do not provide adequate amenities like running water, sanitation, and access to electricity. These conditions have contributed to an environment that is unsafe and full of health risks for TCNs. In general, a worrying reduction in healthcare provision in all RICs on the islands has been observed (Médicins Sans Frontières 2017a). TCNs' current squalid living conditions in Greece are inadequate (for example, in Samos' Vathy camp, in Chios' Vial camp, and in Lesvos' Moria camp). During consultations, they stress that uncertainty about their future, the threat of deportation, and their lack of access to appropriate healthcare negatively affect their mental well-being (Médicins Sans Frontières 2017b). The abovementioned situation of poor living conditions is encountered in accommodation facilities in the mainland and in the housing environments of TCNs in Greek cities.

Unveiling Perceptions of Racial and Ethnic Discrimination During the COVID-19 Pandemic in Greece

In Greece on the Athens-Thessaloniki train route, when at the Lianokladi station, a legal migrant from Cameroon was forced off the train, because they believed that he had coronavirus. During the inspection of his ticket, it was found that he had purchased a ticket to Livadia and bore a document stating that he had contracted coronavirus in May 2020, four months previously. The passengers panicked and demanded he get off the train. The inspector asked him to sit on the floor until they reached the next station, where he left the train, while the police and the National Center for Emergency Care (EKAV) were informed (iEfimerida 2020). Another incident took place on the Athens-Thessaloniki route on November 2021, when the train was stopped to disembark 27 Bangladeshi nationals, as the rest of the passengers were disturbed by their presence and asked the specific people to be checked for the mandatory health certificate (iEfimerida 2021).

Protection measures against COVID-19 were applied in the RICs and in the accommodation centers, and administrative actions were implemented (Fouskas 2020): (a) suspension of asylum applications, (b) extension of residents' permits, (c) suspension of reception and administrative actions (recordings, interviews, filing of an appeal, etc.), (d) suspension of all special activities in the accommodation facilities, and (e) forced lockdown and restriction on movement periodically extended. This approach was problematic, as there was concurrently a lifting of restrictions only for the public and for international visitors, so this paved the way for anti-immigration attitudes and mobilizations. Other measures included the suspension of all special activities and amenities in the facilities, while new arrivals were checked for fever and other COVID-19 symptoms and subjects were confined to quarantine if found to be ailing (Kathimerini 2020c). Sanitation measures were implemented to ensure that all common areas were regularly cleaned and modernized, and instructions in multiple languages were distributed twice a day in the island camps (Kathimerini 2020a). TCNs in camps were discouraged from strolling around the facilities or going outside the RICs, even to get provisions. Moreover, controlled entry and exit in previously open facilities was implemented, so they functioned as closed centers (Kathimerini 2020d). In addition, preventive measures against the spread of COVID-19 in RICs and accommodation centers of TCNs were launched, via a National Action Plan of Crisis Management in Refugee Structures entitled AGNODIKI. It also included delivery points by companies and the installation of ATMs within the structures (GOV.GR 2020). Several COVID-19 cases were detected in accommodation centers in mainland Greece (see Figure 5.1). During the first cases of COVID-19, multiple attempts to enter Greece via the Greek-Turkish land borders were recorded. The State implemented measures of prevention of entry and border sealing policies, followed by the suspension of asylum applications.

In the context of the COVID-19 pandemic, inequalities emerged particularly regarding marginalized and racialized populations (Abedi et al. 2021). Strong

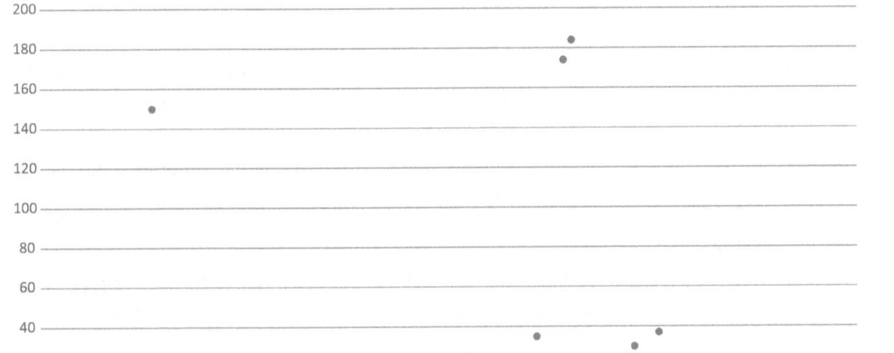

FIGURE 5.1 COVID-19 cases among migrants in Greece.
Source: Fouskas 2020

differences existed concerning mortality and infection rates by age, gender, ethnicity, work status and conditions, housing, and geographic residence. Racism involves a disadvantaged position in society where consistent disparities arise along with institutional exclusion (Balibar 1991; Banton 2018) in employment, education, housing, healthcare, and everyday interaction. It is articulated via xenophobic behaviors and discriminatory practices due to social identification of racial and ethnic origin with precarious, low/status/low wage work, poor housing and living conditions. Immigrants, asylum seekers, and refugees are subject to aggression and false characterizations, negative behaviors, lack of work advancement and access to education and healthcare. All these lead to poor life opportunities and unfavorable exclusion regarding healthcare, employment, and housing, and place migrants on the receiving end of multiple forms of violence (verbal, physical, and psychological) and increasing disparities (Fouskas and Koulierakis 2022). Racism and xenophobia against migrants, in particular, are on the rise (Esses and Hamilton 2021). Anti-migrant sentiments and mobilizations, social exclusion, and xenophobia have intensified as governments, local societies, communities. and individuals react to fears and challenges related to the disease, regarding migrants as a threat to public health. This anti-migrant political and social media hateful rhetoric is targeted at migrants (Farro and Maddanu 2022; Yerly 2022). Xenophobia entails attitudes, prejudices, and practices that cast off, exclude, and frequently denigrate individuals based on the belief that they are outsiders or foreigners (Essed 1991). Racism entails practices and norms that allocate lower value and determine prospects according to the external looks or skin color of individuals. Racism, being a conceptual construct, assumes a position of power over others based on physical and cultural attributes, e.g., skin color, origin, and language (Wimmer 1997). Although these are separate ideas, they overlap as phenomena, since one triggers the other. The media play a catalytic role in boosting racist and xenophobic narratives. During the pandemic, prejudice and disdain against migrants offer an emotional outlet for anxieties driven by fear and ignorance. Both racism and xenophobia against migrants have been established in clandestine and unconcealed ways (clearly visible verbal and physical abuse, hateful rhetoric, practices, and behavior) and varied forms at all levels, regenerating from each other and ultimately creating barriers to integration.

COVID-19 Pandemic Impact on Social Determinants of Migrant and Refugee Health and Their Integration

Social determinants of health contribute to racial and ethnic groups being disproportionately affected by COVID-19 (Centers for Disease Control and Prevention 2020):

a Living environment: they face difficulties finding inexpensive, quality housing (Wilder 2021). This limits their options to neighborhoods and residences with other racial and ethnic groups, and/or crowded conditions that may also lack access to reliable transportation. Under such conditions, illnesses, diseases, and injuries are more common and more severe. Access to nutritious affordable food may be limited and they may be exposed to environmental pollution within their neighborhoods. Older adults are at increased risk due to living in overcrowded conditions.

b Healthcare: they are disproportionately affected by lack of access to quality healthcare, health insurance, and linguistically and culturally responsive healthcare, resulting in their distrust of State healthcare systems and considering health, health promotion, preventive care and hygiene as unimportant (Turner-Musa et al. 2020).

c Occupational conditions: they are disproportionately represented in precarious, low-status/low-wage work due to the unequal division of labor. Hence, it entraps migrants almost exclusively into the informal sector of the economy, where employers benefit financially by avoiding social security contributions and hiring people without contracts. Migrants exercise manual labor in agriculture, construction, crafts, domestic work, restaurant and hotel services, personal care, nursing, factory work, fishery, food production, public transportation and in itinerant trade. These jobs are not attractive, offer no social prestige and are socially inferior (Fouskas 2021). In such settings, they are at an increased risk of being exposed to COVID-19 due to close contact with the public or other workers, as they are involved in activities that cannot be done from a distance, or they lack benefits such as health insurance and paid sick leave.

d Income: they face barriers in accumulating funds, have greater debts and are unable to send remittances to their country of origin, pay for health coverage in cases of uninsured individuals, cover medical bills and access housing, nutritious food and childcare.

e Education: they are disproportionately affected by inequities in access to formal education. This can lead to lower literacy, limited school completion rates, barriers to university-level education, poor access to quality job training and language courses, thus restricting future job choices and leading to inferior pay or unstable jobs.

Failure to deal with social determinants of health disparities increases vulnerability of these racial and ethnic groups to infectious diseases; thus combating social inequalities needs to be a priority in both policy and practice (Dalsania et al. 2022). For example, there have been reports of racism against Chinese individuals and other groups in response to the way the origins of the virus were stated (Wang et al. 2021); there are documented occurrences of xenophobic responses where racial and ethnic groups were marginalized. They are perceived by societies as "unwanted individuals" or as a "threat", a "health time-bomb", "criminals and dangerous", "invaders/intruders", individuals who "alter the homogeneity of the host country", people who are "uneducated, uncultured and do not want to attend school", and who "take the jobs of native-born workers", a threat to democracy, and draining of public resources and during COVID-19, a threat to public health (Moreno Barreneche 2020). All these descriptions have been used by political leaders and the media (Vega Macías 2021).

Once infected with SARS-CoV-2, individuals who have been marginalized are in greater need of hospitalization, because they often have chronic comorbidities (Gravlee 2020). The prevalence of chronic diseases is higher among low-income, minority populations. Racial or ethnic minority patients in the European Union (EU) often lack health insurance, suffer from comorbidities, live mostly in low-income and unsafe neighborhoods, and are dependent on care from low-funded safety-net institutions. Patients with limited English-language skills and especially limited health literacy are more likely to suffer worse health outcomes (Fouskas et al. 2019). Disparities in socioeconomic conditions across racial lines have intensified during the COVID-19 pandemic (Laster Pirtle and Wright 2021; Pirro et al. 2022). Amid the state pandemic measures, the rhetoric on pandemic uncertainty, anti-vaccination movements, and vaccine hesitancy, migrants have been among the worst hit by the pandemic and migrant workers have been at a higher risk of infection. This is due to their precarious employment and legal status, while still being considered essential workers throughout the public health crisis in both low- and high-skilled jobs in the EU (Fassani and Mazza 2020). Additionally, while residing in confined and crammed spaces in accommodation facilities, squalid housing, and unsanitary conditions with inadequate access to healthcare, migrants have been vulnerable to COVID-19 infection.

Methodology

The chapter attempts to address the following central question: has the COVID-19 pandemic raised barriers against integration and allowed space for anti-migrant attitudes? The results are based on findings from the project "Local Alliance for Integration" (LION/General Secretariat for Research and Innovation (GSRI)/University of West Attica (UNIWA)/81018): "Migrant and refugee integration into local societies during the COVID-19 pandemic in Spain and Greece", carried out by the Department of Public Health Policy at the School of Public Health of the University of West Attica and funded by the General Secretariat for Research and Innovation,[1] implementing a qualitative methodology under the National Funding 2019 with Scientific Director/Principal Investigator (PI) Theodoros Fouskas, Assistant Professor at the Department of Public Health Policy at the School of Public Health of the University of West Attica (UNIWA). The interviews were conducted in person during the first half of 2022 (between 18 March 2022 and 28 May 2022). In the current chapter, research results from Greece are presented. A total of 32 in-person, semi-structured interviews were conducted in Greece with adult male and female TCNs (immigrants, refugees, and asylum seekers) from Afghanistan, Congo, Iraq, Kuwait, Morocco, Somalia, Syria, and Uganda (see Table 5.1), living in open accommodation facilities for migrants and refugees in the wider region of Attica (Greece). Additionally, 15 semi-structured interviews were conducted in Spain with adult male and female TCNs from Colombia, Venezuela, El Salvador, Romania, and others in the greater Andalusian region, along with 47 in-depth interviews regarding the experiences of immigrants and refugees in Spain and Greece. The research unveils increased barriers towards integration during the COVID-19 pandemic, which function as a means of perpetuating exclusion in healthcare and posing obstacles to their integration. Thematic analysis was implemented. The study was conducted in accordance with the Declaration of Helsinki, and the methodological design and the information collection instruments were designed by the Scientific Director and approved by the Research Ethics Committee of the University of West Attica (UNIWA) (approval ref. no. 22354/08-03-2022). Participants were informed of the procedure and purpose of the study; participation of the sample and continuation in the research were voluntary; the investigation was carried out under the principle of confidentiality of data provided, ensuring the correct use of the same; and the research participants signed the informed consent. All personal data obtained in the study is confidential and will be treated in accordance with Law 4624/2019 on data protection.

Precarious Conditions, Barriers to Integration, and Perceptions of Racism

Employment

Some Congolese men, one Iraqi woman and two Somali women had work experience in their home country: house painters, an English teacher, a housekeeper and a street vendor, respectively. One participant (interviewee 6, female, Somalia) stated that she had never worked in her life, while one participant (interviewee 24, male, Syria) stated that he had never worked in his country but had worked part-time in Greece. Others had worked in Greece, one in low-skilled and informal work (interviewee 29, male, Syria) and two as female volunteers (interviewee 26, female, Congo, Red Cross volunteer in a facility on an Aegean island; and interviewee 4, female, Iraq, volunteer English teacher at a refugee accommodation facility on an Aegean island). Participants reported finding it difficult to find work in Greece or lacked access to employment for a variety of reasons, unrelated to the pandemic. An interviewee from Congo (interviewee 3, male) said:

> I lost my job at the moving company. My boss said “We don’t have work now. It’s the pandemic. It’s difficult to find a job now.”

TABLE 5.1 Characteristics of the sample

Interview Code	*Nationality*	*Gender*	*Age*	*Entry Year in Greece*	*Reasons for Entry*	*Way of Entry*	*Education*	*Family status*	*Children*	*Employment*	*Residence*	*Community Association Participation*	*Healthcare via NHS*	*Healthcare via NGOs*	*COVID-19 Positive*	*COVID-19 Vaccinated*
1	Syria	Male	23	2019	Warfare	Irregularly/Sea	ISCED 2: Lower secondary education or second stage of basic education	Married	1	No	Container in Open Accommodation Facilities for Migrants and Refugees	No	No	No	No	No
2	Congo	Male	36	2019	Warfare		ISCED 2: Lower secondary education or second stage of basic education	Single	0	No		No	No	No	No	No
3	Congo	Male	34	2019	Warfare		ISCED 1: Primary education or first stage of basic education	Single	0	No		Yes	Yes	No	No	No
4	Iraq	Female	55	2018	Warfare		ISCED 6: Bachelor's or equivalent level	Married	3	No		No	Yes	No	No	No
5	Iraq	Female	21	2020	Warfare		ISCED 3: Upper secondary education	Married	1	No		No	Yes	No	No	Yes
6	Somalia	Female	28	2018	Warfare		ISCED 2: Lower secondary education or second stage of basic education	Married	1	No		No	Yes	No	No	Yes
7	Somalia	Female	20	2018	Warfare		No formal education/below ISCED 1	Married	0	No		No	Yes	No	No	Yes
8	Morocco	Male	44	2019	Economic		ISCED 6: Bachelor's or equivalent level	Married	2	No		No	Yes	No	No	No
9	Congo	Male	21	2019	Economic		ISCED 5: Short-cycle tertiary education	Single	0	Yes		No	Yes	Yes	No	Yes
10	Syria	Male	30	2020	Warfare		ISCED 1: Primary education or first stage of basic education	Married	3	Yes		No	Yes	Yes	Yes	No
11	Somalia	Male	19	2021	Economic		No formal education/below ISCED 1	Single	0	No		No	No	No	No	Yes
12	Congo	Female	29	2017	Family		No formal education/below ISCED 1	Married	2	No		No	Yes	Yes	No	No
13	Kuwait	Male	57	2019	Economic		No formal education/below ISCED 1	Widowed	3	No		No	Yes	No	No	Yes
14	Congo	Female	39	2019	Economic		ISCED 2: Lower secondary education or second stage of basic education	Single	0	No		No	No	Yes	No	Yes
15	Iraq	Female	70	2018	Warfare		No formal education/below ISCED 1	Single	2	No		No	Yes	Yes	No	Yes
16	Congo	Male	41	2018	Political		ISCED 6: Bachelor's or equivalent level	Married	3	Yes		No	Yes	Yes	No	No

Interview Code	*Nationality*	*Gender*	*Age*	*Entry Year in Greece*	*Reasons for Entry*	*Way of Entry*	*Education*	*Family status*	*Children*	*Employment*	*Residence*	*Community Association Participation*	*Healthcare via NHS*	*Healthcare via NGOs*	*COVID-19 Positive*	*COVID-19 Vaccinated*
17	Congo	Female	36	2019	Political	Irregularly/Sea	ISCED 1: Primary education or first stage of basic education	Single	1	No	Container in Open Accommodation Facilities for Migrants and Refugees	No	No	Yes	No	No
18	Congo	Male	20	2019	Economic		No formal education/below ISCED 1	Single	0	No		No	Yes	Yes	No	Yes
19	Congo	Male	29	2019	Warfare		ISCED 6: Bachelor's or equivalent level	Single	2	No		No	No	Yes	No	No
20	Syria	Female	23	2019	Warfare		ISCED 3: Upper secondary education	Married	2	No		No	Yes	Yes	No	No
21	Syria	Male	24	2019	Warfare		No formal education/below ISCED 1	Married	3	No		No	Yes	Yes	No	Yes
22	Somalia	Female	19	2019	Warfare		No formal education/below ISCED 1	Single	0	No		No	Yes	Yes	No	No
23	Uganda	Male	28	2018	Warfare		ISCED 2: Lower secondary education or second stage of basic education	Married	2	No		Yes	Yes	Yes	No	Yes
24	Syria	Male	20	2019	Warfare		ISCED 2: Lower secondary education or second stage of basic education	Married	1	Yes		No	Yes	Yes	No	Yes
25	Somalia	Male	19	2020	Political		No formal education/below ISCED 1	Single	0	No		Yes	No	Yes	No	Yes
26	Congo	Female	39	2019	Economic		ISCED 2: Lower secondary education or second stage of basic education	Single	0	No		No	No	Yes	No	Yes
27	Kuwait	Male	37	2019	Economic		No formal education/below ISCED 1	Widowed	4	No		No	Yes	Yes	No	Yes
28	Congo	Female	29	2020	Economic		ISCED 2: Lower secondary education or second stage of basic education	Separated	2	No		No	No	Yes	No	No
29	Syria	Male	30	2020	Warfare		ISCED 1: Primary education or first stage of basic education	Married	3	Yes		No	Yes	Yes	Yes	No
30	Afghanistan	Female	43	2019	Warfare		ISCED 1: Primary education or first stage of basic education	Married	3	No		No	Yes	Yes	No	No
31	Afghanistan	Male	37	2019	Warfare		ISCED 3: Upper secondary education	Married	2	No		No	Yes	Yes	No	Yes
32	Afghanistan	Female	29	2019	Warfare		No formal education/below ISCED 1	Married	3	No		No	Yes	Yes	No	Yes

Another interviewee, a male, from Afghanistan (interviewee 31), said:

> I was in Athens looking for a job in a restaurant and the man asked me, "Are you vaccinated? Show me proof. Is everyone vaccinated at the place you live?" He had asked me if I was staying in a camp. I felt strange like being interrogated again.

Another interviewee from Morocco (interviewee 8, male) said:

> He [employer] told me that I have to work 4 hours not 8 hours. He said he cannot pay more. But I agreed. I could not stop, as I needed the money, also due to the pandemic.

For example, one participant (interviewee 2, male, Congo) stated, "I do not have a Tax ID [AFM] number, I do not have the documents I need to [find] a job ... but I want to work." Another participant (interviewee 15, female, Iraq) focused on language barriers: "In order to work I have to know the [Greek] language and they do not offer us language classes." One participant (interviewee 6, female, Somalia) focused on her family responsibilities and the lack of a relevant support network that would allow her to work: "I am not able to look for a job – who will take care of my child? I do not feel safe; I feel very unsettled." Finally, another participant (interviewee 22, female, Somalia) gave a gender dimension to barriers in accessing employment, noting that as a woman it is even more difficult to find a job. Finally, in terms of job seeking, most participants seemed to have given up due to insurmountable obstacles, some of which are mentioned above. One of the participants (interviewee 19, male, Congo) stated that many migrants were actively seeking informal work. Specifically, he has sought to find a job by approaching his Greek colleagues who are in the house-painting business, giving them his personal telephone number (mobile) to call him, but "so far nothing."

Education

Some participants noted that there are no opportunities for educational activities for the children in the accommodation facilities. They also mentioned the inhospitable living conditions that children in the accommodation facilities, and/or in the country in general, are subject to. An interviewee from Somalia (interviewee 7, female) added:

> I remember once, when I left my child at school some parents kept staring at me. One man came and asked me where I was from, if I was fully vaccinated, where I lived and if my son had been sick. I felt I was being interrogated.

In particular, one participant (interviewee 1, male, Syria) stated that his child is "not at all happy" with life in the refugee facility, as they "have no money", and his material and other needs cannot be met. Another participant (interviewee 7, female, Somalia), whose child passed away in Greece, noted, "This refugee camp is not good for children; it is not good for people." An interviewee from Congo (interviewee 12, female) said:

> In the camp my daughter did not have access to online lessons because we had a weak wifi signal, while others did not have a tablet. She was disappointed.

Another interviewee from Congo (interviewee 28, female) mentioned:

> When I went to pick up my daughter from school a woman, a parent, asked me if I and my child are vaccinated. I said we were not, but were planning to. She responded: "Why? Are you not afraid? How can you bring your child to school?" I said, "We wear masks and my husband and I will be vaccinated."

Regarding educational, recreational or creative adult employment opportunities, only one participant (interviewee 6, female, Somalia) referred to such activities within the facility, which are not provided by the facility staff but by a well-known humanitarian organization. In particular, an NGO organizes activities in which they participate, such as painting and art classes: "They take us on excursions outside the camp, we are given sewing machines and we sew." The rest of the participants noted the complete absence of such opportunities. As one participant (interviewee 29, male, Syria) bluntly stated, "There is nothing for us to do here!" while in the same spirit, a participant (interviewee 25, male, Somalia) stated, "We do not have a job, we do not have a school, we just sit here." Finally, once again there is a difference between the opportunities provided by different accommodation facilities: in particular, one participant (interviewee 2, male, Congo) mentioned that in the accommodation facility where he was originally located on an Aegean island, Greek lessons were held, unlike the accommodation facility where he now lives. Another participant (interviewee 18, male, Congo) argued that, despite the existence of such options in the Moria facility where he was located, the conditions of confinement and the insecurity he experienced did not allow him to participate in educational or recreational activities:

> It was like a prison there [in Moria]. We were not free; the place was not very safe. I want to learn something, to do something. But it was a confined space and the situation on the island was not good. Everyday life was so stressful; it was not a good learning environment.

Housing

All participants lived in metal containers within the accommodation facilities. Almost everyone expressed their strong dissatisfaction with the living conditions in the facility, the majority of whom focused on the quality of the meals: "The food is not edible" (interviewee 21, male, Syria), "I either give it to someone else or throw [the food] away" (interviewee 15, woman from Iraq), "Honestly, the food we are given is not edible! I do not eat it. It's cold and the fruit [given to us] is rotten" (interviewee 4, female, Iraq), "the food has gone off by the time it reaches us" (interviewee 22, female, Somalia). In addition, other participants also mentioned: (a) lack of room in the cooking and showering facilities; one must take turns (interviewee 9, male, Congo), (b) the absence of heating – it was so cold and they were not allowed to have an open fire heater for safety reasons (interviewee 19, male, Congo), (c) power outages or reduced meals (interviewee 18, male, Congo), (d) lack of cleanliness (interviewee 5, female, Iraq). One of the participants (interviewee 1, male, Syria) described the living conditions in the accommodation facility where he had originally been placed (Moria facility, Lesvos) in the worst possible terms. He referred to the presence of rats and water inside his tent, concluding that "My wife and I lived on the island. It was like a Syrian prison." Once again, there are differences between the accommodation facilities, this time in terms of living conditions: in particular, a participant (interviewee 4, female, Iraq) stated that, in the accommodation facility in Samos where she was originally located, the living conditions were better and sanitation was satisfactory: "Now [in the Facility] I cannot even take a walk inside this camp [in Attica]." At the level of State social protection and/or support from other bodies and services, three participants (interviewee 21, male, Syria; interviewee 9, male, Congo; interviewee 25, male, Somalia) pointed to the pre-pandemic termination of the financial "allowance" for asylum seekers/refugees, a development that resulted in the deterioration of their living conditions. As one participant (interviewee 29, male, Syria) characteristically stated:

> My wife will have a caesarean section in two days. I do not have 100 euros in my pocket for the child; he may need milk – who knows? She [the mother] may not have milk to breastfeed. I only have the blessings of God. I have no money, no salary. Life is very difficult.

Additionally, one participant (interviewee 14, female, Iraq) stated that she could not afford to buy her medication. Finally, only one participant (interviewee 18, male, Congo) reported that another non-State body promised to help him improve his living conditions.

Healthcare

The majority of interviewees reported that, while in Greece, they had visited a public hospital at least once – for themselves or their children – and received medical care and/or medication. One of them (interviewee 15, female, Iraq) reported taking medication for hypertension and diabetes, while another participant (interviewee 9, male, Congo) admitted being treated by a psychiatrist to whom he was referred to by a psychologist, as he had previously been residing under stress in Moria (Lesvos).

They usually mad an appointment with the assistance of officials of the facility in which they lived. However, two participants (interviewee 2, male, Congo; interviewee 19, male, Congo) reported that, since they did not possess Tax ID (AFM/Tax Identification Number and/or Medical ID/National Insurance Number (AMKA)/PAAYPA), they had limited access to medical services and/or had to pay for the medication they needed. Similarly, another participant (interviewee 5, female, Iraq) stated that she could not afford the prescribed medication.

The same participant additionally stated that the absence of interpreters when in the presence of medical staff hindered communication and created difficulties. In fact, even though she spoke a little English, she could not communicate with the medical staff. Another issue that was mentioned was the tendency of health issues to be downgraded by the medical staff. One participant (interviewee 4, female, Iraq) said that she went to hospital not feeling well, but the doctors insisted she was healthy: "I went to the hospital because I was not well; there they told me, 'There's nothing wrong with you.'" In fact, she added that officials of the refugee facility formally complained to a hospital about this practice, but she received the answer that the patient was well or that they should visit the hospital again – "She has nothing" and "Come next week" – something not always feasible due to family obligations ("I cannot leave the girl [her minor daughter] alone every day to visit doctors").

On the other hand, when asked about it, none of the participants reported discriminatory behavior towards them by medical staff, and some said that the behavior of the staff towards them was "good". Regarding the protective measures against the spread of the coronavirus pandemic, almost all participants stated that they adhered to the personal protection measures and specifically the use of masks and antiseptic lotion, adding that they were provided with these items within the facility.

However, it seems that the provision of information on COVID-19 is not the same in all the facilities: for example, as one participant (interviewee 26, female, Congo) reported, while in the refugee facilities on the Aegean islands, the executives informed the refugee population about the COVID-19 protective measures, which apparently was not the case in the facility he where he was currently residing. There was also a difference in the reports by the participants regarding the provision of personal protective equipment, as some of them stated that they were given "only" masks within the facility, while others stated that they had access to other materials such as antiseptic hand lotion. One possible explanation is that the relevant items of personal protection were not sufficient to cover the needs of the entire refugee population living in the facility. An interviewee from Kuwait (interviewee 27, male) said:

> I was in fear. I did not have a mask. Later they gave me a few. We did not have many doctors.

Additionally, three participants (interviewee 15, female, Iraq; and interviewees 6 and 7, two females from Somalia) had already been vaccinated against coronavirus. Of the others, one participant (interviewee 4, female, Iraq) stated that her vaccination had been scheduled, one participant (interviewee 10, male, Syria) stated that he did not wish to be vaccinated, one participant (interviewee 16, male, Congo) stated that he intended to be vaccinated, while another (interviewee 2, male, Congo) wondered how he could be vaccinated not having a National Insurance Number (AMKA or PAAYPA/Provisional Social Security and Health Care Number).

The lack of adequate or effective information is also highlighted via the reservations expressed by some of the participants regarding the safety of coronavirus vaccines. In particular, one participant (interviewee 1, male, Syria) stated that, despite the fact that he feared the coronavirus pandemic, he did not intend to be vaccinated because he did not know what the vaccine contained, while, to strengthen his argument, he referred to the corresponding refusal or reservations of several Greek citizens:

> [I am not vaccinated] because I do not want to be injected with something [the vaccine] that I do not know. Not all Greeks have been vaccinated.

Another participant (interviewee 18, male, Congo) reported that, although initially afraid, he finally decided to get vaccinated because his friends had done so. One (interviewee 29, male, Syria) participant also expressed the view that the coronavirus pandemic and the consequent restrictive measures were simply an excuse to justify his poor living conditions. Specifically, when asked how the pandemic and the restrictive measures affected his life, he replied:

> Excuses! Everyone talks about coronavirus. I have not seen a [case] of coronavirus. I have not had it either; and I undergo tests regularly. I have nothing.

Another interviewee (19, male, Congo) added that the problems he faced before the pandemic were the same as those he faced during the pandemic. As for the other participants, one participant (interviewee 32, female, Afghanistan) focused mostly on the effects of the pandemic and the resulting restrictive measures on mental health: as she characteristically stated, because of the pandemic (and the subsequent restrictive measures) "We are like prisoners", "It has deeply affected us psychologically", "We are afraid to go out", "Our already aggravated psychological condition has been affected." In the same vein, another participant (interviewee 7, female, Somalia) noted that their daily lives were difficult, as they had been under "too much pressure" and were forced to wear masks. An interviewee from Syria (interviewee 24, male) highlighted: "One day I couldn't find my mask. I looked everywhere. I was afraid to go out. Another participant (interviewee 6, female, Somalia) focused on the difficulty of meeting daily needs while she dwelled on the conditions of confinement, but also expressed the hope for better days:

> I cannot go to the supermarket, I cannot go out on the street, I cannot buy anything, but now we have had the vaccinations and I hope things will change.

Finally, another participant (interviewee 23, male, Uganda) stated that he was having a "difficult" time due to the restrictive measures, adding, however, "I thank God that I am alive." An interviewee from Congo (interviewee 26, female) emphasized:

> Now, when we meet, we will be able to talk with each other, because we have been vaccinated. Before, it was difficult because we were afraid to approach one another and spend time together because of COVID-19.

Overall, of the 32 participants, 17 (53.13 percent) had been vaccinated and 2 (6.25 percent) tested positive for COVID-19. Some participants reported feelings of fear, insecurity, and isolation as a result of the pandemic and the restrictive measures that had been implemented. In addition to the effects of the pandemic and the restrictive measures on participants' mental health, they had had a negative impact on their lives at multiple levels. For example, one participant (interviewee 5, female, Iraq) referred to the lengthy postponement of her asylum application process (interview):

> [The pandemic] changed my life 100 percent. I waited two years for my interview [asylum application]. When the interview date came, it was postponed by 1–1.5 years. That was very difficult for me.

Another participant (interviewee 7, female, Somalia) referred to the cessation of educational and creative opportunities within the refugee facility – in particular, before the outbreak of the pandemic, there was an "English-language school" in the facility which closed down at the outbreak of the pandemic. Other participants expressed their dissatisfaction with the required use of masks (interviewee 7, female, Somalia; interviewee 23, male, Uganda; interviewee 25, male, Somalia; interviewee 32, female, Afghanistan), the inability to visit shops (e.g., supermarkets) for basic necessities (interviewee 6, female, Somalia; interviewee 25, male, Somalia). In two cases (interviewee 19, male, Congo; interviewee 21, male, Syria), it was pointed out that pre-existing problems and challenges still existed.

The life of TCNs (immigrants, asylum seekers, and refugees) in Greece is full of challenges: living in accommodation facilities under often unsuitable conditions, time-consuming procedures for international protection applications or appeals, job and education prospects for themselves and their children, lack of access to even basic services (e.g., healthcare), and finally limited or non-existent alternative support networks. The coronavirus pandemic, and the application of restrictive measures aimed at curtailing its spread, have had an additional negative impact on their life in the country: exacerbation of their mental health (widespread feelings of fear and/or isolation due to segregation), additional delays in asylum applications, and restriction of their daily activities.

Despite these adversities, many of them took an active stance against the pandemic threat and the difficult conditions of their lives: they were vaccinated or had scheduled vaccination, adhered to the individual protection measures and, above all, made plans for the future, both for themselves and their children, even in the same country that had not always been hospitable to them.

Intercultural Coexistence and Community Participation

The pandemic resulted in some participants being forced to remain within the facility and to cease their social contacts. Indicatively – and as mentioned above – due to the coronavirus pandemic, one participant (interviewee 15, female, Iraq) stopped socializing with members of her community, while adding that the fear of the pandemic kept them constantly within the Facility, where they felt like "prisoners." Even in the case of one participant (interviewee 29, male, Syria) who refused to be vaccinated, and regarding the pandemic and the restrictive measures as an excuse to cover up other problems, the "fear" of the pandemic – as he argued –had kept him inside the Facility. Regarding the possible existence of discriminatory attitudes towards them during their stay in Greece, one participant (interviewee 19, male, Congo) clearly referred to racist attitudes. In particular, after initially stating that Greece, in general, "is not [considered] good" and that "the country has not helped [him]", he added that, in Lesvos (facility of Moria), where he was initially, he had faced racist behavior due to the color of his skin. An interviewee from Somalia (interviewee 11, male) mentioned:

> One time I feared for my life; there was a guy, I don't know where he was from, but I know he was someone in charge of the camp, who asked me: why are you here? I don't see any refugee who seeks asylum. He said, "This is my country! Go back to your country! I don't want to see you again." I told him he was right and then I left; I was scared for my life.

An interviewee from Iraq (interviewee 4, female) stated:

> I have often experienced racism on public transport. When I sit next to someone, they don't want to be so close. Once there was an elderly lady

> and I was on the train, with my baby, and she started shouting at me to get up and give her my seat. Everybody was looking at me. I gave her my seat.

An interviewee from Syria (interviewee 24, male) said:

> One day, while I was at the bus stop with lots of people, I removed my mask for a minute and a woman told me put it back on. "You carry diseases! Do you want to get us all sick?"

Two other women from Somalia (interviwees 7 and 22) reported harassment by facility staff without any clear evidence of racist motive or some other need ("They do not even talk to you", "They do not help you") – behaviors that may be due to skin color. Along the same lines, another participant argued that, within the refugee facility, the staff were often rude to them. Finally, one participant (interviewee 3, male, Congo) reported armed attacks (with a knife) and muggings (theft of his mobile phone) by refugees/asylum seekers of different nationalities, without the existence of a racist motivation.

The majority of participants mentioned the existence of a friendly environment and lack of participation in organized collectives, either of the same ethnic community or different ones. One participant (interviewee 4, female, Iraq) claimed that, because of the pandemic, she severed social contacts with people from her community, while another (interviewee 16, male, Congo) stated that he had no friends. They performed their religious duties – when they did so – within the facility. When they needed information or advice on key issues (such as jobs, healthcare, housing, paperwork, education), they turned to either NGOs operating within the facility or the facility staff. One participant (interviewee 5, female, Iraq) referred positively to the staff of the facility, noting, "Thank God [the staff of the facility] helps." However, not all participants had the same opinion (or experiences): in particular, another participant (interviewee 4, female, Iraq) stated that, when she asked for information/advice on key issues, she was told, "That is not within our responsibilities." Finally, another participant (interviewee 2, male, Congo) claimed that he did not seek advice and information and focused his efforts on finding a job through his Greek colleagues (house painters).

Conclusions

Integration describes an individual or group process that seeks to adapt to a new country and the reality of immigrants, applicants, and beneficiaries of international protection. It is a dynamic, two-way process of mutual accommodation by both immigrants and residents of EU member states, and the promotion of fundamental rights, non-discrimination, and equal opportunities, for all are key integration issues (European Migration Network 2018). One of the main indicators for examining the degree of integration of immigrants, asylum seekers, and refugees is their access to healthcare services, both at the level of institutional framework and in challenges they face when accessing and utilizing the said services. Moreover, their concentration in precarious, low-status/low-wage jobs contributes to this, especially in the case of irregular migrants, who are severely affected. Precarious work is employment that lacks all the standard forms of labor security, typically takes the form of wage work, and is characterized by exceptionally limited social benefits and legal rights, job insecurity, low wages, and high risk of ill health (Vosko 2006). Migrants form a social category with particular needs in the health sector, given their generally poor living conditions (both in sending and receiving countries), but also due to additional problems caused by difficulties adapting to a new social and cultural environment (Sassen 2016; Fouskas et al. 2019). Thus, the relationship between social exclusion and the health status of migrants works in a bidirectional manner. On the one hand, the experience of social exclusion – as reflected via poor living conditions, low income, difficulties in communication, institutional or actual exclusion from health and other services, and the phenomena of racism and xenophobia – has detrimental effects on the health of immigrants; while, on the other hand, a possible health disorder leads to social exclusion due to difficulty in finding formal employment, since immigrants are mostly employed in casual, informal occupations, in precarious, low-status/low-wage jobs, and experience deterioration of their real income.

What emerges in the post-COVID-19 era is the prevalence of the image of migrants as a threat to public health, which is reinforced by the relevant policy measures. There was an extension (to 14 November 2022) of the Joint Ministerial Decision on emergency measures to protect public health from the risk of further spread of COVID-19 throughout the territory (Government Gazette 2022). It includes RICs, Closed Controlled Structures (CCS), controlled facilities for the temporary accommodation of asylum seekers, as well as any kind of structure and place of reception and accommodation for TCNs.

Taking into account the specific characteristics of the location of the facilities or structure, entry and exit options are being implemented. Based on the identified needs of the participants in this research, and in order to promote the social inclusion of TCNs, the following are proposed: (i) the acceleration of procedures for requests for international protection, but also for appeals and the issuing of the relevant documents in cases of a positive outcome, (ii) the learning of the language (e.g., in cooperation with civil society organizations, adult educational institutions), (iii) the design and implementation of targeted promotion programs in employment and vocational training (e.g., through the Public Employment Service (DYPA)) and/or in the context of corporate social responsibility of private companies/enterprises and vocational training providers).

Regarding the improvement of living conditions, the following are proposed: (i) re-granting a Medical ID/National Insurance Number (AMKA); (ii) improvement of living conditions in accommodation facilities (e.g., through improved utilization of the relevant European funds, the participation of private sponsors when and where possible, and the active – and voluntary – involvement of the guests themselves, through which they will put to use any technical knowledge they have, improve skills and abilities, acquire new ones, and possibly earn a basic income as compensation for their work); (iii) provision of special care for the needs of mothers and children in the accommodation facilities (e.g., opportunities for creative employment and entertainment, parallel support for refugee children so that their parents can participate freely in training/education activities or work); (iv) continuous training and awareness of the accommodation facility staff in order to improve efficiency; and (v) provision of information on the coronavirus pandemic among the refugee population in order to address misinformation or fears that act as deterrents to vaccination.

During the COVID-19 pandemic, migrants experienced: (i) different frequency in testing or treatment; (ii) mobility restrictions; (iii) segregation or quarantine in overcrowded and unhygienic conditions; (iv) delays in vaccinations and exclusion from general response programmes; (v) delays in the issue of residence permits, applications, as well as lack of access to migration/asylum services, driving them to precarity and vulnerability while experiencing covert ways in which racism and xenophobia operate in everyday interactions with nationals. What was observed is a negative stereotypical association between migration and fear; an equation "migrants = dangerous individuals who bring or carry diseases and spread COVID-19" was embedded in social consciousness, leading to erroneous suppositions (Webb Hooper et al. 2020). These suppositions, often reinforced via the construction and standardization of otherness in discourse, are embedded in everyday discussions among nationals. As a consequence, they segregate and exclude migrants as a means of "protecting" themselves, leading to negative characterizations and hatred, along with expulsions and quarantine measures. The above thought process formed the perception that migrants posed a risk, and fear is weaponized in the name of spreading SARS-CoV-2, leading to restriction of their mobility in favor of protecting nationals. However, administrative policy responses intensified the risk of exposure to SARS-CoV-2, as well as to violence, abuse, and stress, thus impacting their physical and mental health beyond the pandemic. All these strengthened public perceptions that migrants pose a risk to public health, which intensified their precarity and vulnerability to health risks, feeding a vicious cycle of precariousness and racism and have had severe repercussions on their integration.

Note

1 Funding: the project "Local Alliance for Integration" (LION/General Secretariat for Research and Innovation (GSRI)/University of West Attica (UNIWA)/81018): "Migrant and refugee integration into local societies during the COVID-19 pandemic in Spain and Greece", carried out by the Department of Public Health Policy at the School of Public Health of the University of West Attica (Greece) and funded by the General Secretariat for Research and Innovation (GSRI) under the National Funding

2019 with Scientific Director/Principal Investigator (PI) Theodoros Fouskas, Assistant Professor at the Department of Public Health Policy at the School of Public Health of the University of West Attica (UNIWA). Research team: Theodoros Fouskas (PI). Researchers in Greece: George Koulierakis, Fotini-Maria Mine, Athanasios Theofilopoulos, Sofia Konstantopoulou, Dimitrios Georgiadis, and Georgia Pantazi. Researcher in Spain: Fabiola Ortega-de-Mora.

References

Abedi, Vida, Oluwaseyi Olulana, Venkatesh Avula, Durgesh Chaudhary, Ayesha Khan, Shima Shahjouei, Jiang Li, and Ramin Zand. 2021. "Racial, economic, and health inequality and COVID-19 infection in the United States". *Journal of Racial and Ethnic Health Disparities* 8, 3: 732–742.

Balibar, Etienne. 1991. "Racism and nationalism". In *Nations and Nationalism: A Reader*, edited by P. Spencer and H. Wollman, 163–172. Edinburgh: Edinburgh University Press.

Banton, Michael. 2018. "The concept of racism". In *Race and Racialism*, edited by S. Zubaida, 17–34. Milton: Routledge.

Centers for Disease Control and Prevention (CDC). 2020. "*COVID-19 racial and ethnic health disparities*". Accessed June 1, 2023. www.cdc.gov/coronavirus/2019-ncov/community/health-equity/racial-ethnic-disparities/index.html#income&education.

Dalsania, Ankur K., Matthew J. Fastiggi, Aaron Kahlam, Rajvi Shah, Krishan Patel, Stephanie Shiau, Slawa Rokicki, and Michelle DallaPiazza. 2022. "The relationship between social determinants of health and racial disparities in COVID-19 mortality". *Journal of Racial and Ethnic Health Disparities* 9, 1: 288–295.

Essed, Philomena. 1991. *Understanding Everyday Racism:. An Interdisciplinary Theory*, Vol. 2. Newbury Park: Sage.

Esses, Victoria M., and Leah K. Hamilton. 2021. "Xenophobia and anti-immigrant attitudes in the time of COVID-19". *Group Processes & Intergroup Relations* 24, 2: 253–259.

European Migration Network (EMN). 2018. "Asylum and Migration Glossary 6.0". Brussels: European Migration Network (EMN). https://home-affairs.ec.europa.eu/system/files_en?file=2020-09/interactive_glossary_6.0_final_version.pdf.

Farro, Antimo, and Simone Maddanu. 2022. *Restless Cities on the Edge: Collective Actions, Immigration and Populism*. Cham, Switzerland: Palgrave Macmillan.

Fassani, Francesco, and Jacopo Mazza. 2020. *A Vulnerable Workforce: Migrant Workers in the COVID-19 Pandemic*. Luxembourg: Publications Office of the European Union.

Fouskas, Theodoros. 2018. "Repercussions of precarious employment on migrants' perceptions of healthcare in Greece". *International Journal of Human Rights in Healthcare* 11, 4: 298–311.

Fouskas, Theodoros. 2020. "Migrants, asylum seekers and refugees in Greece in the midst of the COVID-19 pandemic". *Comparative Cultural Studies – European and Latin American Perspectives* 5, 10: 39–58.

Fouskas, Theodoros. 2021. *Lives (Un)Maid in Greece: Migrant Filipina Live-In Domestic Workers*. New York: Nova Science Publishers.

Fouskas, T., P. Gikopoulou, E. Ioannidi, and G. Koulierakis. 2019. "Health inequalities and female migrant domestic workers: accessing healthcare as a human right and barriers due to precarious employment in Greece". *Collectivus* 6, 2: 71–90.

Fouskas, Theodoros, and George Koulierakis. 2022. "Demystifying Migration Myths: Social Discourse on the Impact of Immigrants and Refugees in Greece". *Urbanities* 12, 5: 9–28.

Fouskas, Theodoros, Symeon Sidiropoulos, and Athanassios Vozikis. 2019. "Leaving no one out? Public health aspects of migration: health risks, responses and accessibility by asylum seekers, refugees and migrants in Greece". *International Journal of Health Research and Innovation* 7, 1: 13–28.

GOV.GR2020. "Preventive measures to avoid the spread of coronavirus disease in reception and identification centers and third country nationals' accommodation centers". https://covid19.gov.gr/proliptika-metra-gia-tin-apofy-gi-tis-diasporas-tou-koronoiou-se-kentra-ypodochis-ke-taftopiisis-ke-domes-filoxe-nias-politon-triton-choron/ [in Greek].

Government Gazette. 2022. "D1a/GP.ok.61055/27.10.2022 Extension of the validity of the D1a/GP. co. 51236/ 8.9.2022 Joint Ministerial Decision on Emergency Measures to Protect Public Health from the Risk of Further Spread of the COVID-19 Coronavirus throughout the Territory until Monday, November 14, 2022 at 06:00". Athens: National Publishing House. www.taxheaven.gr/circulars/41050/d1a-gp-oik-58309-14-10-2022 [in Greek].

Gravlee, Clarence. 2020. "Systemic racism, chronic health inequities, and COVID-19: a syndemic in the making?" *American Journal of Human Biology* 32, 5: e23482.

iEfimerida. 2020. "Unthinkable: a 48-year-old immigrant was thrown out of the train in Lamia because they thought he had coronavirus", August 5. www.iefimerida.gr/ellada/ton-petaxan-apo-treno-nomizan-oti-eihe-koronoio [in Greek].

iEfimerida. 2021. "Lianokladi: incident with unvaccinated irregular migrants on the train from Thessaloniki to Athens", November 2. www.iefimerida.gr/ellada/anembolia stoi-metanastes-treno-thessaloniki-athina [in Greek].

Jalbout, Maysa. 2020. "Finding solutions to Greece's refugee education crisis". London: TheirWorld. https://reliefweb.int/sites/reliefweb.int/files/resources/RefugeeEducation-Report-240420-2.pdf.

Kathimerini. 2019. "Oxfam report details inhumane conditions at Greek migrant camps", January 9. www.ekathimerini.com/236377/article/ekathime-rini/news/oxfam-report-details-inhumane-conditions-at-greek-migrant-camps.

Kathimerini. 2020a. "Fire destroys warehouse at Lesvos migrant center", March 8. www.ekathimerini.com/250368/article/ekathimerini/news/fire-des-troys-warehouse-at-lesvos-migrant-center.

Kathimerini. 2020b. "Fires erupt amid unrest at Samos migrant camp", April 28. www.ekathimerini.com/252108/article/ekathimerini/in-images/fires-erupt-amid-unrest-at-samos-migrant-camp.

Kathimerini. 2020c. "Migrant camps on islands put on lockdown", March 17. www.ekathimerini.com/250739/article/ekathimerini/news/migrant-camps-on-islands-put-on-lockdown.

Kathimerini. 2020d. "Entrance, exit with cards in closed structures", April 14. www.kathimerini.gr/1073748/article/epikairothta/ellada/eiso-dos-e3odos-me-kartes-se-kleistes-domes (in Greek)

Laster Pirtle, Whitney N., and Tashelle Wright. 2021. "Structural gendered racism revealed in pandemic times: intersectional approaches to understanding race and gender health inequities in COVID-19". *Gender & Society* 35, 2: 168–179.

Médicins Sans Frontières. 2017a. "A dramatic deterioration for asylum seekers on Lesbos". Athens: Médicins Sans Frontières. https://msf.gr/sites/default/files/msfpublica-tions//msf_report_vulnerable_lesvos_en.pdf.

Médicins Sans Frontières. 2017b. "Confronting the mental health emergency on Samos and Lesvos: why the containment of asylum seekers on the Greek islands must end". Athens: Médicins Sans Frontières. https://msf.gr/sites/default/files/msfpublica-tions//2017_10_mental_health_greece_report_lowres_spreads.pdf.

Moreno Barreneche, Sebastián. 2020. "Somebody to blame: on the construction of the other in the context of the COVID-19 outbreak". *Society Register* 4, 2: 19–32.
Oxfam. 2019. "Vulnerable and abandoned". Accessed June 1. www-cdn.oxfam.org/s3fs-public/file_attachments/2019-01_greece_media_briefing_final.pdf.
Pirro, Fabrizio, Emanuele Toscano, Daniele Di Nunzio, and Marcello Pedaci. 2022. "When school 'stayed home': a sociology of work approach on the remote work of teachers during the lockdown for the COVID-19 pandemic: the case of Italy". *International Review of Sociology* 32, 3: 529–540.
Sassen, Saskia. 2016. "A massive loss of habitat: new drivers for migration". *Sociology of Development* 2, 2: 204–233.
Turner-Musa, Jocelyn, Oluwatoyin Ajayi, and Layschel Kemp. 2020. "Examining social determinants of health, stigma, and COVID-19 disparities". *Healthcare* 8, 2: 168.
Vega Macías, Daniel. 2021. "The COVID-19 pandemic on anti-immigration and xenophobic discourse in Europe and the United States". *Estudios Fronterizos* 22, e066. https://doi.org/10.21670/ref.2103066.
Veizis, Apostolos. 2020. "Leave no one behind and access to protection in the Greek islands in the COVID-19 era". *International Migration*, 58, 3: 264–266.
Vosko, Leah F. 2006. "Precarious employment: towards an improved understanding of labour market insecurity". In *Precarious Employment: Understanding Labour Market Insecurity in Canada*, edited by Leah F. Vosko, 3–39. Montreal: McGill-Queen's University Press.
Wang, Simeng, Xiabing Chen, Yong Li, Chloé Luu, Ran Yan, and Francesco Madrisotti. 2021. "'I'm more afraid of racism than of the virus!': racism awareness and resistance among Chinese migrants and their descendants in France during the Covid-19 pandemic". *European Societies* 23, suppl. 1: S721–S742.
Webb Hooper, Monica, Anna María Nápoles, and Eliseo J. Pérez-Stable. 2020. "COVID-19 and racial/ethnic disparities". *Jama* 323, 24: 2466–2467.
Wilder, Julius M. 2021. "The disproportionate impact of COVID-19 on racial and ethnic minorities in the United States". *Clinical Infectious Diseases* 72, 4: 707–709.
Wimmer, Andreas. 1997. "Explaining xenophobia and racism: a critical review of current research approaches". *Ethnic and Racial Studies* 20, 1: 17–41.
World Health Organization (WHO). 2020. "Coronavirus disease 2019 (COVID-19) Situation Report – 72". Accessed June 1, 2023. https://apps.who.int/iris/bitstream/handle/10665/331685/nCoVsitrep01Apr2020-eng.pdf.
Yerly, Grégoire. 2022. "Right-wing populist parties' bordering narratives in times of crisis: anti-immigration discourse in the Genevan borderland during the COVID-19 pandemic". *Swiss Political Science Review* 22, 4: 675–695.

6

THE IMPACT OF THE COVID-19 PANDEMIC ON DISABILITY SERVICES IN JAPAN

Analysis of Administrative Panel Data

Kenjiro Sakakibara

Introduction

This chapter statistically explores the changing patterns of social services for adults with disabilities after the COVID-19 outbreak. Social services for persons with disabilities include support inside and outside homes, day and residential services, and training. The analysis of such service provisions is important in light of COVID-19, which threatens social interaction and the copresence underlying personal assistance and group support. This study examines whether the assumed pandemic impact on disability services actually occurred, using statistical analysis.

Disability services have long been a social concern. Early debates focused on residential institutions, whose living arrangements were heavily criticized. Deinstitutionalization (Lerman 1982) formulated the actual trend and the ideal of reduced use of residential institutions. Normalization (Nirje 1969; Wolfensberger 1994), which means providing living conditions that are normal in society for persons with disabilities, preferred replacement of congregated living arrangements with individual or smaller group residences where possible. The independent living movement (DeJong 1983), emphasizing the self-determination of persons with disabilities, sought to develop services that would enable community living rather than living in residential institutions. This movement established independent living centers, which spread worldwide and advocated the rights of persons with disabilities and provided them with resources and information regarding community living and self-directed support.

The personalization policy (Power and Bartlett 2018) realized a part of the ideal of self-directed support with personal budgets for users to purchase services of their choice. However, personalization had both advantages and disadvantages. It emphasized the will of persons with disabilities, which was often

DOI: 10.4324/9781003459682-7

overlooked; nevertheless, it was criticized for insufficient resources, due to austerity measures and spending cuts to reduce government debt. Some even argued that personalization, including personal choice and personal responsibility, was only rhetoric and did not work for marginalized people (Cardona 2021).

Personalization affected both residential and day services (services provided in the daytime). Traditional day services were building-based and gathered persons with disabilities in day centers. They provided opportunities for engaging in activities, including work-related activities that differed from competitive employment. Such services were often inflexible rather than personalized, and drew criticism. Day activities were reported to be primarily passive group activities with fewer individual activities (Vlaskamp et al. 2007). In addition, quality of life was reported to be worse for users of these activities than for users of alternative daytime opportunities (Beyer et al. 2010; similar research concerning respite services by Nicholson et al. 2019). Partly due to their inflexibility, some day centers were closed in the UK. However, this was also a result of spending cuts that limited local governments' financial capacity to maintain day centers. Day services remained important sources of collective support for persons with disabilities and their families (Power and Bartlett 2018). In addition, alternative day opportunities could not compensate for the decrease in day centers (Hatton 2017).

After the COVID-19 outbreak, persons with disabilities faced various challenges, including the absence of caregivers (Colon-Cabrera et al. 2021; Pranshu 2022); in addition, women and children with disabilities experienced intersectional difficulties (Pranshu 2022). In Ireland, day services closed in mid-March 2020, affecting users and their families (Doyle 2021).

Schwartz et al. (2021) conducted a survey of service disruptions experienced by persons with disabilities during the pandemic. There were 119 respondents, who were recruited through organizations concerning disabilities and social media. Although the respondents used few services, 54 percent of service changes were attributed to the service being discontinued. This type of survey has the advantage of abundant demographic information (e.g., education) and self-reported causes of the changes. However, in addition to using a non-representative sample,[1] the survey data lacked detailed and accurate information regarding service changes (e.g., monthly service use). In contrast, by analyzing administrative panel data the present study identified precisely when, and to what extent, changes occurred.

The present chapter addresses social services for persons with disabilities during the pandemic. Disability services vary between countries; therefore, it focuses on the Japanese context. The disability policy in Japan has traditionally been characterized by dependence on family care. Consequently, an early independent living movement called for defamilialization (Okahara 1995). Disability services gradually developed, first locally and then nationally (Yamashita 2019). The Support Funding Scheme in 2003 was adopted as the basis for nationwide disability services, which has been part of the Basic Structural Reform of Social

Welfare System since 1998. One of the major characteristics of the reform was shifting "from placement to contract", which enabled the service users to choose among service providers. Service provision increased rapidly under the Support Funding Scheme, exceeding the budget. The scheme was soon replaced by the Services and Supports for Persons with Disabilities Act (2005), which introduced 10 percent user payment but then added payment reduction for users with low incomes after sharp criticism from the disability movement. The act was amended in 2012 and renamed the Act on Providing Comprehensive Support for the Daily Life and Life in Society of Persons with Disabilities, which covered persons with rare diseases in addition to people with physical, intellectual, and psychiatric disabilities.

Figure 6.1 presents the number of deaths caused by COVID-19 in Japan (NHK 2022). As of 23 September 2022, there were 20,896,814 total cases, which roughly correspond to one-sixth of the population, 44,169 deaths, and seven waves of infection. The sixth and seventh waves were larger than the previous waves in the magnitude of infection; nonetheless, the first waves had a strong social impact. Schools were closed in March 2020 (Ministry of Education, Culture, Sports, Science and Technology 2020). Request-based lockdown was adopted four times – 7 April–25 May 2020, 8 January–21 March 2021, 25 April–20 June 2021, and 12 July–30 September 2021 – with differing periods for different areas. The measures included requests for stay-at-home, event cancellations, closure of facilities not deemed essential to maintaining everyday life (e.g., bars and gyms), and remote work. Social welfare facilities were not closed down; however, staying at home was recommended, if and when possible.

The basic statistics of disability services in Japan are collected by the government (Ministry of Health, Labour and Welfare of Japan 2022). The monthly user numbers for each service are available; however, at present, data before the pandemic are averaged by year, and detailed changes are not disclosed. The statistics still offer an important clue to understanding the impact of COVID-19

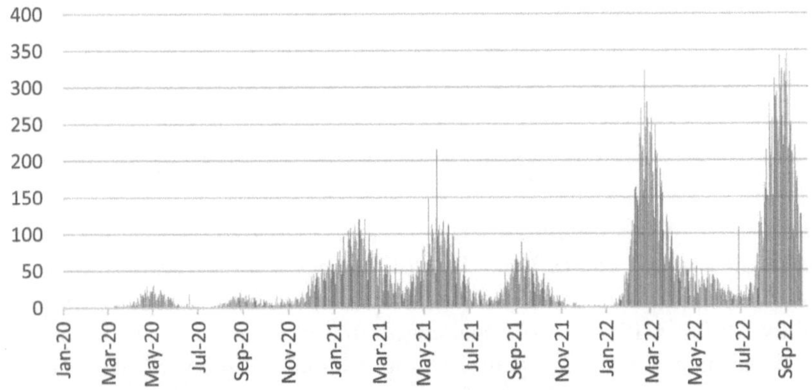

FIGURE 6.1 Deaths caused by COVID-19 in Japan.
Source: Author (data from NHK (2022))

on disability services, and indicate that the use of disability services was largely static post-outbreak. However, a decline was noticed in certain services, such as short-term accommodation (there were 57,075 users, on average, in FY 2019, and only 47.33 percent of this number remained in May 2020). Nonetheless, these statistics have certain limitations. The total numbers have not been disaggregated by demographic attributes, such as gender, age, and type and severity of disability. This leaves unanswered the question of which groups of people were most affected. Furthermore, population changes, such as being newly disabled and death, are not considered, which must be controlled for to derive the COVID-19 effect. These limitations can be addressed by panel data (information of different individuals at different points in time) of service use.

Data regarding care services have been analyzed in the context of elderly persons (Nambu and Sugahara 2004; Hirano 2012). Although some analyses of disability service data have been conducted (Sato et al. 2009; Nakane 2020; Imahashi et al. 2021), the data were cross-sectional, meaning that they only reflected the situation at a point in time or were pooled over a short period. Panel data with a longer time span are required to analyze the influence of the pandemic.

Using panel data, the following research questions are addressed in this study:

1 Did COVID-19 affect the use of social services for persons with disabilities, controlling for demographics?
2 If yes, were there any differential impacts as per individual attributes?

Hypotheses based on these questions are as follows:

1 The use of certain types of social services concerning disabilities decreased after the COVID-19 outbreak.
2 Regarding changes in service use,
    a Service use of persons with severe disabilities was less affected by the pandemic.
    b Other demographics, including gender and age, were involved in the changes in service use.

The definition of "disability" has been highly controversial. Traditionally, disability has been equated with an inherent defect of body function and structure (impairment), which causes the plight of persons with disabilities. However, British disability studies, based on a framework called the "social model of disability" (Oliver 1983, 1990), challenged this assumption to shift the focus from impairment to social exclusion and barriers (disability). Although the strength of the social model arose from the severance between impairment and disability, this undermined the model's definitional capacity, because disability and social exclusion on other grounds cannot be distinguished without reference to the body. This was not necessarily the case when disability was regarded as social exclusion of people with impairment as abnormality (UPIAS and DA 1976; Thomas 1999). However, conceptualizing impairment as abnormality is stigmatization of the bodily condition, even in the context of the social construction of abnormality. Defining impairment as a statistical deviation from the norm (WHO 2001) avoids value judgment; however, there arises the problem of irrelevant deviance, such as the abilities of top athletes statistically deviating from the population mean, which can be considered an impairment according to this definition.

A systems theory definition of disability (Sakakibara 2016), building on Niklas Luhmann (1984, 1997), whose components are introduced before being assembled into a definition, enables a reference to impairment while avoiding treating it as an abnormality inherent in the body. Following the social model, disability is conceptualized as a type of social exclusion. This can be broadly interpreted as a limitation in social participation opportunities. However, a certain form of reference to the body is essential to distinguish disability from general social exclusion. Although the reference to the body is subjected to social construction, it is "external reference" or "information" for social systems that assumes the body as an organism outside the social systems. A distinction between disability and exclusion on the basis of gender and race can be made by the mode of the reference; it is fragmented in the context of disability and restricted to details of body function and structure, while reference to body function and structure in the context of gender and race is synecdochal, merely a marker to group people. Thus, disability can be closely associated with "political anatomy" (Foucault 1975). Social barriers, including actions, are incorporated as social treatment. The causal relationships between the body and exclusion must be replaced by attribution, observation of causality, if impairment as an inherent abnormality of the body cannot be a premise of the definition. This is instrumental in the indirect discrimination and the gray area of disability. Hence, disability can be defined as "social exclusion attributed to a link between fragmented body information and social treatment", where the fragmented body information incorporated in the disability definition corresponds to impairment. This definition allows one to refer to impairment and examine the relationship between social opportunities and body function/structure and the involvement of social treatment in the relationship. In addition, this definition demonstrates that disability is an important topic of sociological inquiry.

Materials and Methods

Anonymized monthly disability service data, which include all use of nationwide services (excluding local support services) of a middle-sized city (hereinafter City X) with a population of approximately 100,000, were analyzed. These data included anonymized history of "disability certificates", including the type and gravity of the disability, gender, age, and status, such as new certificate, return of certificates, transfer, and the demise of the certificate holder. Disability certificates in Japan are certificates of disability in different contexts of social welfare and employment. Although the disability service data contain the "disability support category", which is directly linked to the amount of services funded, disability certificates were adopted as disability indicators, because information about the disability support category could be obtained only at the time of service use.

The target population was limited to service users who had a disability certificate, were present in the city throughout April 2018–March 2021, and used each service at least once in the mentioned period. This enabled us to disregard the effect on service use of newly experiencing disability, moving in and out of the city, and death. The period of April 2018–March 2021 was chosen because the public funding system remained unchanged during this period, including the pandemic outbreak. For each user in each month, the amount of service provision, measured by hours or days, was aggregated, omitting additional payments. Only services with more than 100 users that were not transitional were analyzed: home help (physical assistance), day care,[2] short-term accommodation,[3] and work activities ("continuous support for work, Type B").[4]

The amount of service provision, which reflected all the service use by the target population, was analyzed in two ways. First, changes in the aggregated amount of service use by the same population were examined. Since the length of a month may be involved, service use adjusted for the number of days in a month was also calculated. Second, panel regression, a method to explain a quantity in data (a "variable") by other variables, considering the panel structure with multiple individuals and time points, was applied. Although the data were characterized by complete enumeration, statistical inference still made sense, assuming that service use was affected by disturbance factors, such as being absent for some reasons. Consequently, significance tests of models and coefficients were conducted. The analyzed data were limited to the above-mentioned population without missing values in the variables throughout the period, such that the data were balanced panel data. The analysis cannot be generalized beyond City X, although the situation in the city is closely connected with the national policy.

Panel regression analysis (Equation 1) decomposed the explained variable (i.e., the dependent variable) into: (1) a part that is explained by the explanatory variables (or independent variables, $\mathbf{x}_{it}\boldsymbol{\beta}$), (2) a part that reflects each individual's time-invariant characteristic, which is not observed as a variable (individual effects, c_i), and (3) error (u_{it}):

$$y_{it} = \mathbf{x}_{it}\boldsymbol{\beta} + c_i + u_{it} \quad (1)$$

where y_{it} denotes a dependent variable, $\mathbf{x}_{it}$ indicates a vector of independent variables, and $\boldsymbol{\beta}$ is a vector of coefficients of the independent variables.

There are two basic models – fixed effects (FE) and random effects (RE) models. The former allows arbitrary correlation of the individual effects with the explanatory variables, while the latter assumes the individual effects to be uncorrelated with the explanatory variables. Estimates from the FE models are unbiased under certain assumptions, while estimates from the RE models become biased when the assumption of zero correlation between the individual effects and explanatory variables is violated. However, the effects of time-invariant variables cannot be estimated in the FE model.

Mundlak's approach (Mundlak 1978; Wooldridge 2010; handling of the interaction terms in Schunk 2013), or the correlated random effects (CRE) model, relaxes the assumption of zero correlation while retaining time-invariant variables, which is adopted in this study. This approach appends individual means of time-variant variables to the RE model. The model has the advantage of the estimated coefficients for time-variant variables coinciding with the FE estimators (Equation 2)

$$y_{it} = \mathbf{x}_{it}\boldsymbol{\beta} + \bar{\mathbf{x}}_i\theta + c_i + u_{it} \tag{2}$$

where $\bar{\mathbf{x}}_i$ denotes the mean of $\mathbf{x}_{it}$ for individual $\mathbf{i}$ over time and $\boldsymbol{\theta}$ is a vector of coefficients of $\bar{\mathbf{x}}_i$.

The variables of particular interest in this chapter are the interaction effects with the COVID-19 waves and demographics on service use; that is, the differential impacts of demographics, such as gender and disability, during the pandemic and the main effects of COVID-19, both of which can be estimated by the FE model. However, the main effects of the demographics are required to interpret the estimators and know the base levels from which the changes will be measured. Accordingly, the CRE model was adopted.

The CRE models were constructed for each nontransitional service with more than 100 users in the city, with the amount of service use as a dependent variable. The period concerning the pandemic was classified into (1) 2018–2019, (2) the first wave (April–May 2020), (3) the second wave (August 2020), (4) the third wave (November 2020–January 2021), and (5) the rest of the months during 2020–2021. The time periods, their interaction with the demographics, and the demographics were entered as explanatory variables while controlling for linear trends throughout the period (months from January of year "zero") and dummy variables for 12 months of a year (with the aim to adjust different numbers of days in a month[5] and seasonal effects). Following Mundlak's approach, the individual mean of time-variant demographics and interaction terms of the periods' dummy variables and demographics were entered. However, the individual mean of the interactions of the periods and the time-invariant variables were not entered, because the means were completely correlated with the time-invariant variables; thus, without these terms, the estimates agreed with the FE model. Since a particular variable with only a couple of fluctuations, that is, the severity of intellectual disability, rendered the estimates unstable, it was replaced with its individual means. Similarly, certain variables and interactions were dropped from the models to obtain stable estimates. Consequently, models with only intellectual disability were analyzed, omitting physical and psychiatric disabilities as variables but retaining persons with these conditions. The models were estimated by the xtreg command of Stata.

The data were made available through an official agreement between governmental bodies (the city and institute). Ethical approval and funding were obtained from the National Institute of Population and Social Security Research, Japan.

Results

Figures 6.2(a–d) illustrate the total amount of service use in City X concerning home help (physical assistance), day care, short-term accommodation, and work activities (dashed lines denote values adjusted for the number of days in each month). The use of short-term accommodation dropped to 63.4 percent in April 2020 (ratio of original values), 30.3 percent in May 2020, and 74.4 percent in January 2021, compared to December 2019. Regarding home help, although service use in May 2020 was similar to that in December 2019, it temporarily decreased to 87.6 percent of the previous month amidst an increasing trend. Graphs for the other two services do not display clear tendencies. The monthly fluctuations in these two figures are comparatively large, possibly due to seasonal effects.

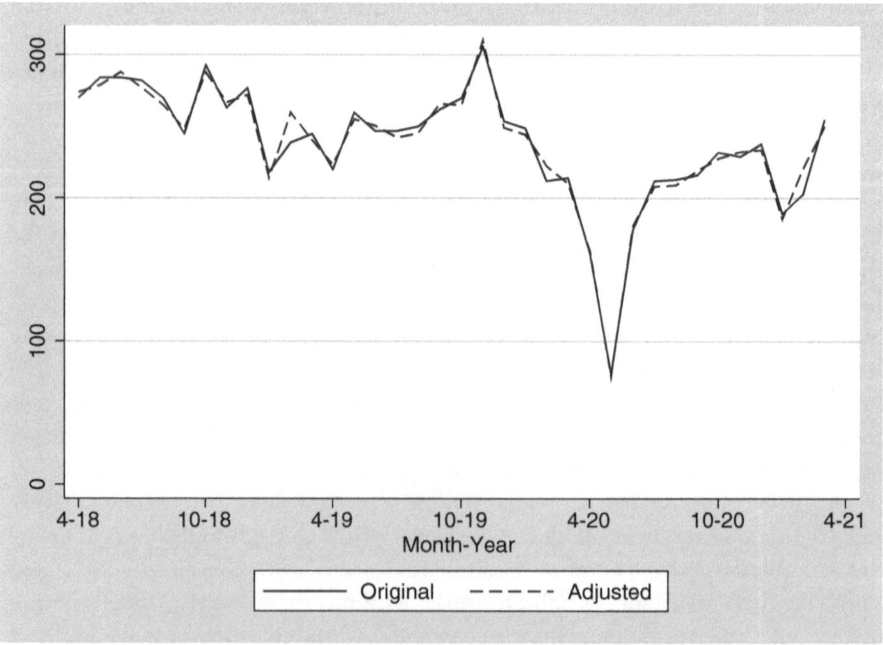

FIGURE 6.2A Monthly use of short-term accommodation (in days) (N=114).

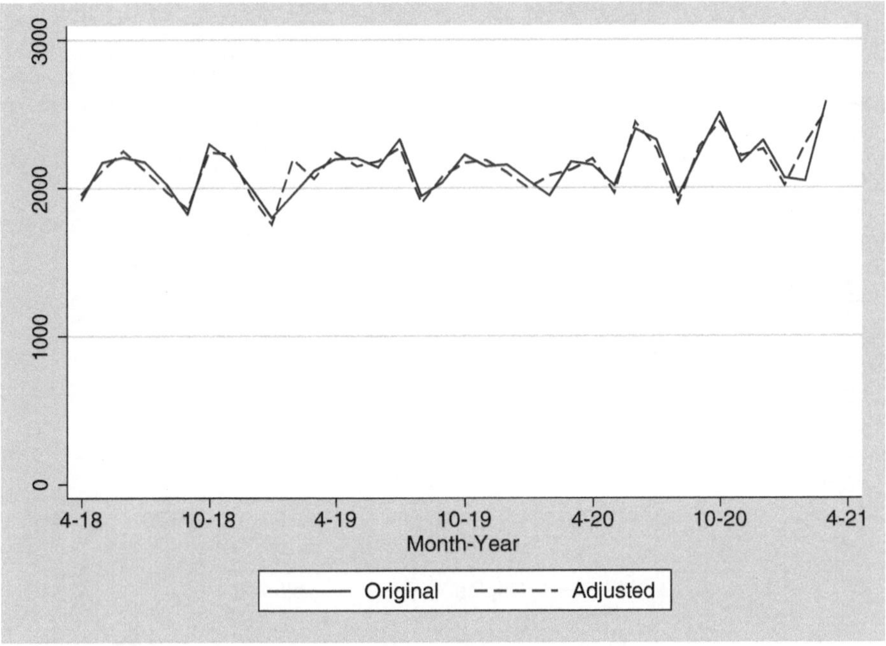

FIGURE 6.2B Monthly use of day care (in days) (N=141) .

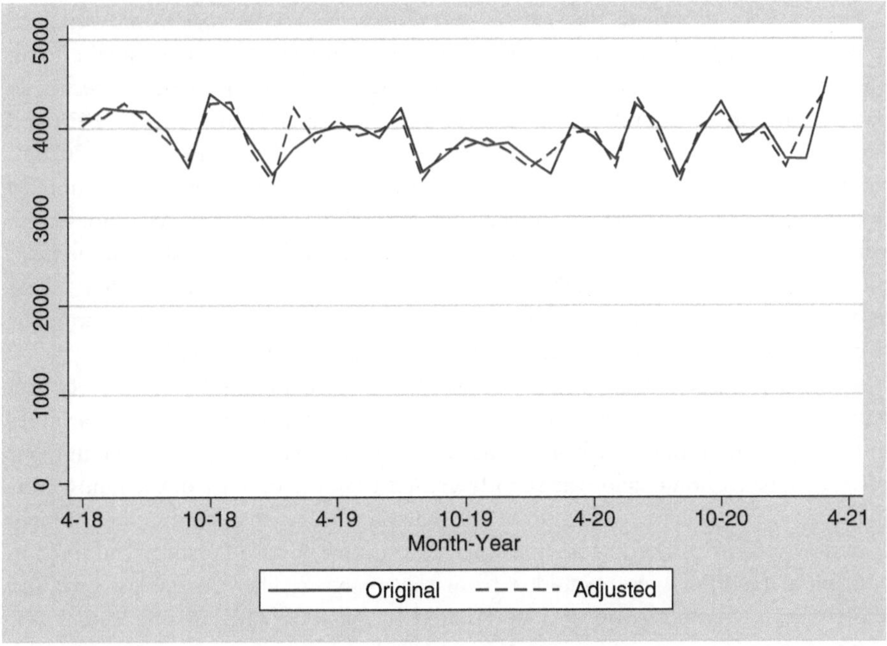

FIGURE 6.2C Monthly use of work activities (in days) (N=308).

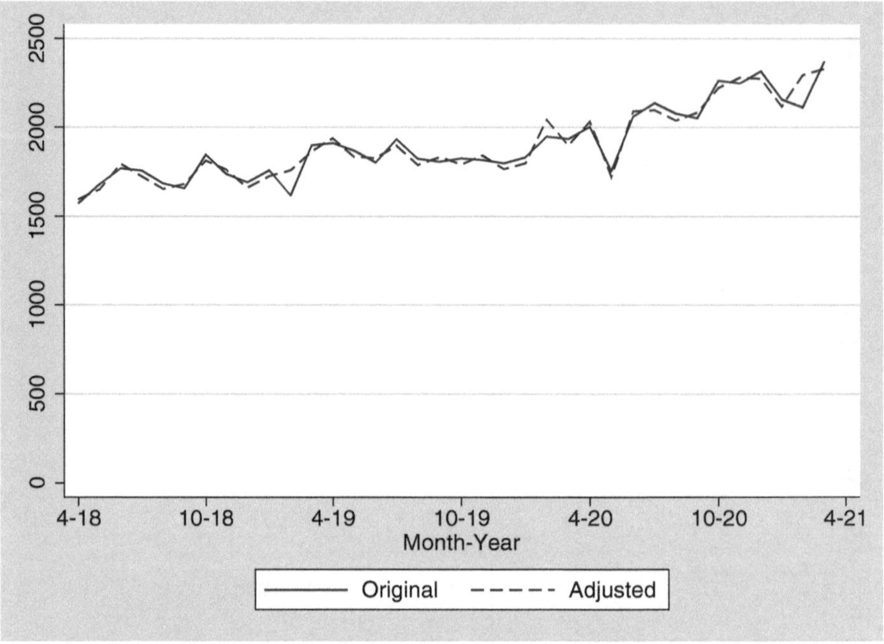

FIGURE 6.2D Monthly use of home help (physical assistance) (in hours) (N=175).
Source: Author (data from City X)

Figures 6.3(a–d) provide the year-on-year difference in service use from April 2019 to March 2021. Negative values indicate decline, while positive values smaller than previous values denote the slowing down of increase. The figures reveal a decline in day care use in April and May 2020 and stagnation in July and August 2020 and January 2021 (referring to the previous year). The ratio of decrease in May 2020 to the unadjusted service use of the previous year was 8.49 percent. Furthermore, a decline in May 2020 was noted in work activities; however, similar reductions were witnessed in February 2020 and in the pre-pandemic period. Regarding home help, the increasing trend around 2020 partially stagnated in January and February 2021 and declined in May 2020. Short-term accommodation presented a continuous decline from the previous year, from February 2020 to February 2021.

To further analyze the impact of the pandemic and demographics on service use, panel regression was applied. Table 6.1 provides the basic statistics of the variables in the regression models corresponding to the service types analyzed. The number of women using home help was slightly greater than the number of men; however, in the other three services, the number of women was less than the number of men. A majority of users lived at home rather than group homes. Persons who lived in residential facilities were excluded from the analysis. The use of day care and short-term accommodation was dominated by persons with an intellectual disability certificate with a severe grade. The numbers of users with severe and mild/moderate intellectual disability were approximately equal for home help; however,

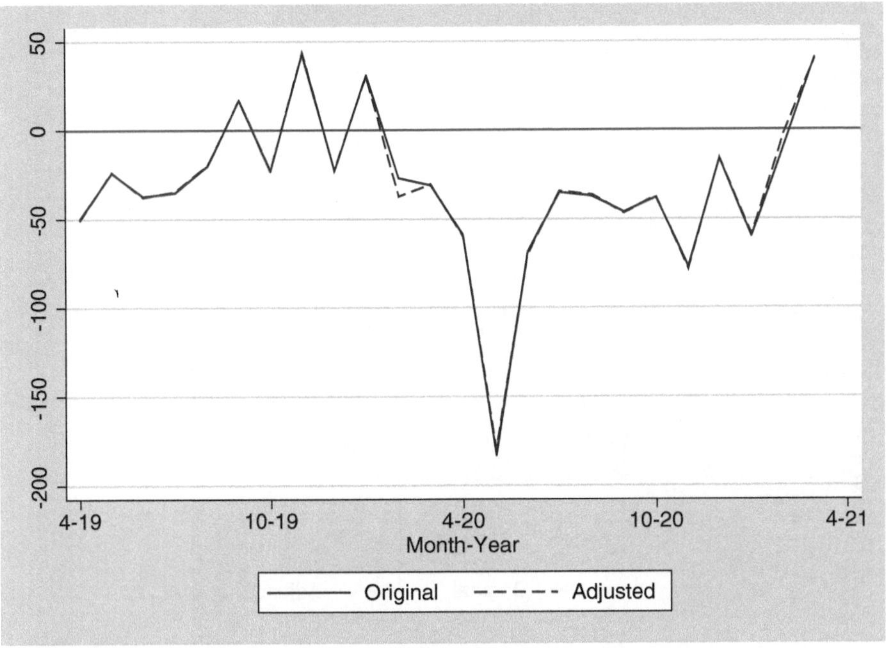

FIGURE 6.3A Year-on-year difference in monthly use of short-term accommodation (in days) (N=114).

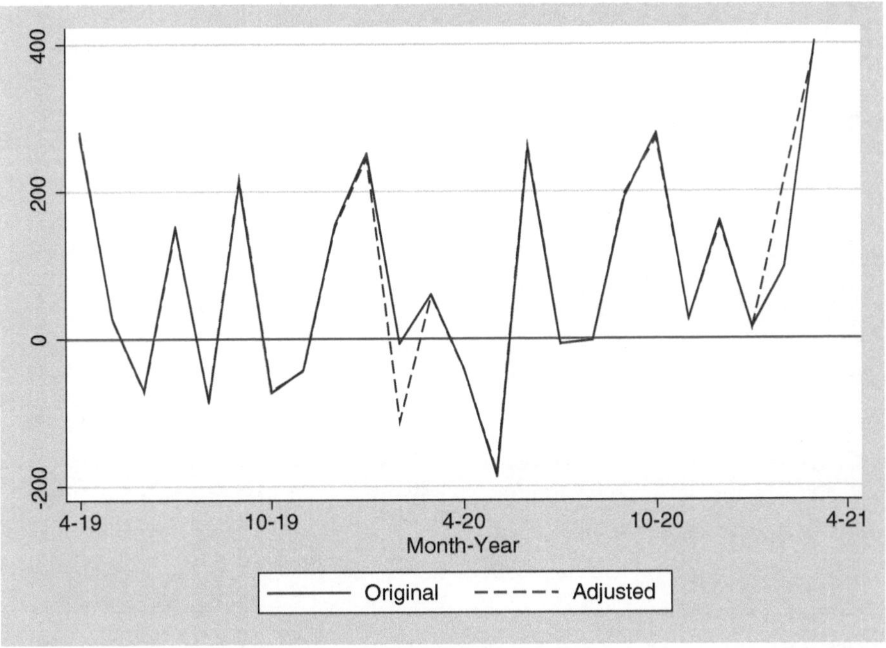

FIGURE 6.3B Year-on-year difference in monthly use of day care (in days) (N=141).

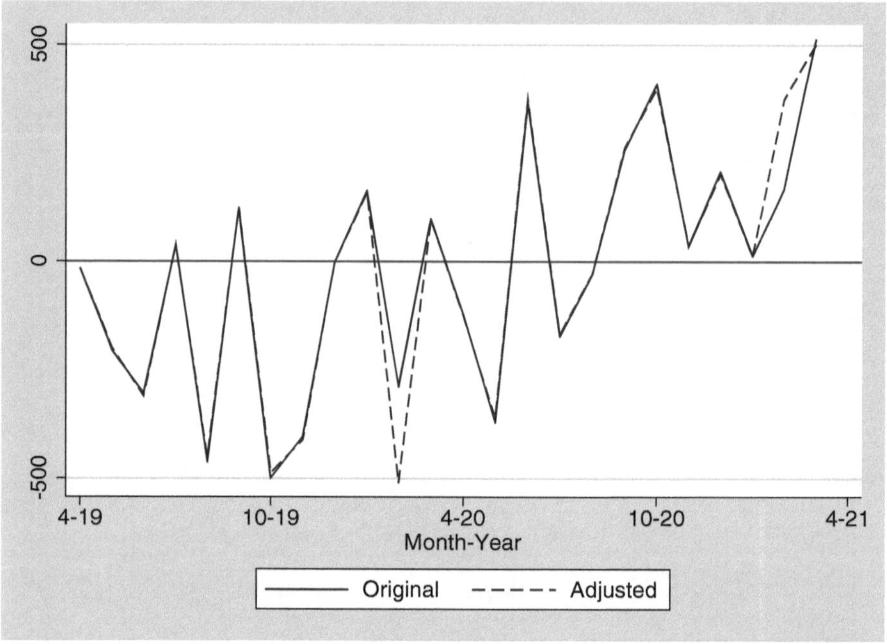

FIGURE 6.3C Year-on-year difference in monthly use of work activities (in days) (N=308).

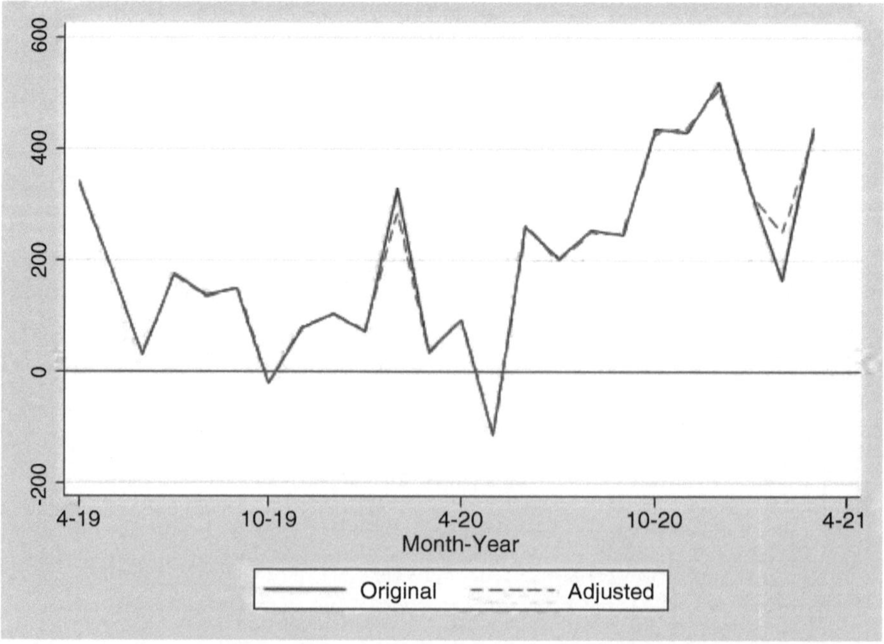

FIGURE 6.3D Year-on-year difference in monthly use of home help (physical assistance) (in hours) (N=175).

Source: Author (data from City X)

TABLE 6.1 Basic statistics

	Short-term accommodation	*Day care*	*Work activities*	*Home help (physical assistance)*
Service use	2.09 days (2.79)	15.17 days (7.51)	12.73 days (8.77)	10.88 hours (18.03)
Months	24236.5 (10.39)			
Wave 1	5.56%			
Wave 2	2.78%			
Wave 3	8.33%			
Other 2020^{+}	25.00%			
Jan … Dec	8.33%			
Women	39.47%	44.68%	38.96%	52.00%
Age	34.09 (11.08)	34.86 (12.02)	39.41 (12.84)	43.15 (12.59)
Group home	1.95%	10.03%	10.58%	2.81%
Intellectual disability				
Severe	72.05%	77.11%	13.78%	25.41%
Mild/moderate	15.67%	7.29%	48.46%	25.30%
N (obs.)	4,104	5,076	11,088	6,300
N (persons)	114	141	308	175

Source: Author (data from City X)

Notes: Standard deviation in parentheses for continuous variables. "Months" refers to months from year "zero". "Jan … Dec" denote the 12-month dummies. Wave 1, Wave 2, and Wave 3 denote April–May 2020, August 2020, and November 2020–January 2021, respectively. Only persons from age 18 to 64, throughout April 2018–March 2021, were included. Persons who had never used each service or lived in a residential facility during the period were excluded. "Work activities" denotes continuous support for work (Type B).

almost half of the users did not possess an intellectual disability certificate. Persons with severe intellectual disability were the minority among users of work activities.

Table 6.2 provides the CRE estimators. The model for short-term accommodation (Table 6.2a) demonstrates that, while the overall use of the service by persons with severe intellectual disability was significantly higher than that by persons without intellectual disability, the amount significantly declined during the first wave of the pandemic. Having mild or moderate intellectual disability, however, was not significantly correlated with either the base level or change in the period of use of short-term accommodation. People living in a group home were more likely to use short-term accommodation than people who lived at home. Gender was uncorrelated with service use or its change at the significance level of 0.05. Even at the significance level of 0.1, gender was correlated with the overall level but not with the change during the pandemic.

TABLE 6.2A Correlated random effects estimators for short-term accommodation

	Main effect	*Wave 1*	*Wave 2*	*Wave 3*	*Other 2020*†
Trend (month)	–0.002 (0.011)				
Time period (main effect)		0.127 (0.869)	–1.066 (1.087)	–1.129 (0.957)	–0.530 (0.654)
Women	0.791† (0.443)	–0.434 (0.315)	0.601 (0.409)	0.423 (0.335)	–0.014 (0.249)
Age	–0.077 (0.088)	–0.010 (0.018)	0.002 (0.020)	0.009 (0.017)	0.004 (0.013)
(Mean)	10.856 (6.754)	–27.710 (23.965)	–78.206† (43.025)	–21.728 (18.178)	–21.033 (14.800)
Living in a group home	3.802** (0.852)				
(Mean)	–2.630 (1.658)				
Intellectual disability (ref: None)					
Severe	2.139** (0.528)	-0.885* (0.403)	0.554 (0.500)	0.543 (0.438)	0.268 (0.325)
Mild/ moderate	0.346 (0.571)	-0.049 (0.437)	0.278 (0.577)	0.367 (0.459)	0.259 (0.366)
Constant	67.803 (269.283)				
N Obs.	4,104	Persons	114		
R^2 Within	0.079	Between	0.210	Overall	0.158
X^2	282.97**	d.f.	43		

TABLE 6.2B Correlated random effects estimators for day care

	Main effect	*Wave 1*	*Wave 2*	*Wave 3*	*Other 2020*†
Trend (month)	0.041 (0.027)				
Time period (main effect)		2.933 (1.982)	2.683 (2.065)	4.699* (2.299)	4.073** (1.562)
Women	0.229 (0.947)	–0.531 (0.622)	–0.507 (0.763)	–0.682 (0.788)	–0.530 (0.555)
Age	–0.037 (0.159)	–0.039 (0.028)	0.027 (0.034)	–0.001 (0.035)	–0.015 (0.024)
(Mean)	–1.005 (14.862)	40.038 (52.020)	26.260 (117.901)	43.373 (52.261)	–22.124 (26.157)
Living in a group home	7.461** (2.384)				
(Mean)	–2.516 (3.061)				

	Main effect	*Wave 1*	*Wave 2*	*Wave 3*	*Other* $2020^{\dagger}$
Intellectual disability (ref: None)					
Severe	11.854^{**} (1.736)	-3.180^{*} (1.429)	-5.879^{**} (1.337)	-5.455^{**} (1.455)	-3.586^{**} (0.955)
Mild/ moderate	5.719^{*} (2.780)	−2.048 (1.545)	−3.341 (2.113)	−2.400 (2.526)	−1.648 (1.467)
Constant	−996.418 (650.224)				
N Obs.	5,076	Persons	141		
R^2 Within	0.178	Between	0.394	Overall	0.342
X^2	1282.57^{**}	d.f.	43		

TABLE 6.2C Correlated random effects estimators for work activities

	Main effect	*Wave 1*	*Wave 2*	*Wave 3*	*Other* 2020^{+}
Trend (month)	−0.032 (0.022)				
Time period (main effect)		1.729 (1.100)	$2.260^{\dagger}$ (1.216)	3.829^{**} (1.347)	3.083^{**} (1.087)
Women	−1.213 (0.807)	−0.080 (0.562)	−0.588 (0.669)	−0.801 (0.721)	−0.400 (0.567)
Age	0.096 (0.147)	−0.036 (0.024)	−0.040 (0.027)	-0.059^{*} (0.028)	$-0.042^{\dagger}$ (0.023)
(Mean)	−8.134 (14.080)	57.988 (56.142)	85.127 (99.856)	52.771 (41.830)	−7.486 (25.962)
Living in a group home	7.206^{**} (2.542)				
(Mean)	−3.184 (2.873)				
Intellectual disability (ref: None)					
Severe	11.155^{**} (1.157)	-2.132^{**} (0.795)	-1.780^{*} (0.835)	−1.041 (0.916)	−0.868 (0.703)
Mild/ moderate	7.638^{**} (0.943)	−0.997 (0.639)	−1.186 (0.722)	−0.622 (0.809)	−0.658 (0.645)
Constant	767.295 (541.298)				
N Obs.	11,088	Persons	308		
R^2 Within	0.062	Between	0.314	Overall	0.255
X^2	1311.44^{**}	d.f.	43		

TABLE 6.2D Correlated random effects estimators for home help (physical assistance)

	Main effect	*Wave 1*	*Wave 2*	*Wave 3*	*Other 2020*†
Trend (month)	0.072† (0.042)				
Time period (main effect)		–0.003 (3.065)	–3.852 (2.884)	-0.604 (4.137)	0.008 (2.564)
Women	–3.681 (2.471)	–1.109 (1.423)	–1.387 (1.408)	–1.344 (1.643)	–1.596 (1.120)
Age	–0.127 (0.257)	–0.002 (0.055)	0.112* (0.056)	0.078 (0.076)	0.037 (0.046)
(Mean)	3.870 (28.067)	–55.910 (108.602)	101.778 (221.146)	–11.465 (103.175)	–9.365 (62.776)
Living in a group home	12.808† (6.992)				
(Mean)	–7.629 (7.419)				
Intellectual disability (ref: None)					
Severe	3.655 (3.259)	–0.161 (1.663)	1.329 (2.381)	–0.169 (2.616)	–0.493 (1.607)
Mild/ moderate	–3.662† (2.113)	0.923 (1.424)	–0.631 (1.453)	–2.092 (1.584)	–0.492 (1.222)
Constant	–1748.291† (1021.960)				
N Obs.	6,300	Persons	175		
R^2 Within	0.059	Between	0.068	Overall	0.066
X^2	123.25**	d.f.	43		

Source: Author (data from City X)

Notes: **p < 0.01, *p < 0.05, and †p < 0.1. Standard error clustered by individual in parentheses. Dummies for months in a year are omitted from the table. The dependent variable is the amount of service use measured in hours for home help and in days for other services. Wave 1, Wave 2, and Wave 3 denote April–May 2020, August 2020, and November 2020–January 2021, respectively. Trend corresponds to the variable of months from the year "zero". Living in a group home is contrasted with living in an individual's home. Dummy variables for intellectual disability were individual means to address few transitions. Only persons from age 18 to 64 throughout April 2018–March 2021, were included. Persons who had never used each service or lived in a residential facility during the period were excluded. "Work activities" denotes continuous support for work (Type B).

In the day care model (Table 6.2b), having intellectual disability was more involved. Compared to having no intellectual disability, having severe intellectual disability was associated with a significantly higher baseline level and a significant decrease in all the periods after the pandemic outbreak. However, mild or moderate intellectual disability was connected with a significantly higher base level but not with changes. The equality test for the main effects of severe and mild/moderate intellectual disabilities rejected the null (chi-squared: 6.39, d.f.: 1, p value: 0.012); thus, the main effect of severe intellectual disability was larger. Living in a group home was associated with higher service use. The positive main effect of the third wave and the dummy for the other months of 2020 indicated an overall increase, which must be added to the other effects to derive the predicted level of service use during each period.

For the work activities model (Figure 6.2c), having severe and mild/moderate intellectual disability was associated with a higher base level of service use than having no intellectual disability. The equality test rejected the null (chi-squared: 11.47, d.f.: 1, p value < 0.001). However, severe intellectual disability interacted with the dummy variables of the first and second waves but not with the dummy of the third wave and of the other months of 2020–2021 for changes in service use. Mild and moderate intellectual disability were not significantly correlated with changes in service use. The amount of service use by persons living in group homes was significantly higher than that by persons living at home. The main effects of the dummy variables of the third wave and the other months of 2020–2021 were also significant, indicating an overall increase during these periods. The effect of the third wave was partially offset by its interaction with age; that is, the service utilization among older people was reduced compared with that among younger people in this period. Gender and its interaction with time period were not significant.

Most coefficients regarding home help (physical assistance) (Table 6.2d), except for month dummies, were not significant at the significance level of 0.05, leading to lower overall R-squared values than those of the other models. Only the interaction term of the second wave and age was significantly positive, suggesting that service use among older people increased compared to younger people.

Discussion

Few services can be regarded as nonessential as long as users choose to use them. During the pandemic, however, essentiality was compromised, owing to prioritizing prevention in the early waves, which may seem less influential than the succeeding waves regarding the total cases and deaths. Nevertheless, the early waves had a major social impact, including a decline in disability services. In particular, the first wave, around April and May 2020, was a period of uncertainty due to the first uncontrollable outbreak of the disease and the subsequent request-based lockdown. It witnessed a notable decrease in services. Although social welfare facilities, in general, were recognized as essential services, stay-at-home was recommended as much as possible. Accordingly, some users chose temporarily to follow the instructions and refrained from using services or suspended the need for service providers.

The compromise of the essentiality of services for disease prevention differed among the service types based on the changing patterns, which may relate to the distinctions of internal/external and individuality/collectivity. A decline in the provision of short-term accommodation in City X during the first wave is of particular interest. While short-term accommodations were considered essential for community living during the emergency and when the need for respite of family caregivers arose, the service provision dropped sharply and continuously during the pandemic. A key to understanding the decrease is that short-term accommodation takes place in residential facilities and utilizes their extra capacity. However, the change implied that long-term residents were prioritized, with their needs being recognized as the most essential.[6] Arguably, short-term use was limited to control the border of the facilities, reduce chances of infection, and protect long-term users. Here, different internal/external distinctions were in operation. Regarding residential facilities, the long-term residents continued to live inside the facilities, which could be characterized by collectivity, while the facilities accepted fewer short-term users from outside. Conversely, the users of short-term accommodations were requested to stay inside their homes, and the opportunities to live temporarily outside their homes, in case of an emergency or necessity for respite, were restricted. This is in contrast with the physical assistance in home help, which witnessed a small decline. This service type aids the basic activities of daily living, such as eating and bathing, that are routinely required and considered essential. This service type takes place inside users' homes and is individual in nature, which fits the stay-at-home recommendation. This differs from day care and work activities, which are forms of collective support outside users' homes. Overall, however, since the essentiality of these services certainly exists, service use recovered after the first wave, except in the case of short-term accommodation.

The detailed analysis demonstrated that the impacts were not homogeneous across service users; rather, heterogeneity among different groups of people was evident. In particular, the effects of severe intellectual disability and, in part, mild or moderate intellectual disability, were confirmed. The main effects indicated that, except for home help, persons with severe intellectual disability had a higher base level of service use than persons with mild or moderate intellectual disability, who, in turn, had a higher base level than persons without intellectual disability. Hence, this posited that disability services were instrumental for persons with intellectual disability in organizing their lives, and the need for services heightened as intellectual disability became severe. After the outbreak, however, the service use of persons with severe intellectual disability dropped, at least in the first wave (short-term accommodation), while the use of day care was affected throughout the pandemic. This indicates that aspects of living conditions were undermined for this population in comparison to other groups. The need for care did not decrease (for instance, day care is targeted at people who have a constant need for care); however, it was assumed that others, particularly family members, would take care of the individuals during the period. Hence, stay-at-home for users of disability services can hardly be discussed without taking care provisions into account.

Persons living in group homes had a higher base level of service use than persons living at home, except for home help.[7] This group could be considered to include people who receive less care from family members than persons with disabilities at home. Thus, living in a group home serves as a proxy indicator of limited family care when information regarding family members is missing. The fact that persons living in a group home use more services in addition to the group home as a service suggests that their daytime and emergent situations need support outside family care. The interaction effects of living in a group home with period dummies were excluded from the abovementioned models because in the FE models that included these interactions, which are not shown here, the interactions were not significant at the significance level of 0.05, and the corresponding CRE models needed to exclude these terms to estimate model fit.[8] The minor interaction significance indicates that the high level of service needs among the population that received less family care continued throughout the pandemic.

Gender was not significantly correlated with the main effects and the interactions. Although this does not preclude a possibility of significance in wider areas, or of intersectional difficulties that women with disabilities may experience, at least, service use in the city did not exhibit gender effects. Age and its interactions with time period were, on the whole, not significant, except for the model for work activities, which included a significantly negative interaction between age and the third wave.

Conclusion

Hypothesis 1 (the use of certain types of social services concerning disability decreased after the COVID-19 outbreak) was supported, albeit to varying degrees among service types. Short-term accommodation service use markedly decreased during the pandemic; however, there was a temporary decline in the use of home help in the first wave. Reduced use of day care and work activities was also observed. Overall, it can be argued that the four service types were adversely affected by the pandemic.

Hypothesis 2a (service use of persons with severe disability was less affected by the pandemic) was partially rejected, except for home help. Although their service use was larger than that of the other groups, its decline during the first wave was larger than the decline observed for the other groups. The absolute decline size, rather than the ratio, is important, because the quantity is connected with the changing gaps with other groups and can be interpreted as the amount of care replaced by other forms, such as family care.

Hypothesis 2b (other demographics, including gender and age, affected service use) was rejected, except that the use of work activities among older people decreased during the third wave. The place of living – namely, group home or an individual's home – was related to the level of service use, but not to changes.

Disability services, when properly organized, facilitate the social inclusion of persons with disabilities, although the services are merely a basis of individuals' lives. This chapter concerns the quantitative sociology of disability in assessing factors involved in attempts at social inclusion. The analysis enabled us to reflect on the largely unintended consequence of the protection measures against the pandemic that undermined daily support for persons with disabilities.

The impact of the reduced use of collective support on users and their family members may be mitigated by temporarily replacing services with individual assistance that covers many hours in a day. Such a service reduces the risk of infection, because workers need not provide care for many different users. Since a decline in service use was notable among persons with severe disabilities, the eligibility criteria for individual assistance must be only partially relaxed. In addition, assisting family caregivers when service users are stuck at home may be necessary. Disability services in Japan serve persons with disabilities and do not directly support family members. Direct assistance can be instrumental in relieving family stress when dependence on family care cannot be avoided.

This study contributed to the literature by analyzing administrative panel data to trace precisely the changes in service use and identify relevant factors. However, this chapter has certain limitations. The data are limited to a city, and the sample size is limited for certain services when the data are decomposed into individual services. However, the service data combined with the disability certificate data indicate certain advantages that service data alone, irrespective of the data size, cannot provide. These include information regarding population change and the population with disabilities, in addition to service users. Some important information is absent, e.g., household types. Nevertheless, the analysis in this chapter offers statistical evidence of the impact of COVID-19 on persons with disabilities who require specialized assistance.

Notes

1 This was also the case with Lunsky et al. (2021).
2 Users living in residential facilities were omitted.
3 Short-term accommodation uses residential facilities, unlike a local service of non-residential respite.
4 Work activities are work opportunities without employment contract, unlike sheltered employment under employment contract ("Type A"). Reasonable accommodation in competitive employment is stipulated under another act.
5 The leap year 2020 cannot be strictly adjusted by this approach.
6 Although residential services were omitted from this chapter, the use of residential facilities in the city was quite stable.
7 Home help can be used in a group home – in which case, personal assistance is primarily commissioned to a provider of home help.
8 Interactions of living in a group home with period dummies were consistently positive for home help, but were not significant.

Acknowledgments

The author would like to thank all the people who were involved in the study, including the staff of City X.

References

Beyer, Stephen, Tony Brown, Rachel Akandi, and Mark Rapley. 2010. "A comparison of quality of life outcomes for people with intellectual disabilities in supported employment, day services and employment enterprises". *Journal of Applied Research in Intellectual Disabilities* 23, 3: 290–295. doi:10.1111/j.1468-3148.2009.00534.x.

Cardona, Beatriz. 2021. "The pitfalls of personalization rhetoric in time of health crisis". *Health Promotion International* 36, 3: 714–721. doi:10.1093/heapro/daaa112.

Colon-Cabrera, David, Shivika Sharma, Narelle Warren, and Dikaios Sakellariou. 2021. "Examining the role of government in shaping disability inclusiveness around COVID-19: a framework analysis of Australian guidelines". *International Journal for Equity in Health* 20, Article 166.

DeJong, Gerben. 1983. "Defining and implementing the independent living concept". In *Independent Living for Physically Disabled People*, edited by Nancy M. Crewe and Irving K. Zola, 4–27. People with Disabilities Press.

Doyle, Laura. 2021. "'All in this together?' A commentary on the impact of COVID-19 on disability day ervices in Ireland". *Disability & Society* 36, 9: 1538–1542.

Foucault, Michel. 1975. *Surveiller et punir: naissance de la prison* (Discipline and Punish: Birth of Prison). Translated into Japanese (1977) by Hajime Tamura. Tokyo: Shinchosha.

Hatton, Chris. 2017. "Day services and home care for adults with learning disabilities across the UK". *Tizard Learning Disability Review* 22, 2: 109–115. doi:10.1108/TLDR-01-2017-0004.

Hirano, Takayuki. 2012. *Data Analysis of Long-term Care Services for Elderly People*. Tokyo: Chuo Hoki.

Imahashi, Kumiko, *et al.* 2021. "Analysis of services and supports for people with disabilities using administrative claims data". *Japanese Journal of Health and Research*. https://doi.org/10.32279/jjhr.202142606.

Lerman, Paul. 1982. *Deinstitutionalization and the Welfare State*, New Brunswick, NJ: Rutgers University Press.

Luhmann, Niklas. 1984. *Soziale Systeme*. Translated into Japanese by Tsutomu Sato (1993–1995). Tokyo: Koseisha-Koseikaku.

Luhmann, Niklas. 1997. *Die Gesellschaft der Gesellschaft*. Translated into Japanese by Yasuo Baba *et al.* (2009). Tokyo: Hosei University Press.

Lunsky, Yona, Nicole Bobbette, Megan Abou Chacra, Wei Wang, Haoyu Zhao, Kendra Thomson, and Yani Hamdani. 2021. "Predictors of worker mental health in intellectual disability services during COVID-19". *Journal of Applied Research in Intellectual Disabilities* 34: 1655–1660. doi:10.1111/jar.12892.

Ministry of Education, Culture, Sports, Science and Technology. 2020. "[COVID-19]: Information about MEXT's measures". Retrieved 20 October 2022, www.mext.go.jp/en/mext_00006.html.

Ministry of Health, Labour and Welfare of Japan. 2022. "Statistical information". Retrieved 20 October 2022, www.mhlw.go.jp/stf/seisakunitsuite/bunya/hukushi_kaigo/shougaishahukushi/toukei/index.html.

Mundlak, Yair. 1978. "On the pooling of time series and cross section data". *Econometrica* 46, 1: 69–85. doi:10.2307/1913646.

Nakane, Naruhisa. 2020. "A quantitative analysis of disincentives for the transition from institutional to community-based living of people with disabilities in Japan". *Journal of Disability Studies* 16: 129–152.

Nambu, Tsuruhiko, and Takuma Sugahara. 2004. "The effect of self-payment rate on demand for long-term care service: an empirical analysis using long-term care receipt data". *Journal of Health and Society* 14, 3: 191–211. doi:10.4091/iken.14.3_191.

NHK (Japan Broadcasting Corporation). 2022. "COVID-19 Cases in Japan". Retrieved 23 September 2022, www3.nhk.or.jp/news/special/coronavirus/data-all/. NHK stopped publishing the data on 27 September 2022, four days after the author downloaded the data. The already downloaded data are still allowed to be used under the terms of use.

Nicholson, Emma, Suzanne Guerin, Fiona Keogh, and Philip Dodd. 2019. "Comparing traditional-residential, personalised residential and personalised non-residential respite services: quality of life findings from an Irish population with mild-moderate intellectual disabilities". *British Journal of Learning Disabilities* 47, 1: 12–18.

Nirje, Bengt. 1969. "The normalization principle and its human management implications". In *Changing Patterns in Residential Services for the Mentally Retarded*, edited by R. Kugel and W. Wolfensberger. Washington, DC: President's Committee on Mental Retardation.

Okahara, Masayuki. 1995. "Love as an Institution". In *Ars Vivendi*, edited by Junko Asaka*et al.*Tokyo: Fujiwara Shoten.

Oliver, Michael. 1983. *Social Work with Disabled People*. London: Macmillan. doi:10.1007/978-1-349-86058-6.

Oliver, Michael. 1990. *The Politics of Disablement*. London: Macmillan Education. doi:10.1007/978-1-349-20895-1.

Power, Andrew, and Ruth Bartlett. 2018. "Self-building safe havens in a post-service landscape: how adults with learning disabilities are reclaiming the welcoming communities agenda". *Social & Cultural Geography* 19, 3: 336–356. doi:10.1080/14649365.2015.1031686.

Pranshu. 2022. "Persons with disability amid COVID-19 crisis". *Journal of Psychosocial Research* 17, 1: 239–247.

Sakakibara, Kenjiro. 2016. *Social Inclusion and the Body: Defining Disability and Rethinking Different Treatments Following Disability Antidiscrimination Legislation*. Tokyo: Seikatsu Shoin.

Sato, Masumi, *et al.* 2009. "Municipal benefits analysis software under services and supports for Persons with Disabilities Act". *Journal of Social Welfare*, 120: 89–106.

Schunk, Reinhard. 2013. "Within and between estimates in random-effects models: advantages and drawbacks of correlated random effects and hybrid models". *The Stata Journal* 13, 1: 65–76. doi:10.1177/1536867X1301300105.

Schwartz, Ariel E., Elizabeth G.S. Munsell, Elizabeth K. Schmidt, Cristina Colon-Semenza, Kelsi Carolan, and Dena L. Gassner. 2021. "Impact of COVID-19 on services for people with disabilities and chronic health conditions". *Disability and Health Journal* 14, 3: 101090. doi:10.1016/j.dhjo.2021.101090.

Thomas, Carol. 1999. *Female Forms: Experiencing and Understanding Disability*. Buckingham: Open University Press.

Union of the Physically Impaired against Segregation and Disability Alliance (UPIAS and DA) (1976) *Fundamental Principles of Disability*, London: UPIAS and DA.

Vlaskamp, Carla, Saskia J. Hiemstra, Linda A. Wiersma, and Bonne J. H. Zijlstra. 2007. "Extent, duration, and content of day services' activities for persons with profound intellectual and multiple disabilities". *Journal of Policy and Practice in Intellectual Disabilities* 4, 2: 152–159.

Wolfensberger, Wolf. 1994. *A Brief Introduction to Social Role Valorization: A High-Order Concept for Addressing the Plight of Societally Devalued People, and for Structuring Human Services*. Revised edition. Syracuse, NY: Syracuse University.

Wooldridge, Jeffrey M. 2010. *Econometric Analysis of Cross Section and Panel Data*. 2nd edition. Cambridge, MA: The MIT Press.

World Health Organization (WHO). 2001. *International Classification of Functioning, Disability and Health*, Geneva: WHO.

Yamashita, Sachiko. 2019. "The disabled people's movement in connection with the institutionalization of care services". *Journal of Welfare Sociology* 16: 135–153.

7

IMAGES OF PANDEMIC INEQUALITY IN BRAZIL

Marianna Knothe Sanfelicio

Introduction – An Objective Approach

Starting with an objective approach means understanding the context in which the research presented here takes place. This is a situated research, with a well-established spatial and temporal cutout. The results it presents are based on this cutout. This means more than introducing the context in which the research was done. It means to understand that anthropology is a science that is done in particularities, based on dense descriptions.[1]

Since March 2020, when the first case of COVID-19 was reported in Brazil, the country has reached more than 684,000[2] pandemic-related deaths. According to the World Health Organization (WHO), Brazil has the third absolute number[3] of deaths globally. The state of São Paulo, located in the southeastern region of Brazil, has the highest absolute number of deaths in the country: approximately 174,000[4] lives have been lost to COVID-19 in just over two years of pandemic. This also happens in the city of São Paulo, the state capital and the largest city in Latin America. T here, the number of COVID-19 deaths exceeded 43,000.[5]

When the Ipea[6] parameters of accumulated number of deaths per 100,000 inhabitants is taken into consideration, the state of São Paulo does not appear as one of the states where most deaths occurred in Brazil, and neither does the city of São Paulo.[7] However, this does not mean that we are talking about a slight number of deaths, or that these casualties can be overlooked. Even in a city the size of São Paulo, with a population of approximately 12.3 million, this is a significant number: approximately one out of 300 inhabitants of the city have died since the pandemic began (March 2020–April 2022).

The starting point of this chapter is the analysis of the national scene. The data also show other important aspects that should be taken into account when working with pandemic data. First, there is a characteristic that not only covers

DOI: 10.4324/9781003459682-8

the pandemic as it happened in Brazil, but all over the world: we are dealing with numbers that always change, increasing or decreasing according to particularities that are not always predictable. We have to deal, then, with the character of novelty given by research with a disease that has just appeared, in a social-historical context that had not yet experienced a pandemic. It is necessary, therefore, to consider the unpredictability that comes alongside the data, because it is not always possible to deal with accurate predictions. The second characteristic relates to the Brazilian scenario, in which working with statistical data was not valued during the pandemic. The difficulty of working with statistical data in a country where it is complicated to find reliable data must be considered when discussing how to do research. Finding the data often becomes a search exercise, as they are sometimes hidden inside bureaucratic spirals. These data should be easily accessible to ensure transparency, and also to ensure that public policies can be proposed based on them. Instead, it takes some effort to find them.

Legally speaking, Brazil is a federative republic. There are, simultaneously, federal, state, and municipal obligations towards health. This means health is a shared competence, and all spheres of power have different obligations on this theme. The numbers shown above, as we can see, were obtained from different sources. This was necessary because, at a certain moment of the pandemic, the federal government decided to stop sharing the data on deaths in the country. This caused a "data blackout", which, in this context, can be defined as a lack of trustworthy data on the pandemic in Brazil. The data blackout obviously caused statistical problems, which made it difficult to understand how many people were dying from COVID in the country.

Shifting from the national to the municipal sphere of competence, the problem is still present. Scaling it down, we are still working with the same problems presented on a national scale, and, we can also work from nuances. The city of São Paulo, the largest in Latin America, is organized into 96 districts, which answer to subprefectures. Understanding the social, political, and economic organization of the space you are working on also means understanding how to read the data you collect from each location. A city the size of São Paulo, approximately 1,500km^2, demands the researcher to watch out for possible differences between districts.

The deaths that occurred in São Paulo did not happen in the same way in all areas of the city. This can be analyzed by looking at two maps of São Paulo, which show the city divided in its 96 districts. Looking at these images, it is possible to notice that the deaths caused by the pandemic were concentrated in the outskirts and in certain central regions. Moreover, it is possible to see that there are correlations between the areas where most deaths occurred and the areas with the lowest average monthly income.

Figure 7.1 shows the average monthly remuneration of formal employment. It was built by Rede Nossa São Paulo, a civil society organization that works mainly with municipal data from São Paulo. In this map, the light-green areas

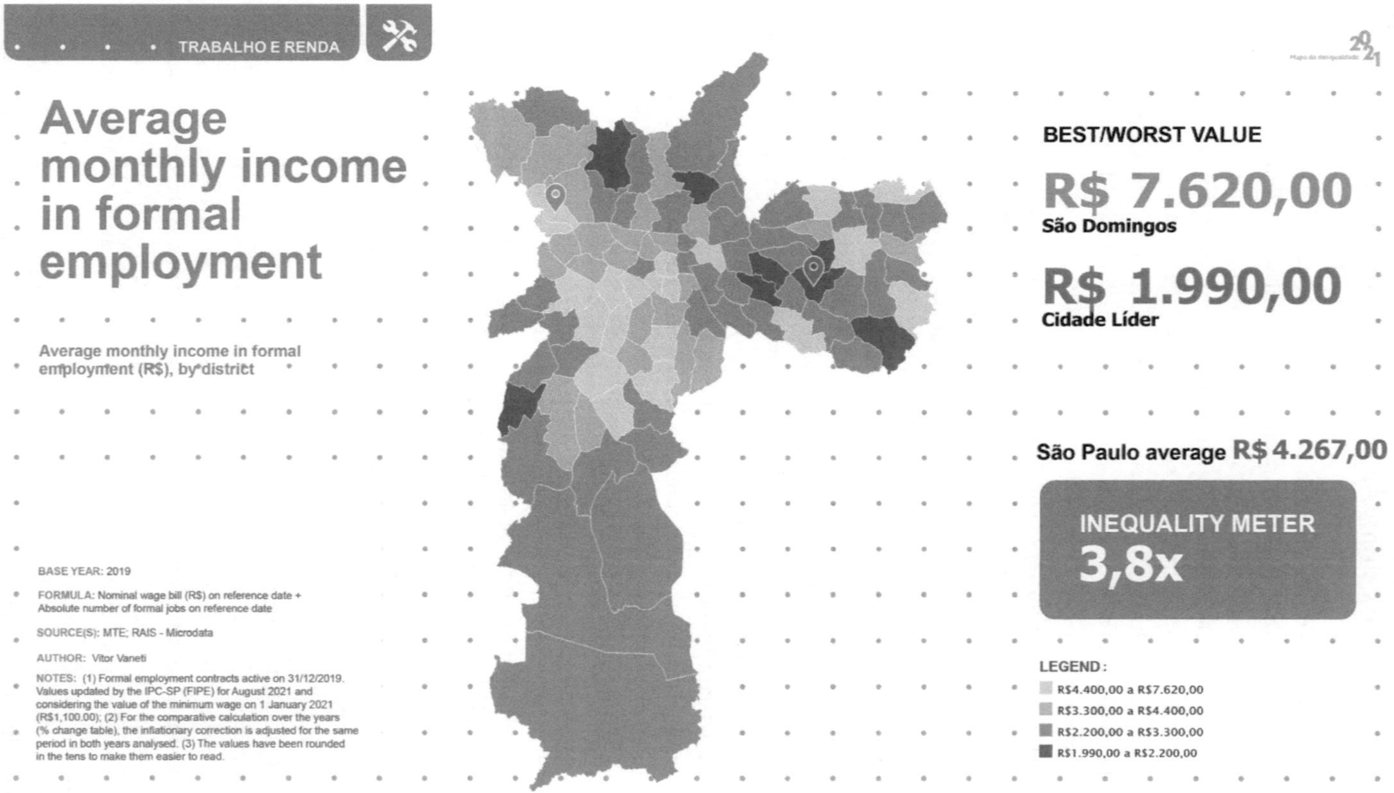

FIGURE 7.1 Average monthly income (in Brazilian Reais) among formally employed people in the city of São Paulo.
Source: Adapted from Rede Nossa São Paulo: www.nossasaopaulo.org.br/wp-content/uploads/2021/10/Mapa-Da-Desigualdade-2021_Mapas.pdf.

represent where the inhabitants earn the highest remuneration (as the shade of green gets darker, the remuneration decreases). Note that the darker shades of green tend to be on the city outskirts.

The map in Figure 7.2 was prepared by a research group of the Faculdade de Arquitetura e Urbanismo da Universidade de São Paulo (FAU-USP), LabCidade, and shows the number of deaths by COVID per 10,000 inhabitants – the darker

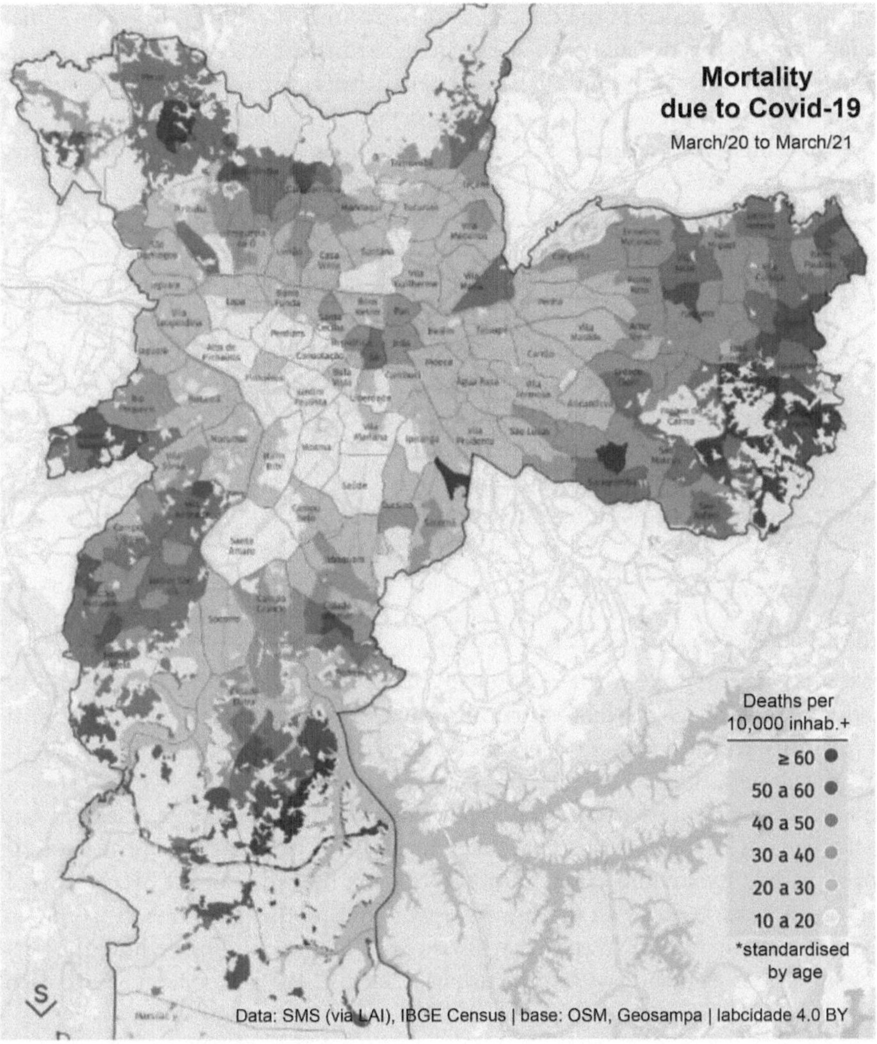

FIGURE 7.2 COVID-19 mortality data in São Paulo, showing deaths per 10,000 inhabitants.

Source: Adapted from LabCidade, www.labcidade.fau.usp.br/prioridade-na-vacinacao-negligencia-a-geografia-da-covid-19-em-sao-paulo/.

the shade of pink, the higher the number of deaths. As can be seen, the highest numbers of deaths are in the outskirts. This map also shows that some data could not be found (represented by the uncolored areas).

It is important to remember that the construction of maps is always social and, in certain ways, also political.[8] Every map is the result of a choice that highlights some aspects and ignores others, taking into consideration the space that one wishes to show. Nossa São Paulo has also produced a COVID mortality map, alongside the map of average monthly income. The decision to LabCidade's map was taken by considering the difficulties of separating the city by districts, something the Nossa São Paulo map does not. Even the monthly remuneration map should be looked at carefully, because some districts are quite large and hold a lot of diversity (which is not taken into account). It is undeniable, however, that we are dealing with a higher number of mortalities in the outskirts of the city, and it is impossible to be more assertive based only in these maps.

Our idea does not work with a pattern of segregation per se, but with one specific pattern of social inequality that appears in the city. In São Paulo, such patterns overlap geographically and build on an opposition between the center and the periphery of the city, in which the center is economically predominant over the periphery. The images produced and published by the press during the COVID-19 pandemic reflect these patterns. Such images make clear how these patterns affect the bodies of individuals living in São Paulo according to their place of origin within the city. In conclusion, in this research the body and its representation in the media will be highlighted for a better understanding of the patterns of social inequality in the city of São Paulo.

A Subjective Approach

Amidst all the production made during these two years of the pandemic, in order to efficiently base their research efficiently, academic work has the task of knowing how to select what is important out of everything that is produced. It is necessary to learn how to select the data so that you don't just build a tangle of information. The selection process towards an answer to a hypothesis or a research question goes a long way. Specifically in the case of this research, our main basis is in the areas of urban anthropology, on the study of cemeterial spaces in São Paulo; and visual anthropology, on the study of the production of images of death used by Brazilian newspapers during the pandemic. It is only in the union of these two strands that it has become possible to see how the various modes of existence within the urban space overlap and dialogue with each other in such a way that life and death deal with the same problems.

Images of Death Produced During the Pandemic

Since the beginning of 2020, Brazilian newspapers have devised narratives about the pandemic in various ways. One of these narratives is through press photographs, considered as objects endowed with structural autonomy, which are both produced by social patterns and responsible for producing them. This is mainly anthropological research based on documents (a collection of photographs), in which we seek to investigate how the analyzed images are an expression of the society in which they were taken. The 232 photographs from the collection built during the research, and brought for analysis here, are treated not as illustrations, but as a way to guide the text (they were taken from Brazilian newspapers), and are therefore what Roland Barthes calls "press photographs":

> the press photograph is an object that has been worked on, chosen, composed, constructed, treated according to professional, aesthetic, or ideological norms which are so many factors of connotation; while on the other, this same photograph is not only perceived, received, it is *read*, connected more or less consciously by the public that consumes it to a traditional stock of signs.
>
> *(Barthes 1983, 198)*

The imagery language related to COVID-19 created from this daily contact with newspapers is unique to our time. Consequently, the relationship we create with these photographs circulating in the media during the pandemic is also unique. These images are, after all, an expression of the society in which they were constructed. In this regard, Barthes says that

> [it] is always developed by a given society and history. Signification, in short, is the dialectical movement which resolves the contradiction between cultural and natural man. Thanks to its code of connotation the reading of the photograph is thus always historical. It depends on the reader's "knowledge" just as though it were a matter of a real language [*langue*], intelligible only if one has learned the signs.
>
> *(Barthes 1983, 206–207)*

Reading, analyzing, and understanding these photographs depends, therefore, on knowing the signs of this era, on understanding how the funeral rites occur at this historical moment, and on realizing how they changed with the pandemic.

It is necessary to say that these images are, no doubt, a result of our times; a historical moment when the death toll could be lower – if not zeroed, at least controlled. And so, the question guiding this research would perhaps be different. That is why the uncontrolled number of deaths in Brazil should also be considered within this analysis – because these photographs are, like it or not, documents that result from political and social choices.as already expressed, "there is no document of civilization which is not at the same time a document of barbarism. And just as such a document is not free of barbarism, barbarism taints also the manner in which it was transmitted from one owner to another" (Benjamin 1968, 245).

It is necessary, therefore, to return to the images the anthropological element that makes them exist, and to treat them as an act, both generated by society and that generates other instances. The images presented in this report represent neither a total illusion nor the unrestricted truth, but rather are part of the very dialectical movement that constructs them. From this, we can ask ourselves how these images dialogue with the urban space. In what ways do they speak about the ways of living in the city of São Paulo?

The production of these photographs, as we will see, happens based on certain patterns. As seen in Figure 7.1, there is an economic cleavage in the city of São Paulo. These images are produced according to this cleavage, and only the bodies of those who live in economically disadvantaged regions are likely to be seen in the images produced during the pandemic. In this sense, the production of these images speaks not only of the space of São Paulo, which in itself is crossed by economic differences, but also of the way people live in the city based on these differences. The bodies, in the construction of this research, become the central point where these differences are highlighted, a place where it is possible to see how the economic factor allows (or not) the right to dignity and mourning.

Images for this research were collected between September 2020 and March 2021. From this research, an online photo archive containing 232 images was created. These images have been added to a table where it is possible to separate them, based on: the source in which they were collected, date of publication, where the photo was taken, and, when possible, other information about the image. From the way the table was organized, it is possible to make correlations between them. It is possible to cross-check relevant information from these images in a variety of ways. The organization and the way the collection is built up is essential so that relevant information can be viewed quickly and cross-referenced. Thus, it makes sense for this collection to be made public, so that its model can be referenced and used by other researchers.[9]

In the first steps of this research, it was possible to cross-reference data about the place where the photo was taken and the publication source. It was possible to see that the photographs reproduced by Brazilian press sources during the period of the COVID-19 pandemic were almost entirely taken in lower-class public cemeteries. These are park cemeteries, located on the outskirts of the city. In these cemeteries there is a policy of exhuming buried bodies three years after burial. The bodies of the dead from the pandemic, rendered invisible during the funeral rites due to the sanitary restrictions imposed by the viral nature of the disease, are present in these photographs in a game of visibility and invisibility: nothing is seen, but everything can be imagined. The double of the dead body is present from the coffins, the graves, the flower crowns.

As an example of our project, we will analyze one photograph from the collection to explain a little of what was found (Figure 7.3). This image was taken at a public cemetery in São Paulo, the largest in the city and located in the east zone. It was published in a newspaper considered to be reputable and competent in its journalistic function, nationally recognized, and with wide public access. These characteristics ensure the public expression of the chosen image. At the same time, however, one must realize that this is a media outlet based in the southeast of the country, a fact that may somehow bias the editorial choice of the photo from the intermediation of editors and the editorial choices of this source itself. It is also important to note that this source is not open access, being a newspaper that uses a paywall and requires readers to pay for access to material. Financial accessibility, in this case, also works as an intermediary characteristic for access to this image.

Considering the intermediations through which photographs pass until they reach readers, those made by photographers at the moment they take the pictures must also be evaluated. Photographs, after all, are frames of a possible real, which pass through the vision of the one who photographs them, and "Even when photographers are most concerned with mirroring reality, they are still haunted by tacit imperatives of taste and conscience" (Sontag 2005, 4). In addition, our own intermediation on the selection of the images that make up this analysis must also be considered. It is, then, about several intermediations: the photographer, the journalistic source, and our own.

At this stage, the decision to work with the analysis of only one image is not accidental: the large number of photographs taken during the pandemic is also a mechanism of dehumanization of the people living in the outskirts of the city. In this sense, to increase the number of images analyzed would be to make the same error. The choice to use a minimum number of images also serves as a reminder that we are not dealing only with numbers, but with people, and that in these images there is more than just their index shows: they are wrapped in a web of relationships that goes far beyond them. If photos are used here, this is despite any pain inflicted on family and friends who survived. This pain will be kept to a minimum. Besides, as is well known, "Photographs shock insofar as they show something novel. Unfortunately, the ante keeps getting raised – partly through the very proliferation of such images of horror" (Sontag 2005, 14).

Figure 7.3 shows a close-up view of a coffin. Inside the coffin, a white cloth covers the body of a dead man. The original caption of this photo, in the newspaper where it was collected, said that this burial was in contradiction with COVID's safety rules. In the background, you can see the feet of a person. It can be assumed that these belong to some relative or friend who is accompanying the burial. The image shows, even if superficially, how the mourning rituals took place during the pandemic in Brazil. Given the contaminating character of the disease, the body of the dead is now seen, itself, as contaminating. With bodies nobody could touch, the collective expression of feelings became, itself, forbidden. If, as Philippe Ariès (2012) teaches, structures of death and mourning were already forbidden in society, the pandemic's role was, then, to reveal these prohibitions and simultaneously to reinforce them.

In the first stage of the research, we could see how the bodies of the dead were depersonalized. The changes in the rites imposed by COVID abolished

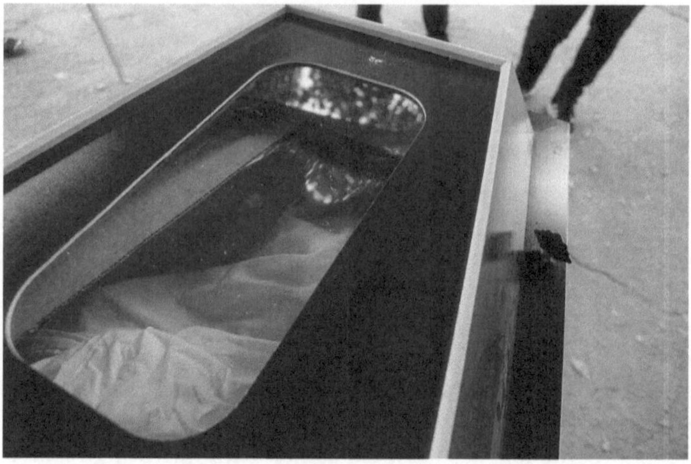

FIGURE 7.3 Close-up picture of a coffin at Vila Formosa Cemetery, São Paulo. Source: Yan Boechat, 1 April 2020.

personalized death and brought death and mourning into the picture as collective social acts. The lack of funeral rites and the impossibility of expressing feelings of mourning create the abolition of personalized death, and this dead person becomes a marginal being.[10] Furthermore, from the tabled collection of photographs, it was also possible to note a hypothesis that gave rise to the research that is now presented here: among the photographs collected, none were taken in cemeteries in the central areas of São Paulo.

As shown in Figures 7.1 and 7.2, most of the deaths occurred in the peripheral areas of the city. These are areas where the average monthly income is lower, and, consequently, are areas of greater social vulnerability. When dealing with these data, we must consider complex issues of the political and economic life of the city. However, what interests us here is to understand why only *these* cemeteries are featured in the newspapers and online sources. Even if the number of deaths in central regions was lower, and even if the number of burials in central cemeteries was lower, why – if deaths happened everywhere – do newspapers publish only photographs of cemeteries on the outskirts of São Paulo? And why do photojournalists seem only to be interested in these spaces? To answer these questions, we must assess how cemeteries are distributed throughout the city, how they fit into the urban landscape, and how they are viewed by those who relate to them.

Photographs and the Urban Landscape

São Paulo has 22 public cemeteries and 18 private ones. Figure 7.4 shows how they are distributed along the city. The 22 public cemeteries are shown in green, while the 18 private ones are shown in red. The only crematorium in the city, which is public, is shown in black.

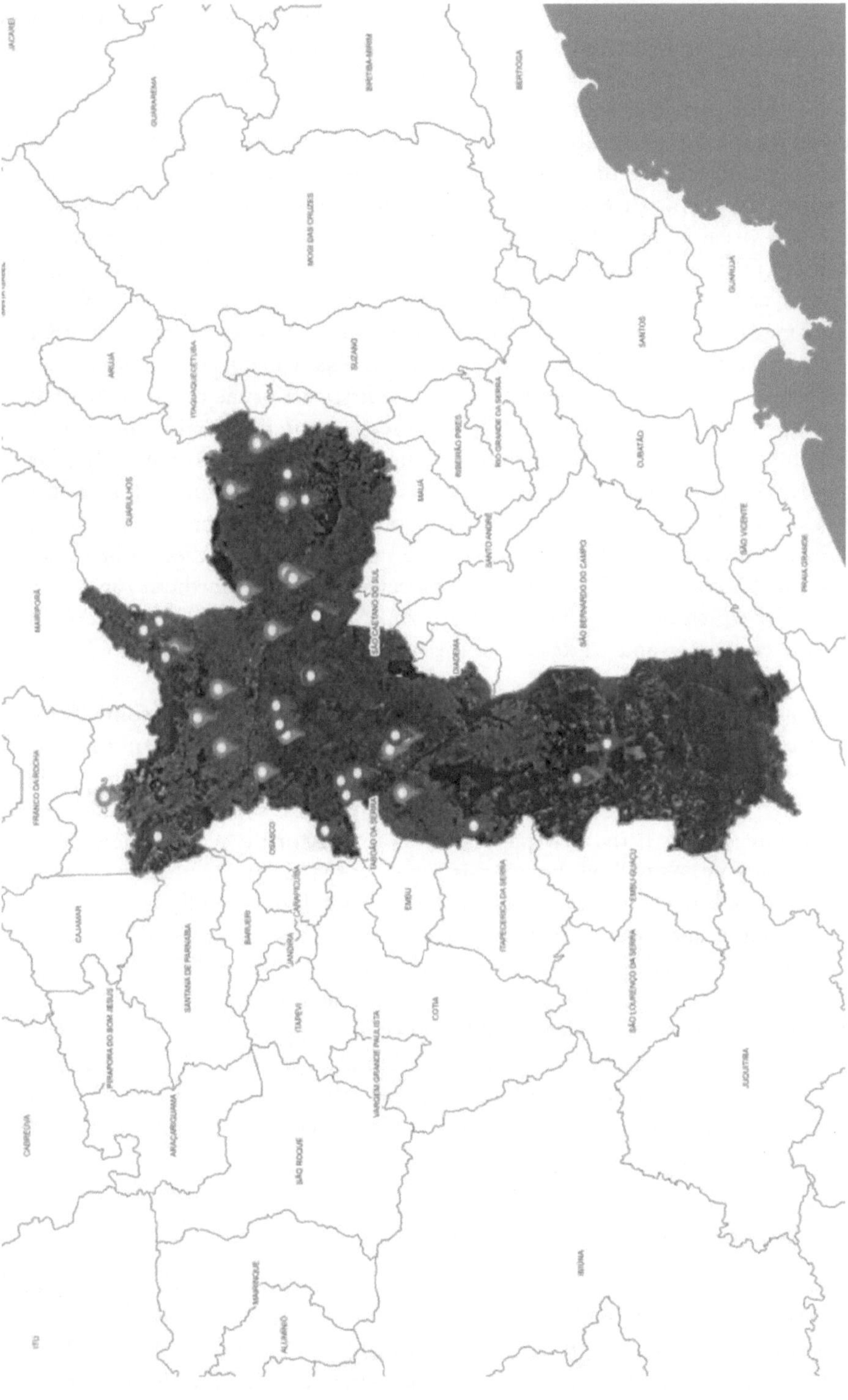

FIGURE 7.4 Map showing all the cemeteries in São Paulo.
Source: Geosampa and Marianna Sanfelicio.

It was possible to establish new criteria that define another research interest from the way the collection was created, which allows information about the photographs to be cross-referenced. If in the first section of the chapter the criterion defined was the source where the photograph was published, without concern for the city or cemetery in which the photo was taken, here the interest is different and, therefore, the criteria for the selection of the photographs are also different. Based on what was perceived in the previous section, the interest here is less in the visual anthropological characteristics that these photographs point to, and more in the places where these photographs were taken. It is in this sense that two criteria were created to be applied in the collection: (a) only photographs made in cemeteries in the city of São Paulo; (b) only photographs that have specified the name of the cemetery where it was made in their caption.

Of the 232 photographs collected during the first part of the research, 105 fall under the first selection criterion. When the second criterion is also considered, this number drops to 96. All of these 96 photographs were taken in only four public cemeteries in the city. Cross-referencing the map in Figure 7.4 with this new stage of the research resulted in the map in Figure 7.5, where it is possible to observe the number of photos that were taken at each of these four cemeteries: one photo at the Nova Cachoeirinha cemetery, in the northern zone; nine at the Vila Alpina cemetery, in the eastern zone; 25 at the São Luiz cemetery, in the southern zone; and 61 taken at the Vila Formosa cemetery, also in the eastern zone.

The narratives built by the newspapers where these photographs come from, as can be seen on Figure 7.5, were created entirely from cemeteries on the outskirts of the city, in places with a lower average monthly income. It is a narrative that corroborates the idea of inequality of deaths seen in LabCidade's map (Figure 7.2), as if the newspapers were looking for the places where more people are dying. As will be shown, this is not all that occurs. Although most of the deaths took place in peripheral cemeteries, this does not fully explain why all the photographs were taken in these places. The narrative of mortuary inequality formulated by newspapers does not come only from the inequalities found on the maps above. Using anthropological methodology, we have carried out semi-structured interviews and informal conversations with photojournalists, and from these it became clear that the narrative cutoff also comes from a preconceived idea within the newspapers that it is easier to photograph in the outskirts' cemeteries – where there is "less likelihood of me being barred by the administration".

The Cemeterial Spaces in São Paulo

As mentioned above, São Paulo has 22 public and 18 private cemeteries. Most of the private places keep their gates closed, which are only opened on special occasions, such as the Day of the Dead and significant emotional dates, such as Mother's Day and Father's Day. Public cemeteries, on the other hand, always

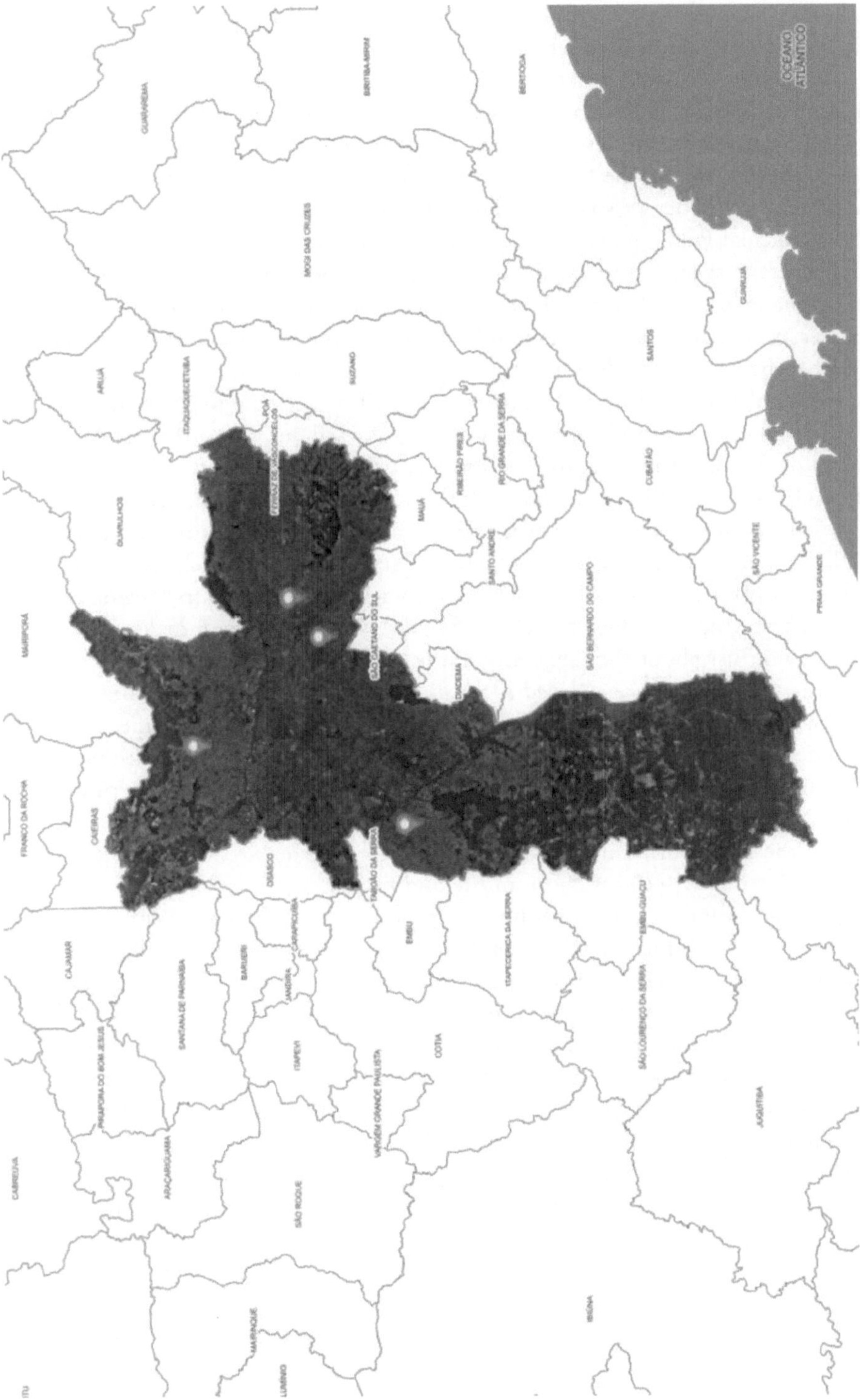

FIGURE 7.5 Map showing the four cemeteries in São Paulo where photographs were taken during the pandemic.
Source: Geosampa and Marianna Sanfelicio, based on information from personal archive.

have at least one gate open, allowing people to enter and leave freely. Research carried out in private cemeteries depends on gaining authorization from each space. In theory, research in public cemeteries should also depend on this.

In practice, we can differentiate between the public peripheral cemeteries and the public central cemeteries. Research on the city of São Paulo's cemetery spaces conducted within the LabNAU research group, found difficulties when it came to entering cemetery spaces in the central regions of the city.

The Municipal Public Power of São Paulo's press office states that research in public cemetery spaces must be done only with authorization. Such a request must be made on the letterhead of the educational institution to which the researcher is affiliated, and contain information about the visit, such as: the cemetery to be visited, the date and time the visit will take place, the visit's purpose, the number of students and teachers who will participate in the visit, who will be responsible, information about the work will be done, the Cadastro Nacional de Pessoa Juridica of the institution, and contact numbers. The request must be filed between 15 and 20 days before the visit, and the authorization – or veto – will be published in the city's official gazette. All this bureaucracy, says City Hall, aims to protect the cemetery space. However, such guidelines are only brought into play when the work is done in cemeteries in the central regions of the city. These kinds of difficulties also affect the work of photojournalists.

So, it is not just about the inequality imposed by class cleavage, but also one regarding *which bodies are allowed to be photographed* and *in which contexts.* Although more deaths have occurred on the outskirts, and more bodies have been buried in cemeteries there, this is not the only reason that there are more photos there. The bodies of the dead who are buried in public cemeteries in districts where pay is higher are given a protection that is not extended to the bodies of the dead buried in public cemeteries in the outskirts. The latter are left visible for public scrutiny, both in life and in death.

Here we ask, along with Judith Butler, "who counts as human? Which lives count as lives? And, finally, what grants a life to be mournable?" (2004, 41). Financially, there is a clear physical and geographical separation in the city of São Paulo. In this sense, the separation between center and periphery is clear when we consider the maps in Figures 7.1 and 7.2. But there is also another kind of separation, shown by the maps in Figures 7.4 and 7.5. The violence of social cleavages shown in Figures 7.1 and 7.2, one of the causes of higher mortality in the outskirts of the cities, is replicated in Figures 7.4 and 7.5, but not exactly caused by social cleavages. In this sense, cemeteries inform us about the social organizations of the living, by showing that the basic values and principles of a "society" are in operation in all planes and activities of that same society. In this sense, the photographs published by newspapers can be considered as "interpretations that societies construct of themselves, impregnated with their values, categories and contradictions" (Hikiji 2012, 69). The distribution of the production of images of the deaths caused by the pandemic throughout the city of São Paulo thus gains a geopolitical meaning. If the distribution of deaths throughout the city goes through a geopolitics of vulnerability that speaks to income distribution, the distribution of the production of images of these deaths goes through a geopolitics of vulnerability of the bodies of the dead.

Thus, the images of death produced in São Paulo during the pandemic reflect the patterns of inequality and segregation present in the city. The images reproduced by the press create a particular representation of death that expresses the social inequalities found in the urban environment. There is a public dimension given to the photographs made in the outskirts, in clear contrast to the attitude of protecting the image of the dead in higher-income districts. We find ourselves again, then, in a problematic of visibility and invisibility: the bodies of the central regions are those that are presented in the newspapers while alive, but are protected in death; the bodies of the peripheral regions, hidden as alive, are those presented to public scrutiny as dead. "Certain lives will be highly protected," Butler says, "and the abrogation of their claims to sanctity will be sufficient to mobilize the forces of war. Other lives will not find such fast and furious support and will not even qualify as 'grievable'" (2004, 32).

The bodies presented in these press photographs are those that Butler classifies as "unreal" – those who suffered the violence of unrealization, and whose very lives were denied. While these bodies are signifiers without real value, dehumanized, objectified to the social gaze, they are also bodies that are visible in the attempts to construct memory and collective mourning created by Brazilian newspapers and media.

At this point, it is still difficult to say how these new findings impact the results obtained previously, when it has been said[11] that photos published in newspapers operate on dual levels. As mentioned above, in this research we argued that photos published in newspapers had results not only from their journalistic function, but also operated from a symbolic function – of a social creation of collective mourning. Funeral rites found new ways to be expressed socially, because they could not operate according to tradition – the human being is, after all, a ritual animal, and "If ritual is suppressed in one form it crops up in others, more strongly the more intense the social interaction" (Douglas 2001, 63). For now, I believe that this new interpretation does not change the results obtained previously, but somehow reinforces the polysemic character of the photographic image, showing that what the image makes us see is multifaceted.

The funeral rites that took place during the pandemic occurred in diverse situations, within the possibilities given by the moment, according to the sanitary measures foreseen for the protection of the collectivity. From the photographs published in the Brazilian press, the narratives created by the newspapers were of extreme publicization of these deaths, especially those that took place in the outskirts, which we are treating here as "unreal". Butler states that

> If there is a "discourse", it is a silent and melancholic one in which there have been no lives, and no losses; there has been no common bodily

> condition, no vulnerability that serves as the basis for an apprehension of our commonality; and there has been no sundering of that commonality.
>
> *(2004, 36)*

The public act of these pandemic deaths, however, is precisely what gives these bodies their marginal character. At a time when there can be no social funeral rite, the publicization of the rites is also transformed, and becomes itself the cause of the dehumanization of these bodies. These overly publicized deaths help in the construction of the depersonalization of the dead. It is precisely in this game of showing and not showing that the dehumanization of the bodies that are shown in the peripheries becomes visible, because the publicizing of these deaths does not have the function of presenting the violence to which these bodies are exposed. Since the rites of the pandemic occur in a veiled way – depersonalized by the very hiding of the dead – the showing of the rite becomes, itself, a source of dehumanization.

If the work of mourning, as Butler says, is about agreeing to undergo a transformation, then, socially, mourning must contain within itself the germ for a transformation of society – even more so when it comes to a situation like the pandemic in Brazil, which has generated so many deaths: "Mourning provides a sense of political community of a complex order, primarily by bringing to the fore relational bonds that have implications for theorizing fundamental dependency and ethical responsibility" (2004, 43). The construction of the rite being made out of dehumanized bodies, one has to wonder how mourning and the memory of the pandemic are actually being built.

Conclusion

Considering our previous topics, we must look at the numbers and remember, just like it was taught by George Didi-Huberman, that to consolidate grief as a social memory we must in fact face it, no matter how small an act looks like. These images are not only objects of study, but they are nevertheless images. The horror they express can often become a source of powerlessness. It is necessary, then, to change the way we look at them. To find a photograph's anthropological character is also to understand it as an image that is "inadequate but necessary, inexact but true" (Didi-Huberman 2008, 39) and, to build from it, what is possible within the context.

It is impossible to say that this type of research does not also have consequences on the researcher. Anthropologically speaking, the process of being affected by a fieldwork like this, where one is working with difficult questions, brings subjective complications that were not always expected at the beginning of the research. To work with a mass killing event as it unfolds is to be immersed in the field, and to be affected by it even in everyday situations where one is not actively doing research. We are not speaking, here, of the inevitable involvement with the object of study, "which does not constitute a defect or imperfection" (Velho 1978, 123), but of experiencing the actual effects brought about by uninterrupted fieldwork on an extreme situation.

To make participation an instrument of knowledge, as Favret-Saada proposes, in the case of the work with the pandemic, becomes an exercise in knowing when to stop. In this sense, one constantly lives the *anthropological blues*. The concept, developed by Roberto da Matta, deals precisely with the unexpected:

> it would be possible, then, to start demarcating the basic area of the *anthropological blues* as that of the element that insinuates itself into ethnological practice, but which was not expected. Like a blue, whose melody gains strength by the repetition of its phrases so that it becomes more and more noticeable. In the same way that sadness and homesickness (also blues) insinuate themselves into the process of fieldwork, causing surprise to the ethnologist.
>
> *(da Matta 1978, 6)*

There is, then, the moment when one misses what was there before the field – and also the awareness that that moment will never be reached again, because the change has also taken place in the anthropologist. "Accepting to be affected supposes, however, that one assumes the risk of seeing one's project of knowledge fall apart. For if the project of knowledge is omnipresent, nothing happens" (Siquera and Favret-Saada 2005, 160). As a member of the society being researched, it remains for the researcher to ask the question of his or her own experience, not only of how the research took place, but how they insert themselves into it – I, a resident of the central area of São Paulo, did not have to go to any cemeteries for personal reasons during the pandemic.

To conclude, the specificities brought about by the intersection between urban anthropology and visual anthropology help us to visualize how the bodies of the dead of the COVID-19 pandemic were caught in a game of visibility and invisibility that speaks of more than just the changes that the funeral rites went through during the pandemic. It was from this intersection that the reflection about how these bodies are treated by society, be it in life or death, unfolded. Starting with the photographs produced and published by Brazilian newspapers between September 2020 and March 2021, we then moved on to an analysis of where these photographs were taken. We began to consider, therefore, the urban space of the city of São Paulo, in Brazil.

We then discussed how these photographs show which bodies can be photographed, in what contexts, and what this publicization of images of the dead means at this historical moment. The way the rites of the pandemic were publicized shows that there are differences in how the bodies of people living in the central regions of the city and people living in the peripheries are seen. The paradox posed by the pandemic is that funeral rites were interdicted by the viral nature of COVID-19, which prevented, in many ways, the rites from being performed in the way society was accustomed to seeing them. In this way, it is precisely the newspapers' publicization of the bodies of the dead during the pandemic that gave them a marginal character, which appears not only in death, but also in life. These bodies are involved in a geopolitics of vulnerability, which affects the people living in the outskirts of São Paulo and allows the photographs of these cemeteries to be publicized in this way.

Notes

1 Geertz (1989).
2 Data from 12 September 2022. Due to the Federal Government's data blackout, this number has been obtained from the National Consortium of Media Sources, which since 8 June 2021 has been reporting figures obtained from state health departments. More information can be found at: https://especiais.g1.globo.com/bemestar/coronavirus/estados-brasil-mortes-casos-media-movel/ (in PT-BR)
3 Absolute number, as it is understood here, is the total number of deaths, not taking into account the number of deaths relative to the population size of each country.
4 Data from 12 September 2022. Source: State Data Analysis System (Seade), www.seade.gov.br/coronavirus/# (in PT-BR). Seade is a data analysis system run by the state of São Paulo government. As a public agency, Seade is connected to the state of São Paulo Secretary of Planning and Management.
5 Data from 18 May 2022. Source: Municipal Health Secretariat of São Paulo, www.prefeitura.sp.gov.br/cidade/secretarias/upload/saude/20220518_boletim_covid19_diario.pdf
6 Instituto de Pesquisa Econômica Avançada
7 Data from Covid-19 Brasil (accessed at https://ciis.fmrp.usp.br/covid19/). This initiative was put together by a team of independent scientists and volunteers from several Brazilian research institutions, with the intention of monitoring in real time the data provided by official sources in the country. One of their main goals was to create mathematical and simulation models to assist in the planning and execution of public policies.
8 On this, see Marino et al. (2021).
9 The link can be accessed at https://bityli.com/KSRWmTCH.
10 Sanfelicio (2022).
11 Sanfelicio (2022).

References

Ariès, Philippe. 2012. *História da morte no ocidente: da Idade Média aos nossos dias*, translated by Priscila Viana de Siqueira. Rio de Janeiro: Nova Fronteira.

Barthes, Roland. 1983. *A Barthes Reader*. New York: Hill and Wang.

Benjamin, Walter. 1968. *Illuminations*. New York: Schocken Books.

Butler, Judith. 2004. *Precarious Life: The Powers of Mourning and Violence*. New York: Verso Books.

Cancian, Natalia, and Renato Machado. 2020. "Brasil tem 141 novas mortes por coronavírus em 24h; total é de 941". *Folha de São Paulo*, 9 April. www1.folha.uol.com.br/equilibrioesaude/2020/04/brasil-tem-141-novas-mortes-por-coronavirus-em-24-h-total-e-de-941.shtmlCovid 19 Brasil. 2022. *Portal Covid-19 Brasil*. https://ciis.fmrp.usp.br/covid19/estado-br/.

Didi-Huberman, Georges. 2008. *Images in Spite of All: Four Photographs from Auschwitz*, translated by Shane B. Lillis. Chicago: University of Chicago Press.

Douglas, Mary. 2001. *Purity and Danger: An Analysis of the Concepts of Pollution and Taboo*. London: Routledge.
Geertz, Clifford. 1989. *A interpretação das culturas*, Rio de Janeiro: LTC Editora.
Hecksher, Marcos. 2021. "Mortalidade por Covid-19 e queda do emprego no Brasil e no mundo". *IPEA*. https://repositorio.ipea.gov.br/bitstream/11058/10877/2/NT_98_Disoc_Mortalidade_por_Covid19.pdf.
Hikiji, Rose Satiko Gitirana. 2012. *Imagem-Violência*, São Paulo: Terceiro Nome.
Marino, Aluízio, Gisele Brito, Pedro Mendonça, and Raquel Rolnik. 2021. "Prioridade na vacinação neglicencia a geografia da Covid-19 em São Paulo". *labcidade*, 26 May. www.labcidade.fau.usp.br/prioridade-na-vacinacao-negligencia-a-geografia-da-covid-19-em-sao-paulo/.
Matta, Roberto. 1978. "O ofício do etnólogo, ou como ter anthropological blues". *Boletim do Museu Nacional*, 27, May: 1–12.
Mauss, Marcel. 1979. "A expressão obrigatória dos sentimentos". In *Marcel Mauss: Antropologia*, edited by Roberto Cardoso de Oliveira, 147–153. São Paulo: Ática.
Py, Ligia and Monteiro, Elisa. 2020. "O direito ao luto no contexto da Covid-19". *Folha de São Paulo*, 31 October. www1.folha.uol.com.br/folha-100-anos/2020/10/o-direito-ao-luto-no-contexto-da-covid-19.shtml.
Rede Nossa São Paulo. 2021. "Mapa da desigualdade". www.nossasaopaulo.org.br/wp-content/uploads/2021/10/Mapa-Da-Desigualdade-2021_Mapas.pdf.
Reis, Thiago, and Vitor Sorano. 2022. "Mortes e casos conhecidos de coronavírus no Brasil e nos estados". *G1*, 12 September. https://especiais.g1.globo.com/bemestar/coronavirus/estados-brasil-mortes-casos-media-movel/.
Sanfelicio, Marianna Knothe. 2022. "Photographing the impossible: rites and images of death produced during the Covid-19 pandemic in Brazil". *Ponto Urbe* 30. https://doi.org/10.4000/pontourbe.11882.
Senado Federal. Comissão Parlamentar de Inquérito da Pandemia. 2021. "Relatório final". https://legis.senado.leg.br/comissoes/mnas?codcol=2441&tp=4.
Siqueira, Paula, and Jeanne Favret-Saada. 2005. "'Ser afetado', de Jeanne Favret-Saada". *Cadernos de Campo* 13, 13: 155–161. https://doi.org/10.11606/issn.2316-9133.v13i13p155-161.
Sontag, Susan. 2005. *On Photography*. New York: Rosetta Books.
Velho, Gilberto. 1978. "Observando o Familiar". In *A Aventura Sociológica*, edited by Edson Nunes, 123–132. Rio de Janeiro: Zahar.
Vernant, Jean-Pierre. 2008. *Mito e pensamento entre os gregos: estudos de psicologia histórica*. Rio de Janeiro: Paz e Terra.

PART II

Pandemic and Youth

8

COVID-19-RELATED LIFE EVENTS AND LIFE SATISFACTION AMONG YOUNG PEOPLE IN FINLAND

Konsta Happonen, Alix Helfer, Lotta Haikkola and Jenni Lahtinen

Introduction

Youth is a stage in life with multiple, overlapping changes that impact life trajectories, such as moving from compulsory schooling to secondary education and graduate studies, transitioning from education to employment and moving from the childhood home to a home of one's own. All these changes are shaped by structural constraints, institutional regulation, individual decisions, and, at times, broad global crises, such as the COVID-19 pandemic. Transitions (Furlong and Cartmel 1997) make youth a particularly vulnerable period for facing broad crises compared to groups with more stable life situations. Thus, whereas the pandemic entailed a health threat and a crisis of isolation and loneliness for older people, for young people it was also a threat to their chances of completing transitions. The pandemic restrictions targeted many important aspects of youth, such as schooling, studying, employment in industries with high proportions of young workers, access to supportive services at school, social and health care, employment services, access to leisurely activities and the possibility of socializing with the peer group. Although some individuals viewed pandemic restrictions, such as school closures, positively (Moilanen et al. 2021), the extensive measures taken have led to concerns regarding a 'pandemic generation'. Consequently, after the peak of the pandemic, the well-being of young people should be monitored closely to detect any lingering or delayed effects of disturbed life transitions.

Studying life satisfaction is one way of understanding the effect of the pandemic on young people. Life satisfaction refers to the subjective dimension of well-being (Ben-Arieh et al. 2014; Vaarama et al. 2010; Haanpää et al. 2020). Current research on young people's life satisfaction and mental health more

DOI: 10.4324/9781003459682-10

broadly during the pandemic has mostly targeted the adult population or specific youth subgroups, such as university students (Rogowska et al. 2021; Sveinsdóttir et al. 2021; Kokkinos et al. 2022; Salmela-Aro et al. 2022). In this chapter, we focus on young people in general (aged 15–24 years). First, we examine changes in young people's life satisfaction during the pandemic compared to the period before the start of the pandemic. Then, we consider the association between pandemic-related life events and life satisfaction. Third, we examine which demographics were most exposed to COVID-19-related life events. This chapter is based on two extensive surveys that targeted the whole youth population in Finland, with questions on well-being, experiences, and the use of services during the pandemic. Our study provides an important contribution to the literature by examining Finland's youth population in total and integrating their personal experiences of lockdowns and pandemic-related life events with their subjective well-being.

Previous Research on the Determinants of Life Satisfaction and Well-being During the Pandemic

Life satisfaction typically decreases from childhood to adolescence to adulthood (Lim et al. 2017; Casas and González-Carrasco 2019; Daly 2022). Despite the dynamic nature of life satisfaction, it has been shown to be connected to experiences of meaning (Vaarama et al. 2010), supportive relationships with family and peers (Proctor and Linley 2014), health and living standards (Vaarama et al. 2010) and socioeconomic situations, such as labor market status and the income level of one's family (Bannink et al. 2016).

In general, compared to older age groups (30–60 years), young people's (15–30 years) life satisfaction declined during the pandemic. However, there are substantial cross-country differences (Henseke et al. 2022). In Finland, young people's life satisfaction decreased during the first pandemic year (Lahtinen et al. 2022). A Norwegian study found that particularly boys' life satisfaction decreased (Von Soest et al. 2020), while no decrease was observed in a Korean study (Choi et al. 2021). Life satisfaction decreased also among university students (Rogowska et al. 2021). Finnish young people experienced more stress and were more concerned about the impact of the pandemic on their mental health, studies, career, and economic situation compared to older groups (Ranta et al. 2020; Prime Minister's Office and Statistics Finland 2022). Those who used social, health, or substance use services were found to be, on average, more stressed and dissatisfied with their lives (Pitkänen et al. 2022).

Female gender has been shown to be both associated (Gonzalez-Bernal et al. 2021) and not associated with lower life satisfaction (Karataş et al. 2021). Moreover, the pandemic increased psychological symptoms, particularly among university students and school-aged girls in Finland (Helakorpi and Kivimäki 2021; Kestilä et al. 2021).

Regarding individual life events during the pandemic, more days spent in confinement and being isolated were associated with lower personal satisfaction (Gonzalez-Bernal et al. 2021). Leisure time activities, such as hobbies, consumption of experiences, and socializing with friends are positively related to life satisfaction (Schmiedeberg & Schröder 2017; Choung et al. 2021), but we found no research specifically examining the experience of interruption of leisure activities. School closures during lockdowns were associated with adverse mental health effects (Viner et al. 2022), as well as improved sleep and health-related quality of life (Albrecht et al. 2022). The perceived negative financial impact of the pandemic was connected to lower life satisfaction among Greek university students (Kokkinos et al. 2022) and to mental health distress in an adolescent cohort in the UK (Knowles et al. 2022).

At the same time, survey research on the relationship between happiness and catastrophic events, such as war, suggests that often it is the specific experiences related to exceptional times rather than the exceptional times themselves that affect the well-being of respondents (Shemyakina and Plagnol 2013; Coupe and Obrizan 2016).

One open question is whether the pandemic has increased or decreased polarization in terms of young people's life satisfaction. On the one hand, it has been argued that the widespread diseases of the past have disproportionately diminished the capital of the rich (Scheidel 2017). Furthermore, the effects of the pandemic restrictions on leisure time activities and possibilities for consumption might have been more severely felt among the more well-off groups with (generally) more money to use on leisure and consumption. On the other hand, economic shocks tend to most strongly negatively affect the groups in the most precarious economic situations, including women (Sabarwal et al. 2013), people with migrant backgrounds (Couch and Fairlie 2010) and 'older' young people (aged 18+) who may not be directly supported by their families any longer and are just entering the labor market (Karonen and Niemelä 2020). This pattern was repeated during the pandemic (Gallacher and Hossain 2020). There are indications that the pandemic has also exacerbated existing barriers to health-care access (Pujolar et al. 2022).

The COVID-19 pandemic in Finland

The Finnish Government declared a state of emergency on 16 March 2020 and adopted the Emergency Powers Act (Government Communications Department 2020), which lasted for three months. During this time, borders were closed, stay-at-home policies were introduced, and people were advised to avoid public spaces and other gatherings.

The second wave hit Finland in autumn 2020 and reached its peak in December (Kotkas et al. 2022). The restrictions continued, for example, in the capital region until the end of January 2021. The third COVID-19 wave (March 2021) brought tightened restrictive measures, as schools in regions with higher epidemic rates switched to distance education (February–April 2021). Restrictions were gradually eased in spring 2021, according to regional epidemic status. The fourth wave peaked in August 2021, and the fifth wave in late 2021. COVID-19 vaccinations for over-16-year-olds started in August 2021. In early spring 2022, the restrictions were gradually lifted, after almost two years of exceptional circumstances (Helfer et al. 2023).

The state of emergency and school closures restricted access to face-to-face education first during the spring semester of 2020, for all pupils and students except for those aged 7–10 years, with special support needs or with parents working in critical sectors (Mesiäislehto et al. 2022). Distance learning was widely used in secondary and tertiary education throughout the pandemic years of 2020–2021. At the same time, the Finnish education field was, in some ways, ready for the digital leap, because resources had already been allocated to the digitalization of schools since the 1980s (Lavonen and Salmela-Aro 2022).

Many services for children, youth, and families were available only in reduced capacity (Lammi-Taskula et al. 2020). Leisure time, organized hobbies, and municipal youth work activities were heavily restricted through 2020 and 2021 (Helfer et al. 2023). However, Finland did not enforce curfews, and citizens were allowed to move freely outside (Saunes et al. 2022).

The pandemic impacted young people's education and employment, often in a gender-specific manner. For example, the pandemic lockdowns affected particularly the hospitality and cultural sectors, which have high proportions of young workers and women, contributing to the economic consequences of the pandemic for young people. The highest monthly youth unemployment rate was almost as high as during the global financial crisis of 2009 (39.3 percent), which shows that, like the financial crises, the pandemic exacerbated the precarious situation of many young people on the labor market. At the same time, both the NEET rate (a statistical category – "Not in Education, Employment or Training") and educational attendance increased between 2019 and 2020, the latter due to the increased enrolment in school, particularly by young women (Statistics Finland 2023a 2023b, 2023d).

In 2021, the government of Finland extended compulsory education to all people under 18 years of age (see, for example, Varjo et al. 2022). This reform effectively forced almost all under-18-year-olds to enter secondary education starting in autumn 2021. The result was that, at the end of 2022, the proportion of young people with NEET status was at its lowest level since at least 2009 (Statistics Finland 2023b). All else being equal, one would expect changes in life satisfaction to be negatively correlated with changes in NEET rates (Henseke et al. 2022).

Research Questions and Hypotheses

Based on the literature review, we posed the following three main research questions along with associated hypotheses:

Question 1: How did the life satisfaction of young people change after the beginning of the COVID-19 pandemic in Finland? We hypothesize the following:

- Life satisfaction will have decreased compared to the situation immediately before the pandemic.

Question 2: If the level of well-being has changed, is this explainable by demographic variables, COVID-19-related life events, or the general effect of the pandemic? We hypothesize that:

- Young women will have experienced the pandemic more negatively than young men.
- COVID-19-related life events and pandemic experiences will have decreased subjective well-being. We expect events that negatively affected the livelihoods of respondents to have had particularly strong effects on life satisfaction.
- The pandemic will not have had an identifiable effect on young people's life satisfaction after the specific COVID-19-related life events have been adjusted for.

Question 3: Which demographics were likeliest to experience COVID-19-related life events connected to lower life satisfaction? We hypothesize that COVID-19-related life events occurred according to the following two principles:

- First, events that have affected the respondents' material well-being, such as loss of livelihood and limited access to health care, will have been experienced more by groups that already have, on average, a more precarious status in society.
- Second, we assume that an experience of distance schooling will have affected young people in secondary and tertiary education the most, because these schools were most affected by pandemic closures.

Materials and methods

Data

Youth Barometer 2020 and the COVID Survey

We used the Youth Barometer 2020 (hereafter YB; Berg and Myllyniemi 2021) as reference data. The YB is a Finnish annual thematic telephone survey on the values and attitudes of young people aged 15–29 years and contains a question about life satisfaction. The data collection for the 2020 survey began in January, right before the start of the pandemic, which means that the YB provides good baseline data.

Data for the YB were gathered by randomly sampling people from the Finnish Population Information System and interviewing them until representative quotas for first languages (Finnish, Swedish, and Other), age groups (15–19, 20–24, and 25–29 years) and registered sex (Male and Female) were met. Out of the people with phone number information available, 7 percent were not interviewed because the relevant quotas had already been filled, 33 percent could not be reached, 52 percent refused to participate in the survey, and 8 percent were successfully interviewed. The total number of completed interviews was 1,921.

The second dataset was a study of young people's (aged 12–24 years) experiences during the COVID-19 pandemic (hereafter the COVID survey, or CS). The survey contained a question about life satisfaction and charted young people's experiences during the pandemic, service use, and opinions on restrictive measures. The data collection consisted of five rounds of telephone surveys. We used the full dataset in the analysis of temporal trends in life satisfaction. Rounds 2 and 3 (June 2021 and November 2021) had the most similar questionnaires, with the most comprehensive sets of questions about COVID-19-related life events. We used these two rounds in our analysis of the causes of pandemic-related changes in life satisfaction.

For CS, a random sample of the target population was extracted from the Finnish Population Information System for each survey round. The CS used quotas similar to those used in the YB, with the exception that the age groups in CS were 12–14, 15–19, and 20–24 years. Out of these samples, 5.2–6.4 percent had phone number information available, answered the phone, were willing to participate in the survey, and could be reached before the relevant quotas were met. The number of successfully completed interviews in each round thus varied between 1,001 and 1,020. The interviews for both YB and CS were conducted in Finnish or Swedish, which are Finland's national languages.

To make the datasets compatible, YB respondents older than 24 years and CS respondents younger than 15 years were removed. For further analyses, we created two datasets. For the analysis of temporal trends in life satisfaction, we retained all CS rounds but removed respondents who did not answer the question about life satisfaction. Thus, 1.25 percent, 0.65 percent, 0.25 percent, 0.25 percent, 0 percent, and 0 percent of the respondents from YB and CS rounds 1–5 were removed, respectively. Consequently, the total number of respondents in the temporal analysis dataset was 5,040 (1,217 + 712 + 778 + 791 + 768 + 774). The other dataset was built for the regression analysis of causes in pandemic-related changes in life satisfaction and included YB and CS rounds 2 and 3. From this dataset, we removed the respondents who did not answer the questions about life satisfaction, gender, primary occupation, and mother tongue, as well as those with a non-binary gender identification. This meant that 1.3%, 0.6%, and 1.2% of the respondents of the YB and CS round 2 and CS round 3 were removed, respectively. The total number of respondents in the regression modeling dataset was 2,766 (1,211 + 774 + 781). It should be noted that, for the analysis of the prevalence of COVID-19-related life events described below, we used the regression modeling dataset but without the YB. Furthermore, when combining the datasets, we assumed that all answers to questions about COVID-19-related life events in YB were "No", because the pandemic had not yet reached Finland.

Analyzed Variables

The response variable in our analysis was life satisfaction, derived from the question, "How satisfied are you currently with your life altogether, on a scale of 4–10?" Finnish schools grade students on a scale of 4–10, which is why many surveys in Finland have also adopted this scale. We treated the response (integers from 4 to 10) as an ordinal response variable.

The binary variables (yes/no) describing COVID-19-related life events that were used as covariates of life satisfaction, along with their prevalence in the different CS rounds, are listed in Table 8.1. The events describe how the respondents were exposed to the disease and its consequences, including the societal response to the pandemic. These events can be broadly classified as applying to the disease itself, movement, leisure, health-care services, and personal finances.

TABLE 8.1 Prevalence of COVID-19-related life events across the COVID survey rounds

		Survey round				
		2020	2021		2022	
Related to	Event	October	June	November	May	December
		1	2	3	4	5
The disease	The respondent or a person close to them catching COVID-19	-	0.26	0.35	0.82	-
Movement restrictions	Experiencing quarantine	-	0.50	0.54	-	-
	Experiencing a period of distance schooling	-	0.68	0.42	-	-
	Experiencing a period of distance work	-	0.17	0.10	-	-
Leisure time	Interruption of hobbies	-	0.59	0.51	-	-
Access to services	Refraining from seeking medical or dental care	-	0.21	0.20	0.17	-
	Cancellation or postponement of medical services	-	0.28	0.24	0.29	-
Personal finances	Job loss, temporary layoff, or reduction in working hours	-	0.23	0.19	-	0.20
	Worsening of personal financial situation	-	0.26	0.35	0.82	-

We used a binary definition of gender (men/women). The YB and CS employed a self-reported non-binary definition, but the respondents with a non-binary identification were removed, as documented above. Questions about main occupation and place of study were combined into the variable "primary occupation" (primary school, upper secondary school, vocational school, university of applied sciences, university, employed/salaried worker, entrepreneur, unemployed, and other). The other group included, for example, people on parental leave and in military and non-military service. In addition, our analysis included age and self-reported first language. First languages besides Finnish and Swedish were used as a proxy for migrant background, although this group includes speakers of national minority languages (for example, the Sámi languages, approximately 0.05 percent of the population; Statistics Finland 2023e) and many people with migrant background have Finnish or Swedish as their first language.

Analyses

Changes in Young People's Life Satisfaction

To demonstrate that the self-perceived well-being of young people in Finland decreased during the pandemic, we provide the distribution of the answers to the question, "How satisfied are you currently with your life altogether?", which was asked in the YB and all rounds of the CS.

Life Satisfaction Model

We modeled answers to the question about life satisfaction to (1) test whether the decrease in respondents' life satisfaction could be due to random sampling variance, and (2) analyze the connections between COVID-19-related life events and changes in life satisfaction.

We treated the response (integers from 4 to 10) as an ordinal response variable and modeled it using a cumulative likelihood model with a logistic link (Bürkner and Vuorre 2019). To analyze whether the decrease in life satisfaction could be due to sampling variance, we built a model with just one categorical predictor variable: the sampling round (YB, CS round 2, and CS round 3). We set the YB as the reference level. The ordinal response model can be understood as quantifying the distribution of latent life satisfaction values that give rise to the observed values. We quantified the posterior probability of whether the average value of this latent life satisfaction had decreased after the beginning of the COVID-19 pandemic in Finland. This model was also fit for all the CS rounds.

We began the analysis of the connections between COVID-19-related life events and life satisfaction by testing for the optimal way to adjust the results for age, gender and data collection time. Many model configurations were compared using approximate leave-one-out cross validation (Vehtari et al. 2017). A model with data collection time and a logit-linear interaction of age and gender had the highest approximate out-of-sample predictive performance; therefore, we chose it as the basis for the next phase of model building.

We then added all the COVID-19-related life events to the model as binary predictors, where the reference level for each predictor was the answer "No". The credible intervals for many of these effects were wide and intercepted zero. We first removed from the model some of the life events with the most uncertain effects on life satisfaction. These life events were experiencing quarantine, catching COVID-19 (self or a close person), and experiencing a period of distance work. We further removed COVID-19-related job losses, layoffs, and reductions in working hours, because employment-related life events were highly correlated with the worsening of one's financial situation. Thus, the effects of employment-related life events on life satisfaction were indistinguishable from zero after accounting for the worsening of the respondents' economic situations. After dropping these variables, the credible interval of the effect of experiencing a period of distance education on life satisfaction still included zero; therefore, this variable was also dropped from the model.

Last, we investigated whether the answers to the two questions on different forms of the reduced use of health-care services could be combined without much loss of information. We thus replaced the two health-care-related life event predictors in the model with the combined variable "hindered access to health care". The new variable assumed a value of "yes" if the response to either of the constituent variables was also "yes". Combining the variables did not decrease the approximate leave-one-out predictive performance of the model. The final model of life satisfaction thus consisted of the above-listed adjustments for respondent age, data collection time, and gender. The model also considered the following effects of COVID-19: interrupted hobbies, worsened financial situation, and hindered access to health care.

Models of the Prevalence of COVID-19-Related Life Events

After identifying the COVID-19-related life events that were most clearly related to life satisfaction, we built logistic regression models to analyze how different demographic variables affected the probability of reporting such events.

In all models, the likelihood contribution of each observation was weighted using survey weights for the sample based on the intersection of age and gender. The weights were calculated by comparing the share of respondents in the age-by-gender groups to their shares in the target population. Information on the target population at the end of 2019 (Statistics Finland 2023c) was retrieved using the PxWeb R package (Magnusson et al. 2022). The survey weights ranged between 0.63 and 2.03.

For all life events, we began the model selection process with the following predictor variables included in the model as simple linear effects: gender, age, language, and data collection time. We then compared this model to another in which the effect of age was modeled using a thin plate spline with basis dimension 5. After this, we built a third group of models in which we added self-reported primary occupation as a predictor. The expected log pointwise predictive density consistently indicated that the last group of models had the highest predictive performance. Therefore, we chose these models for further analysis.

Model Information and Diagnostics

The models were built in the R environment for statistical analysis (version 4.1.2; R Core Team 2021) using the brms package for applied Bayesian regression modeling (version 2.18.0; Bürkner 2017), which is a user-friendly interface to the Stan language for probabilistic programming (Stan Development Team 2023). The models were fit using the CmdStanr backend (Gabry and Češnovar 2023). Intercepts and β-parameters were given a normal prior distribution with a mean of 0 and standard deviation of 1. The standard deviation parameters associated with the splines were given an exponential distribution with a λ parameter value of 1.

All models were run with 16 chains. Each chain was first run for 1,000 iterations to optimize the parameters of the MCMC sampler. These "warmup" iterations were not used for inference. Then, each chain was run for 125 iterations, for a total of 2,000 samples of the posterior distribution of each parameter. The algorithm did not obviously fail to explore the parameter space, as indicated by the lack of divergent transitions and the fact that R-hat convergence diagnostics had values under 1.1 (Vehtari et al. 2021).

Results

Changes in Young People's life Satisfaction

The subjective well-being of young people had decreased since the onset of COVID-19 in Finland in late January 2020, as evidenced by the grades that the respondents gave to their life satisfaction (Figure 8.1). The life satisfaction instrument from the first CS survey round in October 2020 was not directly comparable with the other surveys because the respondents were asked about life satisfaction during the last six months, instead of "currently". Nonetheless, the response distributions showed a marked shift from higher to lower grades. Furthermore, in December 2022 (CS round 5), average life satisfaction was still lower than before the pandemic, with > 99 percent posterior probability.

Effects of COVID-19-Related Life events on Life Satisfaction

The statistical connections between demographic variables, COVID-19-related life events, and life satisfaction in the YB and CS rounds 2–3 are shown in Figure 8.2. On average, young men gave their life satisfaction a higher grade

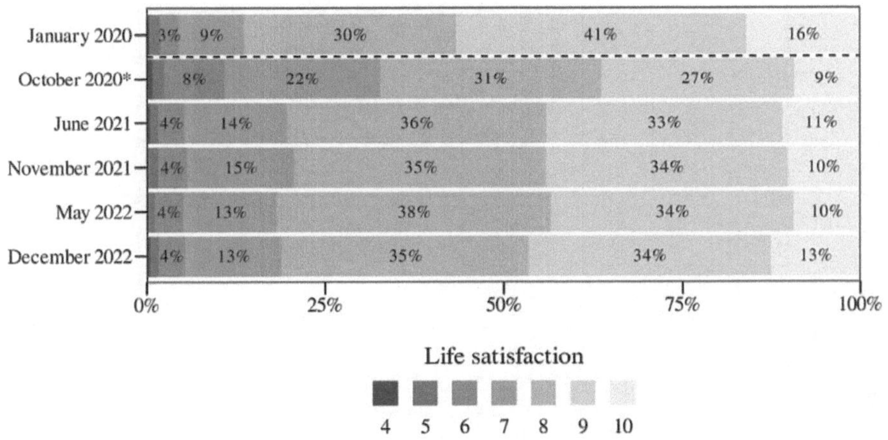

FIGURE 8.1 Life satisfaction among Finnish people aged 15–24 years, 2020–2022. Satisfaction was measured on a scale of 4 (worst) to 10 (best). The percentage points within the bars represent the proportion of the respondents who gave the answer after unsure responses were excluded; these are shown for life satisfaction grades 6–10. The horizontal dashed line marks the beginning of the COVID-19 pandemic in Finland.
* In October 2020, the respondents were asked about life satisfaction "during the last six months" instead of "currently".

than did young women (Figure 8.2a). After accounting for COVID-19-related life events, there were no longer strong and certain differences (i.e., 95 percent credible intervals did not intercept zero) in life satisfaction between 2020 and 2021 for most of the studied demographic groups, except for the oldest (i.e., approximately 24 years old) young women in June 2021 (Figure 8.2b). This means that most of the decrease in life satisfaction after the beginning of the pandemic can be attributed to COVID-19-related life events or the factors related to them. We identified three events that were connected to subjective life satisfaction – in order of absolute effect size, from smallest to largest, interrupted hobbies, hindered access to health care, and worsened personal economic situation (Figure 8.2c).

These life events were not reported evenly among the demographic groups we studied or across time. Women and people who did not have Finnish or Swedish as their first language reported more life events that had a negative effect on their life satisfaction (Figure 8.3a). Older age groups tended to report more life events, but this effect was quite uncertain for hindered access to health care and interrupted hobbies after accounting for primary occupation (Figure 8.3b). Among the occupational groups, young people in upper secondary education had high relative odds of reporting any of the studied events, whereas the situation was more variable in the other occupational groups (Figures 8.3a, c, and e).

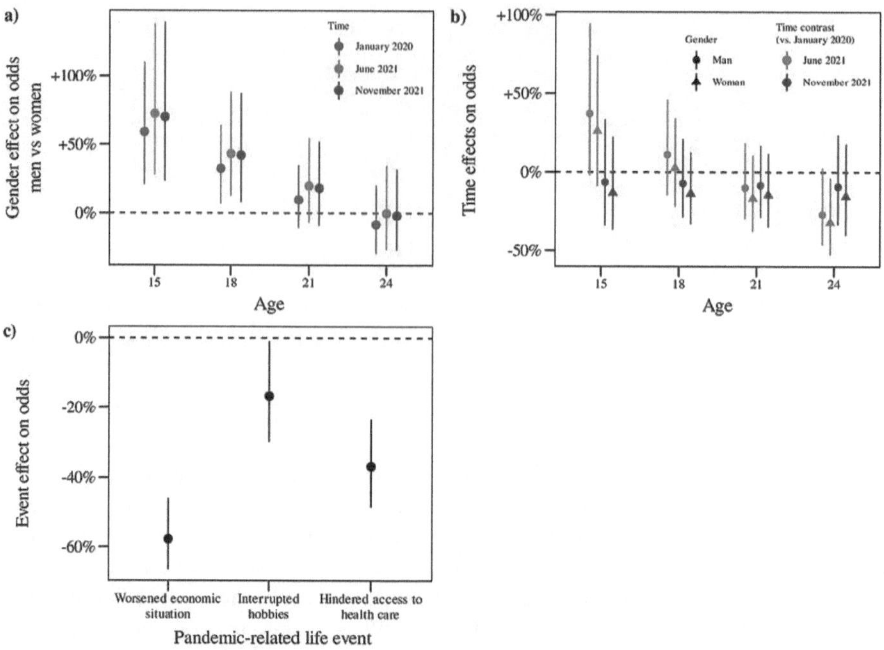

FIGURE 8.2 Effects of gender, time, age, and pandemic-related life events on life satisfaction according to the best-fit model. All effects are displayed as relative changes in the cumulative odds of "positive" versus "negative" answers – that is, the odds of answering 10 (vs. 4–9), the odds of answering 9–10 (vs. 4–8), and so on. Due to the structure of the model, all such odds change similarly. Positive changes indicate a higher probability of giving a high grade to one's life satisfaction and vice versa. Due to statistical interactions, the effects of time, gender, and age need to be displayed simultaneously; for clarity, they are predicted for only four ages. (Figure 8.3a) The effect of being a man versus a woman; (Figure 8.3b) The effect of data collection time. (Note that this subplot does not include the effects of life events, which are displayed in the next subplot.); (Figure 8.3c) The effects of COVID-19-related life events. The points are posterior medians, and the lines show 95 percent credible intervals. The dashed line indicates the point at which the contrast would have a value of zero – that is, where there would be no difference between the studied group and the reference group.

Discussion

In this study, we investigated the development of subjective life satisfaction of young people in Finland before and during the COVID-19 pandemic, along with possible explanations. We found that life satisfaction decreased after the beginning of the pandemic, as shown in other studies. Furthermore, we found that life satisfaction had not returned to pre-pandemic levels by the end of 2022.

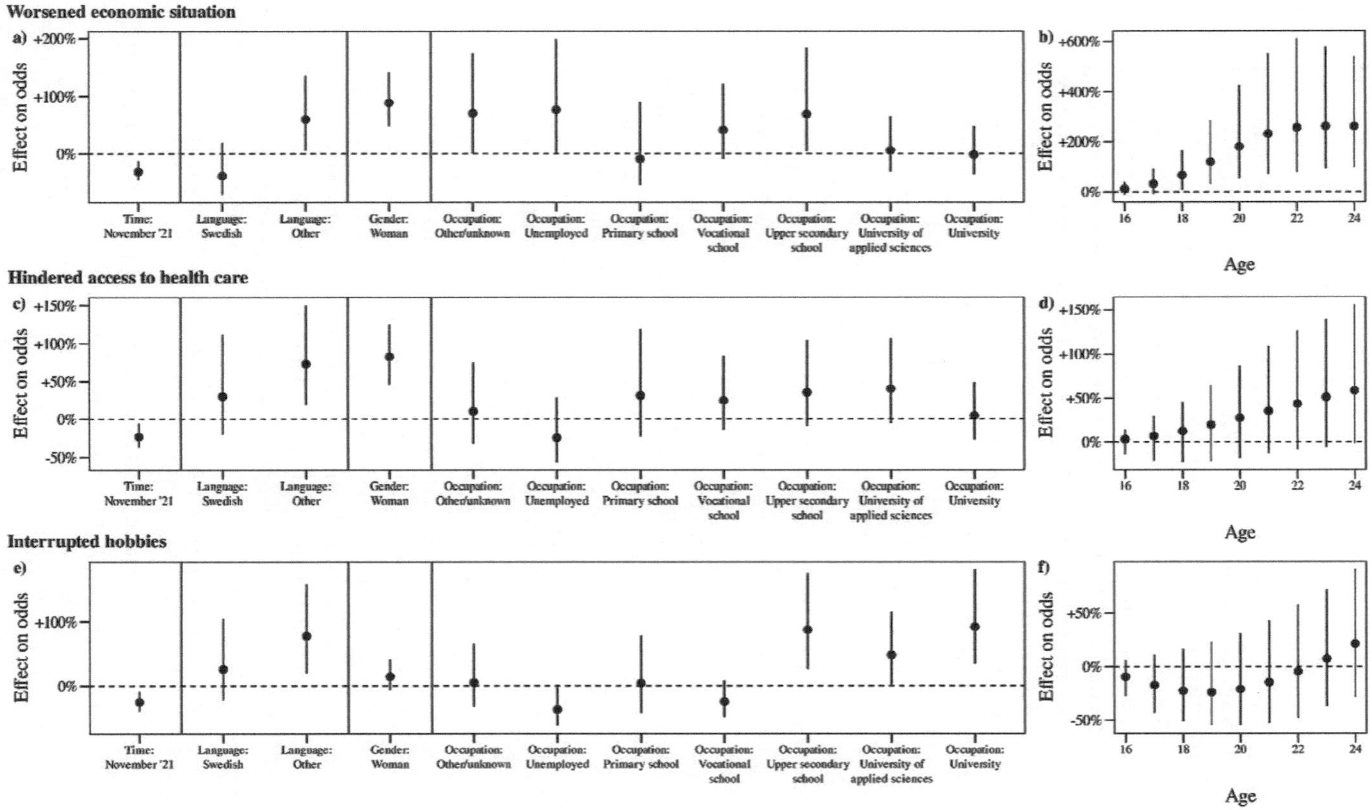

FIGURE 8.3 Effects of categorical predictors (Figures a, c, and e) and age (Figures b, d, and f) on the odds of experiencing COVID-19-related worsened economic situation, hindered access to health care, or interrupted hobbies during the pandemic year 2021. The effects are shown as back-transformed contrasts on a relative odds scale. The reference values for the contrasts in different variable groups are the following: time – June 2021, language – Finnish, gender – male, primary occupation – employed or entrepreneur, and age – 15 years. The points are posterior medians, and the lines show 95% credible intervals. The dashed line represents the odds of the reference group against which all other groups are compared.

This was despite all restrictions having been lifted, which indicates that the effects of the pandemic have been long-lasting. However, the period coincided with the start of the war in Ukraine, which may have had an additional impact on young people's life satisfaction.

Our analysis showed that young women reported lower life satisfaction on average. However, after accounting for COVID-19-related life events we did not identify a direct effect of gender on changes in life satisfaction.

In considering explanations for this decrease in life satisfaction, we found that it was not related to the time of the pandemic itself or to gender, but rather to pandemic-related experiences and life events. Our results suggest that young people who did not experience specific pandemic-related events were, on average, as satisfied with their lives during the pandemic year 2021 as they were before the pandemic. Similar findings about the significance of experiences related to broad societal crises instead of the crises themselves have been discovered in previous research (Shemyakina and Plagnol 2013; Coupe and Obrizan 2016).

The life events linked to lower life satisfaction were interrupted hobbies, hindered access to health care, and worsened economic situation. Our results thus contribute to the evidence that one's financial situation is linked to life satisfaction, both in general (Bannink et al. 2016) and during the pandemic (Kokkinos et al. 2022; Lahtinen et al. 2022). It is noteworthy that experiences of distance schooling or distance work were not related to changes in life satisfaction, but interrupted hobbies were. Distance schooling may have long-term effects on learning, but for young people's well-being the consequences seem to be more varied (Albrecht et al. 2022; Viner et al. 2022). Although Finland did not impose curfews, and young people could still use public and semi-public spaces to hang out and socialize with friends (Laine et al. 2023), this did not compensate for the decrease in life satisfaction caused by interrupted hobbies. Based on these results, it follows that organized free-time activities are an important facet of good life among youth – even, or perhaps especially, in times of societal disruption. This should be considered when planning future large-scale public-health interventions, such as pandemic restrictions.

The above-mentioned life-satisfaction-decreasing events did not affect all young people equally. To make broad generalizations, such events were most frequently reported by women, people whose first language was not Finnish or Swedish, students in upper secondary schools, and the oldest respondents of the study (approximately 24-year-olds). These results suggest that the pandemic effects on the subjective well-being of young people depend on the intersection of gender, ethnicity, and labor market status.

Previous research on the association between gender and life satisfaction during the pandemic had varying results (Gonzalez-Bernal et al. 2021; Karataş et al.2021), but young women have been shown to report more adverse mental health effects (Helakorpi and Kivimäki 2021; Rogowska et al. 2021). In our research, we found that young women were more likely to report that their economic situation worsened. Young women also reported that they had experienced hindered access to health care. In addition, although gender did not have a direct effect on the probability of experiencing interrupted hobbies, attending upper secondary school or tertiary education did. The majority of students in these schools are women (Statistics Finland 2023a). These are some of the reasons why female respondents felt more dissatisfied with their lives. Thus, our study demonstrates that women experienced the pandemic more negatively than men, but this is not due to any difference between the genders' ability to tolerate stress; rather, the restrictions related to the pandemic were likelier to affect women.

Youth whose first language was not one of the national languages of Finnish or Swedish (i.e., who are likely to have a migrant background) were likelier to report all of the life events that were negatively associated with life satisfaction. Although there is great heterogeneity in this group, and the reasons for the clustering of pandemic experiences cannot be conclusively affirmed here, these results resonate with previous research highlighting racism in the Finnish labor market (Ahmad 2022) and barriers to service use among immigrants (Çilenti et al. 2021). Thus, in these areas of society, the pandemic seems to have deepened existing inequalities related to language and migrant backgrounds. It should be noted, however, that respondents to the YB and CS with migrant backgrounds were a selected group, as everyone was able to respond to the survey in one of the two national languages. Thus, it is likely that these COVID-19-related life events were clustered even more clearly towards young people with migrant backgrounds than our analysis indicates. The reasons behind this clustering of pandemic-related negative life events are an important topic for further research.

Conclusions

The study investigated life satisfaction as an indicator of subjective well-being and found that the pandemic did not affect all young people uniformly. Instead, it deepened existing divisions. In the management of broad societal crises, it is key to pay close attention to the intersection of gender, migrant background, and labor market status. Future studies should continue to investigate the inequalities in well-being during and after the pandemic as well as carefully examine the unequal distribution of pandemic-related experiences among young people globally.

Author contributions

Conceptualization: JL, LH, KH, AH; data curation, formal analysis, methodology, validation, visualization: KH; supervision: LH; writing (original draft): KH, AH, LH; writing (review and editing): KH, AH, LH, JL.

Funding

Ministry of Education and Culture, Youth Unit; Academy of Finland, Project Grant 332674.

Acknowledgements

We thank Tuuli Pitkänen, Riku Laine, and Eila Kauppinen, who worked on a previous Finnish-language investigation of the same data. We also thank Sinikka Aapola-Kari for project administration.

References

Ahmad, Akhlaq. 2022. "Does additional work experience moderate ethnic discrimination in the labour market?" *Economic and Industrial Democracy* 43, 3: 1119–1142. https://doi.org/10.1177/0143831X20969828.

Albrecht, Joëlle N., Helene Werner, Noa Rieger, Natacha Widmer, Daniel Janisch, Reto Huber, and Oskar G. Jenni. 2022. "Association between homeschooling and adolescent sleep duration and health during COVID-19 pandemic high school closures". *JAMA Network Open* 5, 1: e2142100. https://doi.org/10.1001/jamanetworkopen.2021.42100.

Bannink, Rienke, Anna Pearce, and Steven Hope. 2016. "Family income and young adolescents' perceived social position: associations with self-esteem and life satisfaction in the UK Millennium Cohort Study". *Archives of Disease in Childhood* 101, 10: 917–921. https://doi.org/10.1136/archdischild-2015-309651.

Ben-Arieh, Asher, Ferran Casas, Ivar Frones, and Jill Korbin. 2014. "Multifaceted concept of child well-being". In *Handbook of Child Well-Being: Theories, Methods and Policies in Global Perspective*, edited by Asher Ben-Arieh, Ferran Casas, Ivar Frønes, Jill E. Korbin, 1–27. Cham: Springer. https://doi.org/10.1007/978-90-481-9063-8_134.

Berg, Päivi, and Sami Myllyniemi, eds. 2021. *Palvelu pelaa! Nuorisobarometri 2020* [Youth Barometer 2020]. Helsinki: State Youth Council and Finnish Youth Research Society.

Bürkner, Paul-Christian. 2017. "Brms: an R package for Bayesian multilevel models using Stan". *Journal of Statistical Software* 80: 1–28. https://doi.org/10.18637/jss.v080.i01.

Bürkner, Paul-Christian, and Matti Vuorre. 2019. "Ordinal regression models in psychology: a tutorial". *Advances in Methods and Practices in Psychological Science* 2: 77–101. https://doi.org/10.1177/2515245918823199.

Casas, Ferran, and Mònica González-Carrasco. 2019. "Subjective well-being decreasing with age: new research on children over 8". *Child Development* 90: 375–394. https://doi.org/10.1111/cdev.13133.

Choi, Jihye, Youjeong Park, Hye-Eun Kim, Jihyeok Song, Daeun Lee, Eunhye Lee, Hyeonjin Kang, *et al.*2021. "Daily life changes and life satisfaction among Korean school-aged children in the COVID-19 pandemic". *International Journal of Environmental Research and Public Health* 18: 3324. https://doi.org/10.3390/ijerph18063324.

Choung, Youngjoo, Tae-Young Pak, and Swarn Chatterjee. 2021. "Consumption and life satisfaction: the Korean evidence". *International Journal of Consumer Studies* 45: 1007–1019. https://doi.org/10.1111/ijcs.12620.

Çilenti, Katja, Shadia Rask, Marko Elovainio, Eero Lilja, Hannamaria Kuusio, Seppo Koskinen, Päivikki Koponen, and Anu E. Castaneda. 2021. "Use of health services and unmet need among adults of Russian, Somali, and Kurdish origin in Finland". *International Journal of Environmental Research and Public Health* 18: 2229. https://doi.org/10.3390/ijerph18052229.

Couch, Kenneth A., and Robert Fairlie. 2010. "Last hired, first fired? Black-white unemployment and the business cycle". *Demography* 47: 227–247. https://doi.org/10.1353/dem.0.0086.

Coupe, Tom, and Maksym Obrizan. 2016. "The impact of war on happiness: the case of Ukraine". *Journal of Economic Behavior & Organization* 132: 228–242. https://doi.org/10.1016/j.jebo.2016.09.017.

Daly, Michael. 2022. "Cross-national and longitudinal evidence for a rapid decline in life satisfaction in adolescence". *Journal of Adolescence* 94: 422–434. https://doi.org/10.1002/jad.12037.

Furlong, Andy, and Fred Cartmel. 1997. *Young People and Social Change*. Berkshire: Open University Press.

Gabry, Jonah, and Rok Češnovar. 2023. "*cmdstanr: R Interface to 'CmdStan'*". https://mc-stan.org/cmdstanr/.

Gallacher, Guillermo, and Iqbal Hossain. 2020. "Remote work and employment dynamics under COVID-19: evidence from Canada". *Canadian Public Policy: Analyse de Politiques* 46: 44–54. https://doi.org/10.3138/cpp.2020-026.

Gonzalez-Bernal, Jerónimo J., Paula Rodríguez-Fernández, Mirian Santamaría-Peláez, Josefa González-Santos, Benito León-Del-Barco, Luis A. Minguez, and Raúl Soto-Cámara. 2021. "Life satisfaction during forced social distancing and home confinement derived from the COVID-19 pandemic in Spain". *International Journal of Environmental Research and Public Health* 18: 1474. https://doi.org/10.3390/ijerph18041474.

Government Communications Department. 2020. "Government, in cooperation with the president of the republic, declares a state of emergency in Finland over coronavirus outbreak", March 16. https://vnk.fi/en/-/hallitus-totesi-suomen-olevan-poikkeusoloissa-koronavirustilanteen-vuoksi/.

Haanpää, Leena, Enna Toikka, and Piia Af Ursin. 2020. "Alakouluikäisten lasten moniulotteinen elämääntyytyväisyys Suomessa" [The multidimensional life satisfaction of primary school-aged children in Finland]. *Yhteiskuntapolitiikka* 85: 519–530.

Helakorpi, Satu, and Hanne Kivimäki. 2021. "*Lasten ja nuorten hyvinvointi – Kouluterveyskysely 2021*" [The well-being of children and youth according to the School Health Promotion Study]. Finnish Institute for Health and Welfare. https://urn.fi/URN:NBN:fi-fe2021091446139/.

Helfer, Alix, Sinikka Aapola-Kari, and Jakob Trane Ibsen, eds. 2023. *Children and Young People's Participation During the Corona Pandemic – Nordic Initiatives*. Helsinki: Finnish Youth Research Society.

Henseke, Golo, Ingrid Schoon, Christoph Schimmele, Rubab Arim, Hans Dietrich, Aisling Murray, Emer Smyth, and Véronique Dupéré. 2022. "Youth life satisfaction during the COVID-19 pandemic in a cross-national comparison". *Economic and Social Reports* 2. https://doi.org/10.25318/36280001202201100002-eng.

Karataş, Zeynep, Kıvanç Uzun, and Özlem Tagay. 2021. "Relationships between the life satisfaction, meaning in life, hope and COVID-19 fear for Turkish adults during the COVID-19 outbreak". *Frontiers in Psychology* 12. https://doi.org/10.3389/fpsyg.2021.633384.

Karonen, Esa, and Mikko Niemelä. 2020. "Life course perspective on economic shocks and income inequality through age-period-cohort analysis: evidence from Finland". *Review of Income and Wealth* 66: 287–310. https://doi.org/10.1111/roiw.12409.

Kestilä, Laura, Merita Jokela, Vuokko Härmä, and Pekka Rissanen, eds. 2021. "*COVID-19-Epidemian vaikutukset hyvinvointiin, palvelujärjestelmään ja kansantalouteen. Asiantuntija-arvio, kevät 2021*" [The effects of the COVID-19 epidemic on welfare, the service system, and national economy. Expert assessment spring 2021]. Helsinki: Finnish Institute for Health and Welfare. https://urn.fi/URN:ISBN:978-952-343-865-1/.

Knowles, Gemma, Charlotte Gayer-Anderson, Alice Turner, Lynsey Dorn, Joseph Lam, Samantha Davis, Rachel Blakey, *et al.*2022. "Covid-19, social restrictions, and mental distress among young people: a UK longitudinal, population-based study". *Journal of Child Psychology and Psychiatry, and Allied Disciplines* 63: 1392–1404. https://doi.org/10.1111/jcpp.13586.

Kokkinos, Constantinos M., Costas N. Tsouloupas, and Ioanna Voulgaridou. 2022. "The effects of perceived psychological, educational, and financial impact of COVID-19 pandemic on Greek university students' satisfaction with life through mental health". *Journal of Affective Disorders* 300: 289–295. https://doi.org/10.1016/j.jad.2021.12.114.

Kotkas, Toomas, Elisa Husu, Hanna Wass, and Anu Kantola. 2022. "Finland: legal response to COVID-19". In *The Oxford Compendium of National Legal Responses to Covid-19*, edited by Jeff King and Octávio L. M. Ferraz. https://doi.org/10.1093/law-occ19/e32.013.32.

Lahtinen, Jenni, Riku Laine, Lotta Haikkola, Eila Kauppinen, and Tuuli Pitkänen. 2022. "Nuorten tyytyväisyys elämään korona-ajan ensimmäisenä vuonna" [Youth life satisfaction during the first year of the pandemic]. In *Poikkeuksellinen nuoruus korona-aikaan. Nuorten elinolot -vuosikirja 2022*, edited by Marjatta Kekkonen, MikaGissler, PäiviKänkänen, and Anna-Maria Isola, 50–61. Helsinki: Finnish Youth Research Society, Finnish Institute of Health and Welfare, and State Youth Council. https://urn.fi/URN:ISBN:978-952-343-937-5/.

Laine, Sofia, Eila Kauppinen, Karla Malm, and Tommi Hoikkala, eds. 2023. *Nuoruus korona-ajan kaupungissa* [Youth in the city during the pandemic]. Helsinki: Finnish Youth Research Society.

Lammi-Taskula, Johanna, Maaret Vuorenmaa, Kaisa Aunola, and Matilda Sorkkila. 2020. "Matalan kynnyksen sosiaalipalvelut lapsiperheiden tukena ja palveluiden käyttö COVID-19-epidemian aikana" [Low threshold social services supporting families with children and the use of services during COVID-19]. Tutkimuksesta tiiviisti 15/2020. Finnish Institute for Health and Welfare. https://urn.fi/URN:ISBN:978-952-343-522-3.

Lavonen, Jari, and Katariina Salmela-Aro. 2022. "Experiences of moving quickly to distance teaching and learning at all levels of education in Finland". In *Primary and Secondary Education during Covid-19: Disruptions to Educational Opportunity during a Pandemic*, edited by Fernando M. Reimers, 105–123. Cham: Springer.

Lim, M., C. Cappa, and G. Patton. 2017. "Subjective well-being among young people in five Eastern European countries". *Global Mental Health* 4. https://doi.org/10.1017/gmh.2017.8.

Magnusson, Mans, Markus Kainu, Janne Huovari, and Leo Lahti. 2022. "Pxweb: R Tools for PXWEB API". http://github.com/ropengov/pxweb/.

Mesiäislehto, Merita, Anna Elomäki, Johanna Närvi, Miska Simanainen, Hanna Sutela, and Tapio Räsänen. 2022. "The gendered impacts of the COVID-19 crisis in Finland and the ffectiveness of the Poplicy responses". Finnish Institute for Health and Welfare. http://urn.fi/URN:ISBN:978-952-343-800-2/.

Moilanen, Johanna, Anna Rönkä, and Päivi Fadjukoff. 2021. "Asiantuntijat pohtivat korona-ajan kotia" [Expert reflections on the home during the pandemic]. *Yhteiskuntapolitiikka* 86: 641–646. https://urn.fi/URN:NBN:fi-fe2021112456758.

Pitkänen, Tuuli, Jouni Tourunen, Helena Huhta, Teemu Kaskela, Janne Takala, Alix Helfer, Susanna Jurvanen, Riku Laine, Meri Larivaara, and Leena Suurpää. 2022. "Nuorten mielenterveyden tukeminen sosiaalihuollossa ja matalan kynnyksen toiminnassa: Työntekijöiden ja nuorten näkemyksiä tarpeista ja toimintatavoista" [Supporting young people's mental health in social services and low threshold operations]. Prime Minister's Office. https://urn.fi/URN:ISBN:978-952-383-169-8/.

Prime Minister's Office and Statistics Finland. 2022. "Citizen's Pulse 11/2022". Finnish Social Science Archive. https://urn.fi/urn:nbn:fi:fsd:T-FSD3736.

Proctor, Carmel, and P. Alex Linley. 2014. "Life satisfaction in youth". In *Increasing Psychological Well-Being in Clinical and Educational Settings: Interventions and Cultural Contexts*, edited by Giovanni Andrea Fava and Chiara Ruini, 199–215. Dordrecht: Springer Netherlands. https://doi.org/10.1007/978-94-017-8669-0_13.

Pujolar, Georgina, Aida Oliver-Anglès, Ingrid Vargas, and María-Luisa Vázquez. 2022. "Changes in access to health services during the COVID-19 pandemic: a scoping review". *International Journal of Environmental Research and Public Health* 19: 1749. https://doi.org/10.3390/ijerph19031749.

Ranta, Mette, Gintautas Silinskas, and Terhi-Anna Wilska. 2020. "Young adults' personal concerns during the COVID-19 pandemic in Finland: an issue for social concern". *International Journal of Sociology and Social Policy* 40: 1201–1219. https://doi.org/10.1108/IJSSP-07-2020-0267.

R Core Team. 2021. *R: A Language and Environment for Statistical Computing* (version 4.1.2). Vienna, Austria: R Foundation for Statistical Computing. www.R-project.org/.

Rogowska, Aleksandra Maria, Cezary Kuśnierz, and Dominika Ochnik. 2021. "Changes in stress, coping styles, and life satisfaction between the first and second waves of the COVID-19 pandemic: a longitudinal cross-lagged study in a sample of university students". *Journal of Clinical Medicine Research* 10: 4025. https://doi.org/10.3390/jcm10174025.

Sabarwal, Shwetlena, Nistha Sinha, and Mayra Buvinic. 2013. "How do women weather economic shocks? A review of the evidence". World Bank Policy Research Working Paper. https://doi.org/10.1596/1813-9450-5496.

Salmela-Aro, Katariina, Katja Upadyaya, Inka Ronkainen, and Lauri Hietajärvi. 2022. "Study burnout and engagement during COVID-19 among university students: the role of demands, resources, and psychological needs". *Journal of Happiness Studies* 23: 2685–2702. https://doi.org/10.1007/s10902-022-00518-1.

Saunes, Ingrid Sperre, Karsten Vrangbæk, Haldor Byrkjeflot, Signe Smith Jervelund, Hans Okkels Birk, Liina-Kaisa Tynkkynen, Ilmo Keskimäki, *et al.*2022. "Nordic responses to Covid-19: governance and policy measures in the early phases of the pandemic". *Health Policy* 126: 418–426. https://doi.org/10.1016/j.healthpol.2021.08.011.

Scheidel, Walter. 2017. *The Great Leveler*. Princeton: Princeton University Press. https://doi.org/10.1515/9781400884605.

Schmiedeberg, Claudia and Schröder, Jette. 2017. "Leisure activities and life satisfaction: an analysis with German panel data". *Applied Research in Quality of Life* 12: 137–151. https://doi.org/10.1007/s11482-016-9458-7.

Shemyakina, Olga N., and Anke C.Plagnol. 2013. "Subjective well-being and armed conflict: evidence from Bosnia-Herzegovina". *Social Indicators Research* 113: 1129–1152. www.jstor.org/stable/24719554.

Stan Development Team. 2023. "Stan Modeling Language Users Guide and Reference Manual". https://mc-stan.org/.

Statistics Finland. 2023a. "Official Statistics of Finland (OSF): Students and Qualifications". https://stat.fi/en/statistics/opiskt/.

Statistics Finland. 2023b. "Participation of Young People (15–29) in Education and the Labour Market". https://statfin.stat.fi/PXWeb/api/v1/fi/StatFin/tyti/statfin_tyti_pxt_13am.px/.

Statistics Finland. 2023c. "Population According to Age and Sex". https://statfin.stat.fi/PXWeb/api/v1/fi/StatFin/vaerak/statfin_vaerak_pxt_11re.px/.

Statistics Finland. 2023d. "Population by Labor Force Status". https://statfin.stat.fi/PXWeb/api/v1/fi/StatFin/tyti/statfin_tyti_pxt_135y.px/.

Statistics Finland. 2023e "Population 31.12.2022". Population 31.12. by Region, Language, Age, Sex, Year and Information". https://pxdata.stat.fi:443/PxWeb/sq/e243a802-ea4f-4b75-849d-b93442665522.

Sveinsdóttir, Herdís, Birna Guðrún Flygenring, Margrét Hrönn Svavarsdóttir, Hrund Scheving Thorsteinsson, Gísli Kort Kristófersson, Jóhanna Bernharðsdóttir, and Erla Kolbrún Svavarsdóttir. 2021. "Predictors of university nursing students burnout at the time of the COVID-19 pandemic: a cross-sectional study". *Nurse Education Today* 106: 105070. https://doi.org/10.1016/j.nedt.2021.105070.

Vaarama, Marja, Eero Siljander, Minna-Liisa Luoma, and Satu Meriläinen. 2010. "Suomalaisten kokema elämänlaatu nuoruudesta vanhuuteen" [The Finns' experiences of their quality of life from youth to old age]. In *Suomalaisten hyvinvointi 2010*, edited by Marja Vaarama, PasiMoisio, and Sakari Karvonen, 126–149. Helsinki: Finnish Institute for Health and Welfare.

Varjo, Janne, Mira Kalalahti, and Tristram Hooley. 2022. "Actantial construction of career guidance in parliament of Finland's education policy debates 1967–2020". *Journal of Education Policy* 37: 1009–1027. https://doi.org/10.1080/02680939.2021.1971772.

Vehtari, Aki, Andrew Gelman, and Jonah Gabry. 2017. "Practical Bayesian model evaluation using leave-one-out cross-validation and WAIC". *Statistics and Computing* 27: 1413–1432. https://doi.org/10.1007/s11222-016-9696-4.

Vehtari, Aki, Andrew Gelman, Daniel Simpson, Bob Carpenter, and Paul-Christian Bürkner. 2021. "Rank-normalization, folding, and localization: an Improved R^ for assessing convergence of MCMC (with discussion)". *Bayesian Analysis* 16: 667–718. https://doi.org/10.1214/20-BA1221.

Viner, Russell, Simon Russell, Rosella Saulle, Helen Croker, Claire Stansfield, Jessica Packer, Dasha Nicholls, *et al.*2022. "School closures during social lockdown and mental health, health behaviors, and well-being among children and adolescents during the first COVID-19 wave: a systematic review". *JAMA Pediatrics* 176: 400–409. https://doi.org/10.1001/jamapediatrics.2021.5840.

Von Soest, Tilmann, Anders Bakken, Willy Pedersen, and Mira Aaboen Sletten. 2020. "Life satisfaction among adolescents before and during the COVID-19 pandemic". *Tidsskrift for Den Norske Legeforening*. https://doi.org/10.4045/tidsskr.20.0437.

9

GENERATIONAL INEQUALITIES IN MULTIPLE CRISES

Pandemic and Italian Youth on the Edge

Enzo Colombo and Paola Rebughini

Introduction: Pandemic Social Hierarchies

COVID-19, like all epidemics, has not been democratic. Even though every human being is vulnerable to the virus and its mutations, social conditions – such as age, income, work, access to the health system, type of housing – can change the outcome of the disease and its social consequences. Slogans such as "We're all in the same boat" and "It's gonna be OK" were just first rhetorical reactions and expressions of wishful thinking. The pandemic has taught us a great deal about social inequalities, prejudices, social differences, and financial cuts to the health system (Hage 2020). Low-income workers and the working poor, most of them young people, women, and immigrants, have been the most damaged by the consequences of the lockdown policy and the economic impact of the pandemic (Leonini 2020; Saraceno 2020). In the case of Italy, the poverty risk doubled for precarious workers, such as those working in industries and services affected by the lockdown. Overall, the pandemic impacted low-income households more heavily, especially single-income families (Casarico and Lattanzio 2020; OECD 2020).

The pandemic seemed apolitical, but it was in fact hyperpolitical. On the one hand, the drama of the situation and the urgency of safeguarding health and life itself left no room for reflection, dialogue, or political criticism. The immanent and imminent danger required immediate action that left no room for political mediation but, apparently, suspended and postponed it. On the other hand, every decision and every action taken to confront the emergency – apparently on the basis of aseptic technical-specialist reasons or commonsense logic – designed specific social scenarios that distributed resources and burdens in different ways and generated consequences that had lasting effects differentiated according to the social subjects concerned. The state of exception created by the

DOI: 10.4324/9781003459682-11

emergency seems to have dismantled the barriers to accessing the political space. It seems to have given a voice to everyone in the digital world and in the virtual global village, but it muffled or silenced the voices of those who were less able to be heard; it cancelled their experiences; and it did not recognize their interests. This evidently happened to young people during the early stages of the pandemic.

Hence, as happened in many other contexts, also in Italy the pandemic outbreak exacerbated prior critical situations, in terms of social inequalities, isolation, and individualization, but also in relation to more systemic economic difficulties, which were further worsened by the geopolitical instability caused by the war in Ukraine. Italy has been one of the European countries hardest hit by the pandemic. And it has been so at different levels: contagions and deaths; economic consequences of the lockdown on the labor market; conflicts on governance of the crisis; protracted school lockdown; policies of personal control (Di Cesare 2020); fragility of the local health system; and opacity of data concerning the victims of the virus (Carraro 2020; Gerotto 2020).

The aim of this chapter is to highlight the way in which two years of pandemic impacted on the everyday lives, the social mobility chances, and the perceptions of the future of 18- to 30-year-old Italian youths. In light of a general analysis, the chapter gradually narrows its focus from a wider overview of the consequences of the pandemic in the social stratification of youth to a more in-depth qualitative analysis of their lived experiences during the first, and more radical, lockdown of 2020.

Because Italy was one of the first European countries hit by the COVID-19 virus, it was the first western nation to impose a lockdown, doing so at the end of February 2020. At first, this concerned just some areas of northern Italy, but then, a couple of weeks later, the whole country. After an initial emotional state of incredulity, anxiety, panic, but also irony and self-comfort, the time of the first and most stringent lockdown in Italy is the most interesting to analyze. It was characterized by a systemic tension between the necessity to ensure, on the one hand, the health safety and health care of the population and, on the other hand, the continuity of economic production (Colombo and Rebughini 2021). The most fragile categories and the most fragile areas of the country were those hardest hit by the abrupt economic slowdown, and soon became the ones most dissatisfied with the lockdown and other sanitary precautions.

Indeed, in the first year of the pandemic the voices of scientific experts like virologists were ubiquitous in the media. They provoked contrasting emotional reactions, ranging from the hope of saving solutions to the rejection of medical knowledge (Rebughini 2021). Overall, while the first lockdown was characterized by the leadership of scientific experts, the second year of the pandemic was much more conflictual and focused on the economic crisis and its systemic consequences (Colombo 2021). As Michel Foucault noted in his reflection on biopolitics (Foucault 2005), there is a structural contrast between, on the one hand, the governmentality inspired by biomedical knowledge, and its focus on *zoé* – life in itself – as a cornerstone of political decision-making; and, on the other hand, governmentality inspired by economics founded on the cost-benefit balance. The subject of governance is not the same: the first is the biological body, while the second is the active, rational actor pursuing her/his interests. This contrast is part of traditional western dualism, and during the pandemic it became a core conflict, proving the unsustainability of this dichotomy. Rather than a contrast, there is often an overlap between living matter and economic conditions. What the pandemic highlighted is the need to understand – as a certain feminist gaze already emphasized (Ahmed 2006; Alaimo 2010) – how bodies (not only humans, but also those of the natural environment) are shaped by historical events. Bringing economic issues back into the materiality of health and life is a way to overcome a false universalist or neutral point of view on social problems such as a pandemic, as well as an approach to them in terms of contingent emergency. Contesting the separation between health and the economy means supporting a different interpretation of the pandemic, its damages, and its legacies on the bodily, material experience of individuals and on their social positions. This means also conceiving it within the wider framework of the Anthropocene and climate change, and therefore, again, in terms of its material, historical, and social consequences.

In fact, since the first weeks of the contagion, people in the most unfavorable social positions, with low-paid jobs, were also those most exposed to the risk of catching the disease, such as delivery workers. Yet, while in the first months of the pandemic the need to overcome this dualism was discussed in moments of high-quality reflection, enhanced by the lockdown and the shock of the outbreak, in the following months the focus on quality of life, social justice, and climate justice evaporated.

To summarize, the economic side of the pandemic crisis revealed all the pusillanimity, conservatism, and lack of imagination of economic solutions to cope with this historical event, because the main response was that of returning as soon as possible to previous economic habits. On the health side, the emergency was characterized by recognition of the organizational limits of healthcare systems, as well as a renewed trust in the scientific capacity to find rapid solutions such as vaccines, but without a true recognition of the dependency of research on economic interests or the impersonal nature of medical discourse, unable to recognize social inequalities.

Youth Inequalities and Perceptions of the Future in the Pandemic

The poet Horace's famous aphorism "Quam minimum credula postero" – but without the "Carpe diem" – could be a sort of slogan for many Italian young people deeply affected by the structural consequences of the pandemic. While acceptance of uncertainty and a vocation to "presentness" were already well-established cultural and existential characteristics of the Millennial generation in Italy (Colombo and Rebughini 2019), the disruption caused by the pandemic seems to have strengthened this attitude. While some young people actively engaged in local activities of self-help, mutualism, and social assistance during lockdown (Esu and Dessì 2022), a large majority of them only felt damaged by the consequences of the pandemic on their everyday lives, but also in relation to their future opportunities.

According to available research on public opinion, most Italian youths seem to have reacted to the pandemic with pessimism and resignation. According to research by the Istituto Toniolo conducted in the first months of the emergency (see Rosina and Luppi 2020), 75 percent of young people in Italy believed that the pandemic and lockdown jeopardized their plans for the future, with consequences worse than those envisaged by their European peers; while 33 percent abandoned the idea of living on their own or with a partner. Recent data, gathered by the same institution, and by the Italian Institute for Statistics (ISTAT 2022a), have confirmed this pessimistic attitude: trust in the future and in oneself have drastically decreased. Nevertheless, while interviewees seemed to have lost their trust in self-entrepreneurship in a labor market no longer offering good job opportunities, they claimed for an appropriate salary, protection of workers' rights, and sustainable professions. Faced with the false choice between economic recovery and health protection, they seemed to understand that a sustainable economy and care for human life and environment do not inevitably conflict with economic development. Indeed, in the Toniolo annual report 2022, the attention towards the environment in all domains of work ranked first among interviewees' answers.

Certainly, this social attention towards climate, social justice, and workers' rights was mainly an individualized experience (Colombo and Rebughini 2021), and the pandemic seems to have had a negative influence on this attitude, especially among youths. Overall, the lockdowns have exacerbated the individualized experience of injustices, as well as of personal difficulties in relation to education and work, or access to the health system. Individualization – as a historical process whereby institutions, markets, and labor structures are driven by a logic of self-responsibilization of the individuals – has been enhanced by the pandemic, fostering a perception of social life that starts from personalized, rather than collective, events.

Likewise in the field of education, the pandemic had important and not sufficiently discussed consequences on students' careers. Data concerning the Italian case (Eurispes 2022) highlight that the pandemic condition and distance teaching had a negative influence on the academic performance and motivation of students, especially children and adolescents under 18 years old. One out of three students were unable to follow online lessons regularly, and they lost interest in most of the subjects of study. Not only did the lack of suitable digital devices or of a quiet room to attend online lessons have very negative consequences among students living in low-income families, but also individualization in terms of solitude and outage of social relations with peers had a harmful impact on students' concentration and results.

As expected, the individualized experience of social inequalities during the pandemic was more evident among young people living in low-income families. In Italy, a single year of pandemic – from 2020 to 2021 – provoked an around sixfold increase of social inequalities between the richest and the poorest, and around 1.4 million people found themselves below the poverty threshold, raising the total of poor people to 5.6 million on the national level, while families living in absolute poverty increased from 1.6 million to 2 million (Caritas Italiana 2022; Oxfam 2022). A similar trend was registered for the increase of low-wage workers and working poor (with a salary of less than 970 euros per month), as well as involuntary part-time workers, especially among women.

Young people living in low-income families were more likely to have precarious jobs, like their parents. According to research by the Banca d'Italia (Carta and De Philippis 2021), the lockdowns in 2020 and 2021 impacted mainly on the professional activities of self-employed workers and precarious workers, who also had fewer chances to access remote working. This provoked an increase of unemployment and poverty among low-income families, with immediate consequences on the quality of life of their children.

The pandemic provoked a rise of unemployment also among 15–34 year olds, especially during the most stringent lockdown of 2020. Even though precarious and "flexible" jobs were those most quickly recovered during 2022, youths formed the social category hardest hit by the closure of many business activities related to delivery, services, free-time activities, seasonal contracts, and self-employed activities in general. According to data from the Italian Labor Force Survey (ILFS) (Carta and De Philippis 2021, p. 7), from 2020 to 2021 the percentage of unstable and low-qualified jobs involving young people rose from 29.5% to 37.1%, even though specific forms of social insurance and safety nets, such as the "citizenship income", helped to limit the consequences of the labor market crunch. The overrepresentation of youths among temporary workers and self-employed professions was related to the sudden rise of the already high level of unemployment among young people in Italy. Moreover, as precarious workers, they were the least protected by the existing forms of social insurance against income loss.

Hence, although living in an enduring context of crisis, uncertainty, and precariousness had been a generational characteristic of Italian youths for many years (Rebughini et al. 2017; Colombo and Rebughini 2019), the pandemic brought new characteristics related to social relations with peers and loved ones, emotions, and self-trust that we shall explore in the following section. Indeed, while social inequalities can be more easily measured by statistics and data analysis concerning income, consumption or labor status, social inequalities in everyday relationships, emotions, intergenerational relations, friendships, and acquaintances with peers can be more easily explored with local qualitative analysis (Colombo and Rebughini 2019, 2021). We argue that, not only structural and economic inequalities, but also generational ones, should be taken into account by a sociological analysis of the ongoing consequences of the pandemic.

A Generational Experience of the Pandemic: The First Lockdown in Northern Italy

As already mentioned, discussions about the pandemic – at least in the early period, during the first outburst of the virus – focused on medical or economic issues, proposing solutions for restoration of the previous conditions or control and management of the spread of the disease, the prevention of infection, serious illness, and death. The discourses revolved around medical (biopolitics) or economic (economic governance) issues, proposing solutions for restoration, greater control, and management. More rarely, consideration was made of the consequences for sociality – both in everyday experience and people's relationships and identities (friendships, loves, neighborhood, fun, education) – and of the strains caused to the connective tissue on which modern society rests (social relations in public spaces, public opinion, political action from below, volunteering). This secondary interest in relationships and personal experiences of changes connected with containment of the pandemic often hindered understanding of how young people experienced the most restrictive phases of the pandemic and its long-term consequences.

Although young people were least likely to be severely affected if they contracted COVID-19, they were strongly affected by the drastic measures that were taken to slow down the rate of infection. They were required to make substantial sacrifices to protect the health of older adults. They had to change their everyday lives suddenly and radically: schools, bars, discos, gyms, cinemas, and theaters were closed; music concerts, sports events, and birthday parties were canceled, as well as the possibility to travel, study abroad, or meet friends. Confinement in the home became the only option, a new (forced) lifestyle. This radical and forced change in daily routine confronted young people with the need to rebuild a "new normal", the "Covid normal" world (Moretti and Maturo 2021; Carbajo and Kelly 2022), to imagine new forms of being, thinking, acting, and aspiring in a world characterized by a growing awareness of human and social fragility. Probably, the enduring effects of the COVID-19 pandemic are less the fear of illness and personal death and more the growing awareness of the uncertainty and precariousness of human and social conditions (further increased by the intersection of different and pervasive crises: war, degraded environment, and the persistence of the economic crisis aggravated by the energy crisis and inflation).

The "new normal", the normalcy that encompasses the experience and persistence of the COVID-19 pandemic and, more generally, the omnipresence of crises, includes uncertainty as a constant and widespread condition. It is based on the governance of contingency, on the ability to seize the moment, to build and recognize connections, to think and act in situations characterized by precarity, multiplicity, and continuous change. Although young people may have been less affected by the negative effects of the pandemic because they are more used to adapting to situations of precariousness and crisis or because they adopt two-track thinking (Henkens et al. 2022) in which, on the one hand, they recognize the negative impact on society and individuals in general and, on the other, feel that they are not strongly affected by the pandemic, especially in the long term because they value and trust their own ability to overcome difficulties, it is impossible to ignore that they are paying high costs in terms of stress, mental health, and well-being, increasing fragmentation and precarity in education, training, and employment pathways, restrictions on previously taken-for-granted rights such as those to movement, assembly, and sociality (The World Bank, UNESCO and UNICEF 2021; Carbajo and Kelly 2022; OECD 2022; Shanahan et al. 2022).

Analysis of the effects that the pandemic and the actions implemented to counter it have had on young people did not find much space during the emergency period. The voice of young people remained in the background, since they were considered fundamentally little affected by the risk of contagion and by the consequences of the restrictions on social activities. They were often portrayed as unruly, restless, and irresponsible when not ignored by the press and public debate. It has often been assumed, more or less explicitly, that the restriction of social activities – especially the suspension of school activities – constituted a simple period of unexpected holiday for young people, without high costs.

Reading the accounts that young people have provided of their experience during the first lockdown[1] puts these representations to the test, highlighting the costs that young people have paid, also as a consequence of living in a society that "is not a society for young people".

Young people – especially those born between 1990 and 2005 – have already experienced several serious crises in the crucial years of their growth: the global financial crisis of 2008 following the collapse of the American real-estate market and the Lehman Brothers bankruptcy that triggered a downward-spiraling global crisis; the COVID-19 pandemic; and, now, the geopolitical tensions linked to the Russian aggression against Ukraine. Current tensions foreshadow new future crises: the energy crisis, the growing inflation and the risk of recession that are accompanying the scarcity of energy supply, the ecological crisis, and the inevitable further exacerbation of social inequalities. These crises have affected young people both directly, making it difficult for them to enter the labor market and making transition paths to adult life more complex and uneven, and indirectly, due to the repercussions they have had and continue to have on their families (OECD 2020; Caritas Italiana 2022). The situation appears particularly critical in Italy, where young people, compared to their European peers, have historically suffered from lower rates of higher education, higher school dropout rates, higher unemployment, and less economic and housing autonomy.

We can say that living in a crisis has become a generational feature (Rebughini et al. 2017), a constant element of the biographical and existential horizon of contemporary western young adults. But the crisis produced by the pandemic assumes characteristics that are partly different from those of the financial crisis that has characterized the last 15 years. The financial crisis has made young people live within a horizon characterized by a specific space-time experience, by the pervasiveness of uncertainty, and by the constant injunction to be entrepreneurs of themselves, active, creative, flexible, and adaptable, because – so the dominant rhetoric suggests – only they are responsible for their own destinies (Colombo and Rebughini 2021; Carbajo and Kelly 2022). Experience of the economic crisis and experience of globalization converge in creating a specific perception of space, which is dilated and detached from simple geometric dimensions to redefine itself on the basis of relational characteristics.

In the experience of economic crisis and globalization, if space is dilated, time appears to be increasingly compressed and accelerated. People's experience of uncertainty and the speed of change induce them to focus on the contingent, on the immediate. The past and the future are blurred, and interest is reserved for the present. The presentification in which young people find themselves living is characterized by a paradoxical oscillation between fatalism and hyper-realism. On the one hand, the difficulty of selecting and interpreting the complexity of the data and contexts to which young people have access generates a fatalistic attitude, so that they are resigned to accepting the situations in which they find themselves, contenting themselves with navigating in uncertainty without excessive damage. They focus on the opportunities that arise and they try to seize the right moments. On the other hand, the aforementioned difficulty leads to a realistic, disenchanted approach, free from illusions and utopias, focused on results, and based on the obsessive calculation of available options, so that young people are committed to compulsively accumulating qualifications and certified experiences to add to their LinkedIn profiles. Difficulties in making long-term plans, or in predicting the effects of current choices, foster tactical attitudes and require the ability to navigate the instability of the present.

With lockdown, the experience of time and space created by economic crisis and globalization was radicalized and contradicted at the same time. The practices that young people were painstakingly constructing in order to cope with dilated spaces and compressed times required a rapid restructuring amid the experience of confinement and within the experiential horizon opened by the pandemic. With the measures made necessary to contain the spread of the virus, space was limited, confined to the home, while time was slowed down and dilated – the days were all the same and never seemed to pass. Even the injunction on young people to be active, entrepreneurs of themselves, to try to rely only on their own strengths and skills in order to cope with the unpredictability of situations and seize the right moments, seems to have been contradicted by lockdown. The strength of external factors was evident, and their origin and control lay far beyond any individual's will and possibility. Solidarity and mutual help regained value, and awareness of individual fragility grew in the face of systemic problems that could only be addressed by seeking and implementing systemic solutions.

As young people wrote in their diaries, adapting to the new routines imposed by lockdown was not always easy. Having a lot of time available, and having to live in a confined space, constituted a real experiment of social rupture that forced individuals to question the taken-for-granted domains within which daily action unfolds. The radical change in the temporal and spatial frames of experience forced individuals to question themselves about what until a few days previously had been considered normal and banal. As in the case of the stranger analyzed by Alfred Schütz realizing that the habits and categories used previously "no longer work" generated crisis and uncertainty but also stimulated the development of new meanings.

Having overcome the first sensation of an unforeseen holiday and the expectation of being able to enjoy a moment of tranquillity to devote to greater self-care, the difficulty of finding new family balances emerged. For youths living the whole day with parents, brothers, and sisters, the difficulty of finding their own space and a moment of solitude became crucial. The relationship with the space to which they were accustomed and the relationships that developed in it changed radically: from the centrality of the external space to confinement in the domestic space; from the multiplicity and fluidity of friendships to the constraints of family coexistence. The burden imposed by the overcrowding of the domestic space often overlapped with isolation from the outside world. The quality of family relationships and housing conditions were among the factors that most influenced the lockdown experience. Young people who had conflictual relationships with their parents, or who did not have their own room, access to a garden, or a large terrace, generally experienced the lockdown as confinement.

Anxiety, uncertainty, and anger were the moods that emerged with greatest insistence as the situation of domestic isolation continued. The cost imposed on young people by restrictions on their social activities became evident. They felt limited and dispossessed of the experiences that constitute the main texture of adolescence and youth: meeting people and facing new situations, experiencing spaces of independence from family ties, and having opportunities to test one's body, affectivity, and sexuality. The uncertainty that generationally characterizes young people born and raised constantly in a crisis was further amplified by the extreme reduction of the possibilities for action. The present in which they were used to living – a present characterized by speed, constant change, and the need for a constant response – became crystallized, devoid, and empty. The need imposed by lockdown to rework the space-time coordinates of experience further exacerbated the youthful experience of uncertainty. What had been painstakingly elaborated to face the permanent crisis was called into question by a new and sudden modification of daily life. A "new normal" was still being worked out, but it included an attempt to restore some aspects of the previous space-time experience with an increased awareness of the fragility of that experience. It implied "returning" to a normal which could not be entirely what it had been previously. The tools devised to rebuild a "new normal" were always mainly linked to individual initiative, to the ability to be an entrepreneur of oneself, available, dynamic, creative, and flexible. However, the fragility of such tools and increased awareness of the ineffectiveness of individual will and dedication amid collective problems and challenges increased frustration and anxiety (Nocentini et al. 2021; ISTAT 2022a; Korte et al. 2022)

The interruption of school life, relationships with friends, and, in general, the extreme limitation of the social experiences that characterize youth generally had different effects according to the cultural capital of the family. Young people with families possessing high cultural and economic capital often experienced lockdown as a parenthesis which limited their possibilities but did not completely interrupt their educational and experiential pathways. Supported by their parents, they were able to continue their training process, albeit with greater slowness, fatigue, and difficulty. On the other hand, young people in more deprived socioeconomic situations often accumulated further distance and delay. Socioeconomic status and cultural capital, in fact, constituted a second determining factor in defining the experience of the pandemic – a factor that had the most lasting effects and radicalized social differences among young people.

Given the exceptional circumstances of lockdown, the availability of, and the ability to use, electronic technology and social media were important factors in defining the experience of social isolation. For a generation of "digital natives", it is no wonder that during the lockdown the use of digital resources, smartphones, the internet, Instagram, Tik Tok, and other social networks substantially increased.

However, technological skills and the material availability of technology constituted one of the most significant social differences among young people. The negative effects associated with distance learning affected all young people, but they were more marked for those who attended lessons remotely with inadequate digital tools and in unsuitable environments (Brandolini 2022). The need to close schools and start distance learning had to be implemented in a highly differentiated social context: 12.3 percent of children between the ages of 6 and 17 did not have computers or tablets at home; the share was close to 20 percent in the south (470,000 children). Only 6.1 percent lived in families where at least one computer was available for each member (ISTAT 2020b). At the outbreak of the pandemic in Italy, among the 14- to 17-year-olds who could use the internet, two out of three had low or basic digital skills, while fewer than three out of ten (equal to about 700,000 children) had high-level digital skills (ISTAT 2020b). Consequently, 20 percent of Italian children and 27.9 percent of children with immigrant families were unable to follow lessons continuously. Pupils with disabilities who did not participate in video lessons amounted to 23.3 percent (29 percent in the south) (ISTAT 2021). The lack of technological skills and adequate electronic tools made it more difficult for children belonging to contexts with severe socioeconomic difficulties or with disabilities to participate in distance learning. These complexities hindered or completely interrupted the educational pathway, preventing achievement of one of the objectives that an inclusive school sets itself even before learning – socialization (ISTAT 2020b). The accumulated delay, as research is starting to confirm (Favretto et al. 2021; Brandolini 2022), can have lasting consequences on the work, income, and quality of life of these young people.

For the young people who could use them, social networks were of fundamental importance in coping with the sudden isolation of lockdown. Not surprisingly, internet usage increased dramatically, and young people spent more hours on social media during the pandemic. Lockdown did not mean the dissolution of social relations, but their radical reorganization. Direct interactions were reduced and replaced with social relations conditioned by technology, in which communication was mediated by the telephone, social media, and software such as WhatsApp, Telegram, Zoom, and Skype. Social distancing did not translate into distancing from the social and from others, but into communication and sociality at a distance (Granic et al. 2020). Digital technology enabled young people to maintain constant contact with friends and relatives, even though the number of calls often turned out to be a faded substitute for the absence of physical relationships – a surrogate that highlights the lack of direct contact and the ineffectiveness of replacing the quality of relationships with the quantity of calls. However, as the pandemic progressed, there emerged widespread dissatisfaction with the type of relationship that social media made possible – highlighting the incomplete substitutability of face-to-face relationships with mediated relationships. The possibility to have a variety of information and communication technologies available and greater or lesser digital competence constituted a third decisive factor of difference among young people, considerably widening the gap between those who had more material and cultural resources and those who did not.

Conclusion: Uncertainty and the "Politics of the Present" of Italian Youth

Young people today live in the historical framework of neoliberal societies, where individuals confront uncertainty, perform everyday forms of resilience, and are required to adapt themselves to rapid change. The COVID-19 pandemic further underscored the individual vulnerability intrinsic to this state of unpredictability. It highlighted various forms of material and relational poverty, psychological fragility, incapacity to adapt oneself to unexpected situations, in a context where all previous forms of social organization and solidarity – those typical of industrial capitalism and its association with a welfare state system – have been considerably scaled down. In the new "immaterial economy", knowledge and skills, social relations, and personal initiative become resources for the economic system itself (Lorey 2015), and the phase of the repeated lockdowns highlighted the intertwining of biology and biography, health and economy, the production of subjectivities and the production of economic value (Di Cesare 2020).

Overall, the pandemic increased the feeling of *presentification* and changed the younger generation's perception of self-agency and vulnerability. Yet, as research conducted during the lockdown also showed, both agency and vulnerability – physical, psychological, and economic – can be analyzed in the continuous processes whereby social actions and social meanings are produced, in a specific situation and historical context (in this case, that of the pandemic). Young people are engaged in continuous work translating the material, relational, and cognitive resources at their disposal and adapting them to new and changing situations, and the pandemic is one of these. Aside from the various accelerating changes in the economic, productive, and technological fields, the pandemic and the lockdowns have also changed social experience and everyday life, fostering multiplicity, complexity, and uncertainty (Colombo and Rebughini 2019).

The pandemic experience is bound to have lasting effects, especially on young people. They have grown up considering the crisis context to be "normal", have had to adapt to the restrictions imposed by the pandemic by renouncing a significant part of the fundamental experiences of youth. The cost they have incurred is often underestimated. The experiential delay, and the stress of redefining a "new normal" in constant uncertainty, may constitute a further obstacle to inclusion in adult life and a reduction in the chances to obtain education, employment, and social participation. However, the pandemic has not had a leveling effect, nor has it had an equal negative impact on young people in different sociocultural circumstances. Instead, it has widened – and may widen further – the gap between those who have been able to face the pandemic period with adequate material and cultural resources and those who have seen their marginal situation worsen further. Constant attention to the condition of youth, especially of young people with fewer cultural and social resources, is necessary to limit the potential capacity of the pandemic to constitute an experience that confirms the uncertainty and fragility of a generation raised amid crisis and forced to adopt a politics of the present that emphasizes personal initiative but constantly jeopardizes its effectiveness.

Note

1 The following reflections are based on materials produced by students during the lockdown period. We thank Professor Fabio Giovanetti and Professor Marilina Comeglio for providing us with the rich material produced by students attending the State Institute of Higher Education "City of Luino - Carlo Volontè"; We also thank Dr Anna Biffi of the social enterprise 'Spazio Giovani' in Lissone for giving us access to the equally rich material produced by boys and girls at different schools in the province of Monza and Brianza as part of the Peer Education project promoted by ATS Brianza. Retrospective narratives on the lockdown experience were collected in September 2020 from students attending the Culture and Society course at the University of Milan. Other materials were found directly on the internet. Of especial interest are the diaries produced by the students of the Institute of Higher Education "Einaudi-Scarpa" of Montebelluna at the request of Professor Lucio De Bortoli (available at www.iiseinaudiscarpa.edu.it/diario /); the stories published on the website of the State Technical Institute "Marco Polo" in Florence (www.ittmarcopolo.edu.it/scuola-covid); the diaries kept by students of the Liceo Classico "Andrea D'Oria" in Genoa (http://lascuolafanotizia.diregiovani.it/2020/05/30/diario-minimo-del-lockdown-15-marzo-5-maggio-2020/); the diaries of students attending the schools of Biella and published on the website (www.newsbiella.it); the chronicle of

the quarantine of the girls and boys of the State Comprehensive Institute "Sinopoli-Ferrini" in Rome (material available on the website http://lascuolafanotizia.diregiovani.it/; and reflections on the website www.giovanicreativi.it).

References

Ahmed, Sara. 2006. *Queer Phenomenology: Orientations, Objects, Others*. Durham: Duke University Press.

Alaimo, Stacy. 2010. *Bodily Natures: Science, Environment and the Material Self*. Bloomington: Indiana University Press.

Brandolini, Andrea. 2022. "La pandemia di COVID-19 e la disuguaglianza economica in Italia". *Politiche Sociali* 2: 181–210. https://doi.org/10.7389/104616.

Carbajo, Diego, and Peter Kelly. 2022. "COVID-19, young people and the future of work: Rethinking global grammars of enterprise". *The Sociological Review*, 71, 1: 65–84. https://doi.org/10.1177/00380261221093403.

Caritas Italiana. 2022. *L'anello debole. Rapporto 2022 su povertà e esclusione sociale in Italia*. Roma: Caritas.

Carraro, Dante. 2020. "La salute globale come impegno quotidiano". In various authors, *Il mondo dopo la fine del mondo*, 89–97. Roma-Bari: Laterza.

Carta, Francesca, and Marta De Philippis. 2021. "The impact of the COVID-19 shock on labour income inequality: evidence from Italy". *Banca d'Italia Papers* 606. www.bancaditalia.it/pubblicazioni/qef/2021-0606/QEF_606_21.pdf?language_id=1.

Casarico, Alessandra, and Salvatore Lattanzio. 2020. "La democrazia del lockdown". *lavoce.info*. www.lavoce.info/archives/65146/la-demografia-del-lockdown/.

Colombo, Enzo. 2021. "Human rights-inspired governmentality: COVID-19 through a human dignity perspective". *Critical Sociology* 47, 4–5: 571–581. https://doi.org/10.1177/0896920520971846.

Colombo, Enzo, and Paola Rebughini (eds.). 2019. *Youth and the Politics of the Present: Coping with Complexity and Ambivalence*. London: Routledge.

Colombo, Enzo, and Paola Rebughini (eds.). 2021. *Acrobati del presente: la vita quotidiana alla prova del lockdown*. Roma: Carocci.

Di Cesare, Donatella. 2020. *Virus sovrano? L'asfissia capitalistica*, Torino: Bollati-Boringhieri.

Esu, Aide, and Valeria Dessì. 2022. "Recasting solidarity during the COVID-19: a case study". *Social Movements Studies* 22. https://doi.org/10.1080/14742837.2022.2134105.

Eurispes. 2022. "Osservatorio", 14 March. https://eurispes.eu/news/atti-della-presentazione-dellosservatorio-permanente-sulle-politiche-educative-delleurispes/.

Favretto, Anna Rosa, Maturo Antonio, and Stefano Tomelleri (eds.). 2021. *L'impatto sociale del Covid-19*. Milano: FrancoAngeli.

Foucault, Michel. 2005. *The Hermeneutics of the Subject: Lectures at the Collège de France 1981–1982*. New York: Picador.

Gerotto, Luca. 2020. "L'evoluzione della spesa sanitaria". *Osservatorio sui Conti Pubblici Italiani*, 14 March. https://osservatoriocpi.unicatt.it.

Granic, Isabela, Morita Hiromitsu, and Scholten Hanneke. 2020. "Young people's digitals interactions from a narrative identity perspective: implications for mental health and wellbeing". *Psychological Inquiry* 31, 3: 258–270.

Hage, Ghassan. 2020. "The haunting figure of the useless academic: critical thinking in coronavirus time". *European Journal of Cultural Studies* 23, 4: 662–666. https://doi.org/10.1177/1367549420926182.

Henkens, J., K. Visser, C. Finkenauer, S. T. Vermeulen, and G. Stevens. 2022. "'I think it'll all blow over in the end': how young people perceive the impact of COVID-19 on their future orientations". *Young* 30, 4: 309–326.

ISTAT. 2020a. "L'inclusione scolastica degli alunni con disabilità – a.a. 2019–2020". www.istat.it/it/files//2020/12/Report-alunni-con-disabilit%C3%A0.pdf.

ISTAT. 2020b. "Spazi in casa e disponibilità di computer per bambini e ragazzi ". www.google.com/url?sa=t&rct=j&q=&esrc=s&source=web&cd=&ved=2ahUKEwiCk_WO0-76AhWYQfEDHZk-CnsQFnoECBAQAQ&url=https%3A%2F%2Fwww.istat.it%2Fit%2Ffiles%2F2020%2F04%2FSpazi-casa-disponibilita-computer-ragazzi.pdf&usg=AOvVaw0jDTac73rc6y68vIJFl4Jt.

ISTAT. 2021. "L'inclusione scolastica degli alunni con disabilità – a.a. 2020–2021". www.istat.it/it/files//2022/01/REPORT-ALUNNI-CON-DISABILITA.pdf.

ISTAT. 2022. *Rapporto Bes 2021: il benessere equo e sostenibile in Italia.* Roma: ISTAT.

Korte, Ciera, Robert D. Friedberg, Tammy Wilgenbusch, Jennifer K. Paternostro, Kimberly Brown, Anusha Kakolu, *et al.*2022. "Intolerance of uncertainty and health-related anxiety in youth amid the COVID-19 pandemic: understanding and weathering the continuing storm". *Journal of Clinical Psychology in Medical Settings* 29, 3: 645–653. https://doi.org/10.1007/s10880-021-09816-x.

Leonini, Luisa. 2020. "Vite diseguali nella pandemia". *Polis/polis: Ricerche e studi su società e politica* 2: 181–190. https://doi.org/10.1424/97363.

Lorey, Isabell. 2015. *State of Insecurity: Government of the Precarious.* London: Verso.

Moretti, Veronica and Antonio Maturo. 2021. "'Unhome' sweet home: the construction of new normalities in Italy during COVID-19". In *The COVID-19 Crisis: Social Perspectives*, edited by Deborah Lupton and Karen Willis, 90–102. London: Routledge.

Nocentini, Annalaura, Benedetta E. Palladino, and Ersilia Menesini. 2021. "Adolescents' stress reactions in response to COVID-19 pandemic at the peak of the outbreak in Italy". *Clinical Psychological Science* 9, 3: 507–514. https://doi.org/10.1177/2167702621995761.

OECD. 2020. "Youth and COVID-19: response, recovery and resilience". www.oecd.org/coronavirus/policy-responses/youth-and-covid-19-response-recovery-and-resilience-c40e61c6/.

OECD. 2022. "Delivering for youth: how governments can put young people at the centre of the recovery". https://read.oecd-ilibrary.org/view/?ref=1131_1131487-xd5bm4h5h8&title=Delivering-for-Youth-how-governments-can-put-young-people-at-the-centre-of-the-recovery.

Oxfam. 2022. "Disuguitalia". www.oxfamitalia.org/wp-content/uploads/2022/05/WEB_Disuguitalia_2022_CLEAN.pdf.

Rebughini, Paola. 2021. "A sociology of anxiety: Western modern legacy and the Covid-19 outbreak". *International Sociology* 36, 4: 554–568.

Rebughini, Paola, Enzo Colombo, and Luisa Leonini (eds.). 2017. *Giovani dentro la crisi.* Milano: Guerini.

Rosina, Alessandro, and Francesca Luppi. 2020. *Covid-19: rischio tsunami sui progetti di vita dei ventenni e trentenni italiani.* www.google.com/url?sa=t&rct=j&q=&esrc=s&source=web&cd=&ved=2ahUKEwjyh_y57uP_AhUVQ_EDHVqKBuMQFnoECB4QAQ&url=https%3A%2F%2Fwww.rapportogiovani.it%2Fnew%2Fwp-content%2Fuploads%2F2020%2F04%2FReport-PROGETTI-GIOVANI-E-IMPATTO-COVID-def_rev.pdf&usg=AOvVaw05C84WZVmAT4QA7mIxD5s8&opi=89978449.

Saraceno, Chiara. 2020. "Disuguaglianza e povertà in epoca Covid-19". *Pandora Rivista* 2. www.pandorarivista.it/pandora-piu/disuguaglianza-e-poverta-in-epoca-covid-19/.

Shanahan, Lilly, Annekatrin Steinhoff, Laura Bechtiger, Aja L . Murray, Amy Nivette, Urs Hepp, *et al.*2022. "Emotional distress in young adults during the COVID-19 pandemic: evidence of risk and resilience from a longitudinal cohort study". *Psychological Medicine* 52, 5: 824–833. https://doi.org/10.1017/S003329172000241X.

The World Bank, UNESCO, and UNICEF. 2021. *The State of the Global Education Crisis: A Path to Recovery*. Washington, DC, Paris, and New York: The World Bank, UNESCO, and UNICEF.

10

THE COVID-19 EMERGENCY AND UNIVERSITY STUDENTS

An Analysis of Effects from Inequalities in Cultural and Socioeconomic Capital*

Gabriella D'Ambrosio and Barbara Sonzogni

Introduction

Theoretical Framework

The present work aims to investigate the implications of global emergencies in terms of redefining lifestyles, with specific attention to the youth population. In this respect, the COVID-19 pandemic is undoubtedly one of the most important worldwide crises in our contemporary society within the national and international landscape.

Within this framework, the current research is then particularly interested in two aspects of the concatenation of *personality, culture* and *social system*: first, how such intersections result in emotional-perceptual impacts on everyday life, and consequently, on the subjects' visions of the future; and second, how these impacts and feelings are unevenly distributed within the compositional parts of society.

A further specific interest will be to examine the possible consequences of these aspects in exacerbating and increasing the structural inequalities present in society. Starting from this, the chapter explores these aspects in terms of the specific case of consequences arising from global emergencies, such as the COVID-19 pandemic.

Various scholars have already noted how, beginning in 2020, the pandemic has exacerbated poverty and increased gaps in income and gender opportunity. In particular, this study aims to explore how the state of the individual's preexisting cultural and socioeconomic capital can interplay with such consequences in both the personal and social spheres. The chapter continues an established line of research on how the feelings that arise in catastrophic contexts can overwhelm the individual, reducing them to varying states of uncertainty. A particular sociological proposal has been that the "extraordinary"

DOI: 10.4324/9781003459682-12

state provokes destabilizing fears, and then leads people in unpredictable directions, with disruptive effects on "ordinary" everyday life (Sorokin, 2010; Bonolis et al., 2020).

The reference to elements (magnitudes, random variables) that limit intentionality is well represented in a contribution by Elster (2007), who, in this regard, offers an exemplification related to the fall of the Twin Towers in September 2001. In a similar situation, it is evident that we were faced with a case of a disturbance of the daily routine, of a coefficient affecting our inner algorithm that led to a revision of the values of habitual rationality; from the point of view of the pattern of action, this corresponds to a sudden influence on the non-intentional component. In this sense, we would be in the presence of a hypothesis of a depotentiation of the stabilizing networks of behavioural patterns that result from the deconstruction of the priority orders of everyday life. With respect to this, even the "rational choice theory" postulates conditions of system stability that, when they fail due to pantoclastic disruptions, there is reason to believe that they suffer from such suspensions and redirections.

Along these lines, there are many exemplary phenomenal spheres that can show such evidence; among others, the consumer behaviour, the phenomenon of political voting and microcredit activations. All these are case studies based on the logic of rational choice (in its classical and neoclassical sense). This exemplifies how, even in a context ostensibly based on attitudes of rationality, vectors of incidence (emotional, affective domains) come into play in the unconventionally intentional dimension of the scheme of action. This becomes even more evident when attention is turned to investigating the implications arising from cases of global emergency, such as natural disasters, terrorist attacks and pandemic phenomena (Sonzogni and D'Ambrosio, 2022).

The theoretical-interpretative framework assumed is based on the concepts of Parsons (1951), and synthesizing both Weberian (Weber 1922a, 1922b) and Durkheimian (Durkheim 1914, 1925) traditions. So, the scope is to examine and assess: (a) the underlying patterns of action in individual decisions in emergency contexts; and (b) their embedding in a cultural frame of reference. This framework is merely intended to be a starting point, since, starting from classical sociology, the three elements considered by Parsons could be seen as an interpretative key.

Parsons' conception (Parsons and Bales, 1955) is that a social system involves the interaction of three "centres of integration" (Parsons, 1951, p. 34), necessarily functioning in correspondence:

- *Culture*, a system of models, patterns of conduct and responses, projective systems, ways of seeing things, interpretative schemes, etc.;
- *Personality*, the subject acting and developing character, sharing in characterizing culture, and being characterized by structure;

-*Social structure*, affecting personality by certain dispositions, for example, the "golden middle way".

In the current conception, then, all these structures come into play in different dimensions, scopes and capacities.

These elements – as Bonolis (2007, pp. 144-145) points out – illustrate how the concrete performance of actions in the role cannot take place outside a "shared order of symbolic meanings". This common pattern ("cultural tradition") thus serves as a code, and action makes use of it from time to time. This relationship of irreducibility "individual-role", which Goffman called "role distance" (1961), does not only concern the problem of assuming ownership of the role, but is also found in the "practice" ("execution") of the role itself. In this sense it is like something that moves in the role, that is influenced by it, but it retains its own autonomy. In this sense, Parsons concludes on this point,

> the relation of the personality to a uniform role structure is one of interdependence and inter-penetration, not a relation of "inclusion" in which the properties of the personality system are constituted by the roles from which it is composed.
>
> *(1951, p. 25)*

From the Conceptual Dimension to the Identification of the Indicators

Assuming the theoretical framework explained above, in which beliefs, desires and opportunities influence attitudes, behaviours and actions, Figure 10.1 maps the dimensions of relevance in the manner of *Coleman's Boat* (Coleman, 1990). The indicators represented in this figure have thus been examined in the survey stage of the study and, thus, operationalized into measurable variables (Lazarsfeld, 1958), as will be explained in the next sections.

Therefore, after having articulated the theoretical framework in conceptual dimensions, the related indicators could be identified in the survey that was done.

The data are analyzed considering the idea that, within the social structure, the positions occupied by individuals are not evenly distributed in the social space. The cultural resources and the socioeconomic capital at the disposition of the individual are inevitably variable, and this variability influences the individual's position with respect to the future, in terms of their emotions, aspirations (cognitive-emotional dimension), perspectives and desires on the future, and their planning for possibilities (action-intention dimension).

Within this framework, we are interested to discern how emergencies may modify "ordinary social states" (Mangone, 2018) – to what extent the impacts on daily life, requiring adaptations to new situations, then exacerbate pre-existing differences; or, on the other hand, how some differences linked to social and individual characteristics may be cancelled out in the face of a new social state so disruptive that the subjects are all rendered equal in the face of the emergency upheaval.

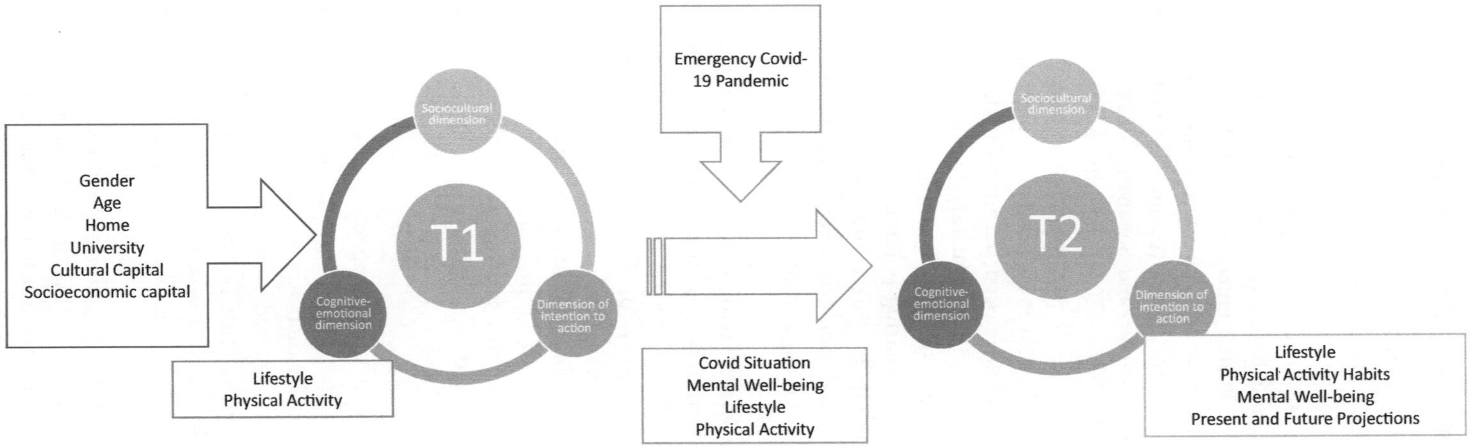

FIGURE 10.1 Relevant conceptual dimensions and reference indicators.
Source: Authors' own elaboration.

How COVID-19 Exacerbates Social Inequalities: A Global Overview

Recent studies have revealed how the spread of the COVID-19 pandemic has exacerbated or created new inequalities in relation to gender (Barnes et al., 2021), age (Łuszczyńska and Formosa, 2021; Khan, 2022), race and/or ethnicity (Solomos, 2021; Navarro and Hernandez, 2022; Thomas et al., 2022), and social and economic status (Deaton and Jones, 2021; Ryan and Nanda, 2022). Unlike other pandemics, this specific health emergency struck both developing and developed countries all around the world, characterizing as a kind of "leveller" but also placing a spotlight on the injustices and inequalities across social, political and economic systems (Michie and Sheehan, 2022).

In this respect, The World Bank (2021) has itself observed contexts of unequal access to vaccines (just over 7 percent of people in low-income countries receiving a dose, compared to over 75 percent in high-income countries), widening income gaps (although losses occurred broadly, the poorest 20 percent experienced the steepest declines) and, in general, disproportionate impacts on the vulnerable and poor people. One of the impacts was in school closures according to the World Bank stimulating potential levels of "learning poverty" of 70 percent in low- and middle-income countries (International Association for the Evaluation of Educational Achievement – UNESCO, 2022; Koehler et al., 2022). So, there is evidence to suggest how

> the economic shock associated with Covid-19, which resulted from the lockdown and severe reduction in economic activity of many sectors of the economy, will not affect all in the same way. Indeed, it is becoming clear that it will interact with many of the pre-existing inequalities along dimensions such as gender, ethnicity, age and geography. Moreover, this pandemic-induced crisis is having impacts across multiple related aspects of life, from health to jobs and to family life, and these impacts are interrelated. The most vulnerable groups by socio-economic background and health status are also those that may be hit the hardest.
>
> *(Blundell et al., 2020, p. 2)*

Moreover, the pandemic-induced crisis impacts across multiple interrelated aspects of the individual's life, from health to work to family life, with varying effects in consideration of the individual's personal and social resources. Other lines of research have thus investigated how, especially for more vulnerable categories (e.g., children, women, elderly, poor), the COVID-19 pandemic could diminish and impair their entire quality of life and psychological well-being (OECD – Organization for Economic Co-operation and Development, 2020; Haas, 2021).

According to Gunter (2022), at the beginning of the COVID-19 pandemic, the major public health concern was the status of public mental health, since several people were clearly fearful of infection while others were made anxious by the threats posed to their livelihoods and access to social support systems by strict behaviour constraints. All these impacts represented a parallel wave of public health crises occurring alongside COVID-19, since people adjusted to their changed circumstances. Also, lifestyle adjustments took a form that could lay the foundations of problematic behaviour down the road. Overall, these restrictions, for many people around the world, represented a major change to their whole quality of life.

In this vein, looking at the statistical available data, in the study *COVID-19 and Well-being: Life in the Pandemic* (OECD – Organization for Economic Co-operation and Development, 2021a), the OECD reported, examining data from April to December 2020, not only an 16 percent increase in deaths, compared to previous data, but also the increasing incidence of depression and anxiety arising from restriction measures and other aspects of the pandemic. In more detail:

a Younger cohorts have experienced some of the most severe job insecurity and disruption arising from the pandemic, and the greatest declines in mental health and social connectedness, as well as facing job disruption and insecurity. For youths aged 15 to 24, data from 12 OECD counties show rates of depression and anxiety at 41.2% and 38.9%, compared to the much lower 27.9% and 26.0% typical of age 25 to 64, and 14.9% and 14.7% for those aged 65 and over.
b Gaps in mental health are variable with race and/or ethnicity (see Smith et al., 2020; Thomeer et al., 2022).
c Mental health outcomes worsened, in particular for women, since, examining data from 16 OECD countries, 29.4% of women were likely to be at risk of depression and 26% at risk of anxiety (compared to 23.9% and 23.7%, respectively, for men).
d Symptoms of depression and anxiety were more common among the unemployed and those experiencing financial difficulties (OECD – Organization for Economic Co-operation and Development, 2021b).

The present research focuses in particular on the cases of last-mentioned groups of the unemployed and financially precarious (Carstairs and Morris, 1989; Goldblatt, 1989; Wilkinson, 1989) considering that this category of people had disproportionately faced the largest challenge during the COVID-19 pandemic in coping with economic shocks due to their low asset base, lack of savings and the informality of their work (Fang et al., 2020).

More specifically, the intention is to investigate whether, in the emergency context, people of lower cultural and socioeconomic conditions experience greater difficulty in daily management and mental well-being, and so "descend" still further. One of the reasons for this would be that, as several studies have shown, the starting conditions of problematic socioeconomic status determine greater exposure to infectious diseases in general, and higher incidence and even case-fatality rates in respect of specific illness.

This has held true in the present context of COVID-19, where sociocultural and socioeconomic features (financial resources, contexts for personal hygiene, access to testing and treatment, possibility of complying with health guidance such as distancing, possibilities of remote working) have been found closely related to rates of diffusion, incidence and mortality (Bambra et al., 2020; Kawachi, 2020; Weill et al., 2020).

In short, the COVID-19 pandemic, like other catastrophic events of the past, ranging from natural events such as hurricanes and earthquakes, to wars and great recessions, has weakened economic resiliency and in particular reinforced disadvantage, principally for people already exposed. Indeed, as pointed out by Papyrakis (2022), the lack of institutional preparedness, the presence of inadequate infrastructures, the limited access to information, and public resources has amplified both health and economic weaknesses; in fact, the combination of the COVID-19 pandemic and widespread poverty has aggravated economic insecurity for vulnerable individuals and communities.

Due to the rising of social inequalities (Adams-Prassl et al., 2020; Sumner et al., 2020), the great challenge in the years ahead will be to prevent the spread of the gaps we observed in this chapter and to offer vulnerable people accessibility to financial, social and psychological support in order to counteract the barriers they faced during the pandemic. To ensure that the crisis does not induce an increase in inequality, the adoption of specific policies is important to consider in both the long and short term; definitely, among the most important policies that can protect the well-being of households and ensure that a minimum level of economic activity is maintained, the following directions are taken into consideration (Vargas Hill and Narayan, 2020):

- compensation for the loss of labour and non-labour income through social protection programmes (including transfers and unemployment benefits);
- support of firms and workers to protect jobs and facilitate recovery;
- investment in safety nets and social insurance programmes.

For this reason, as recommended in Oxfam's *Commitment to Reducing Inequality Index* (2020), by adopting strong anti-inequality policies on public services, tax and labour rights, all governments could contribute to reducing social inequalities and the gap between rich and poor radically, with immediate results (Molina and Ortiz-Juarez, 2020; Oxfam, 2020). According to Vargas Hill and Narayan,

> policy measures need to be adopted during the recovery phase that keep the eye on the long game while also spurring economic recovery in the short run. This requires a strong focus on inclusiveness and building resilience to future disasters, particularly among vulnerable people and communities.
>
> *(2020, p. 23)*

According to this point of view, the upset provoked by the COVID-19 emergency could be seen as an opportunity to reflect on how we might build a better society for the future, for the next generation.

Data Collection and Methodology

During and Post-Pandemic: Feelings and Perception in Challenging Times

In 2021, an internet-based survey was conducted targeting students of Sapienza University of Rome, who during the previous three years had spent a period of academic mobility outside of Italy for the purposes of study or research ("outgoing" students) or who were "incoming" students spending a period of academic mobility at Sapienza. The general aim of the survey was to collect information from these students on their point of view on social issues, living conditions, ideas, and problems of this current historical time, with one of the aims being to identify potential new lines of research in these areas.

The questionnaire was composed of 56 questions, divided into the following eight sections: general beliefs about society, family and individual; COVID situation; housing situation; family relationships; pandemic policy management and information; mental-health-free time; lifestyles, and present and future projections. A final section aimed to collect the respondents' socio-demographic information.

From this survey it was possible to develop indices of both the cultural capital and socioeconomic capital of the respondents, starting with the main variables of parents' educational qualification and professional categories.

The results obtained show how, during the pandemic period beginning 2020, irrespective of whether the comparison was with cultural capital or socioeconomic capital, students with lesser capital resources on average experienced more negative feelings than was the case for those with higher capital resources. As seen in Table 10.1, [1] persons with lower resources are more likely to declare themselves angry, bored, depressed, nervous, powerless and sad, with differences between the two groups sometimes greater than 10 percentage points. Contrarily, during the same pandemic period, people with higher cultural and socioeconomic capital were more likely than lower-resourced persons to state they were amused, confident, proactive and happy. Furthermore, these differences were transversal among the interviewed population – that is, with no differences between those departing and incoming to Italy, nor with respect to any home country. In other words, the effects of resource base, high or low, were transversal in the population, without distinction by country. In addition to this, the information about the COVID-19 situation (i.e., if the interviewee has been diagnosed with COVID-19 and where he or she spent the period of illness) underline no discrepancy among responses.

TABLE 10.1 Emotions experienced during the 2020 pandemic period, by cultural and socioeconomic capital (%)

Types of basic emotions	*Cultural capital*		*Socioeconomic capital*	
	Low	*High*	*Low*	*High*
Afraid	36.9	21.3	27.0	28.2
Amused	10.6	24.5	22.2	25.0
Angry	42.1	26.0	34.9	25.0
Bored	63.1	54.2	61.9	53.9
Confident	28.9	29.8	17.5	26.5
Demoralized	42.2	31.3	38.1	37.5
Depressed	36.9	20.2	35.0	20.3
Happy	15.8	38.8	23.8	39.1
Nervous	44.7	35.6	42.9	37.5
Powerless	55.4	41.0	50.8	43.0
Proactive	23.7	30.3	17.5	31.3
Restless	31.6	30.8	25.4	28.9
Sad	44.7	25.5	39.7	24.2

Source: Authors' own elaboration.

Examining some of the most strongly contrasting aspects between the two subsets of interviewees, it emerges that about 40 and 34.9 percent, respectively, of those with low cultural and socioeconomic capital feel the greatest uncertainty about the future, compared to only 30.3 and 29.7 percent of those who feel this way, respectively, with high cultural and socioeconomic capital.

On the other hand, about 50 percent of students with both high cultural and socioeconomic capital reported suffering feelings of distance from loved ones, compared with only 34.2 percent of those with low cultural capital and 44.4 percent of those with low socioeconomic capital. Students with greater capital resources were also more likely to suffer the loss of freedom of movement (41 percent, against the 26.3 percent for students with low cultural capital; 43 percent against the 41.3 percent for those with high *versus* low socioeconomic capital). This could possibly be explained by the need of higher resourced students to live the pandemic period with fellow students or other cohabitants, rather than taking advantage of more typical options, for this population, of freely returning to the family of origin.

Other results emerging from the analyses underline that persons with low (*versus* high) cultural capital are more likely to report difficulties or dissatisfaction with daily time management in the pandemic context (13.2 compared to 5.9 percent), and dissatisfaction with closure of the school environment (36.8 compared to 23.4 percent); people with low socioeconomic capital are also more likely to feel that during the pandemic period they have been unproductive or "without useful activity" (9.5 compared to 3.9 percent of those with high resources).

Coherent with these last indications, the responses to the question "What do you wish to do in the near future, among the things you have not been able to do because of restrictions related to the COVID-19 emergency?" were particularly interesting. Indeed, the lesser-resourced individuals expressed frustration at the loss of their productive school or work environments. It was the respondents with high cultural capital who were most likely to want to return to the people closest to them (20.7 percent), while those with low socioeconomic capital were least likely to report such longing (13.2 percent). Instead, the persons with low cultural and socioeconomic capital were the most driven to want to continue their studies abroad: 44.7 percent, compared (for example) to those with high cultural capital, of whom only 23.9 percent indicated such priorities.

The states of mind and feelings reported by the students then influence their perspectives and perceptions of the future. Compared to respondents with more cultural and socioeconomic capital, the respondents with lesser resources were clearly more fearful concerning what they viewed as their individual and social futures. Looking at the future, they were more likely to report conditions of fear, anger, demoralization, depression, nervousness, sadness and feelings of being powerless. In this sense, one of the most important findings of the research confirm that financial precarity and insecurity prior to the health emergency made dealing with the pandemic harder, particularly for those in precarious and instable economic conditions (Garthwaite et al., 2022).

Contrarily, those with high cultural and socioeconomic capital were more likely to declare slight optimism in thinking ahead. From Table 10.2[2] it can also be seen that those with low cultural and low socioeconomic capital were more

TABLE 10.2 Feelings concerning the effects about the post-COVID-19 scenario, by cultural and socioeconomic capital (%)

	Cultural capital		*Socioeconomic capital*	
	Low	*High*	*Low*	*High*
The emergency will worsen my economic condition and that of my family	42.1	25.0	41.3	26.6
The COVID-19 will undermine international political relations	44.7	35.1	44.4	32.8
The COVID-19 will lead to the most severe national economic crisis	55.3	43.6	63.5	43.0
The COVID-19 will lead to the most severe worldwide economic crisis	47.4	41.0	61.9	40.6
When the emergency ends, substantial funds will be allocated to adjust the national public health system	50.0	28.2	38.1	28.9
At the end of the emergency more funds will be allocated for scientific research in the medical and pharmacological fields	55.3	35.1	39.7	35.9

Source: Authors' own elaboration.

worried about their financial condition: compared to those with high capital, this group was 40 percent more likely to believe their personal and family financial status would worsen. In general, the lesser resourced group, especially the subset with low socioeconomic capital, was also more likely to believe that COVID-19 would lead to severe national and worldwide economic crises. Moreover, about 44 percent of the lesser resourced students, compared to 32.8 percent of those with greater capital, thought that there would be a deterioration of international political relations.

There were, however, several areas where the lower-resourced group expressed more optimism about social futures. Among these, particularly for the students with lower cultural capital, there was greater anticipation that, after the COVID-19 emergency, more funds would be allocated to the national health system, and medical and pharmacological sectors. Those with low resources, in general, were also more likely to feel there would be greater "individual accountability" (47.4 and 46 percent, compared to 35.1 and 32 percent, respectively, assessing the groups of low cultural and socioeconomic resources compared to high cultural and socioeconomic resources); also, that there would be a greater sense of national belonging (31.6 and 25.4 percent, compared to 22.3 and 21.9 percent, for the groups with high cultural and socioeconomic resources); finally, that individuals would find more support from local communities for personal needs (47.4 and 44.4 percent, compared to 33.5 and 29.7 percent, for those with high resources).

Change in Physical Well-being: A Comparison between Pre- and Post- Pandemic

The questionnaire submitted to interviewees included a specific section on how their physical activity and health might have changed since the onset of the pandemic. From the Figure 10.2, it emerges that those with high cultural and socioeconomic capital were more likely to report an increase in physical activity, engaging in exercise mostly at home, once or twice per week, for aims of maintaining health (45.2 and 54.7 percent shares for those with high cultural and socioeconomic capital, compared to 31.6 and 30.2 percent for those with low capital) or for improving physical appearance (respectively 20.7 and 24.8 percent, compared to 13.2 and 19 percent). Interestingly, not only were the students with lower cultural and socioeconomic status more likely to report a decrease in frequency of physical activity, before and post-pandemic, this was a decrease from an average starting point of lower frequency to begin with, compared to the higher-resourced group. The lower-resourced group was also more likely to report a motivation of "weight loss" for any exercise or sport activity, with frequencies of 23.7 and 23.8 percent for students with low cultural and socioeconomic resources, compared to 12.2 and 7.8 percent reporting this motivation, respectively, among those with high cultural and socioeconomic resources.

For the lower-resourced students, there was more likelihood in general of their overall health situation worsening, in terms of quality of food, consumption of alcohol, smoking and sleeping (Table 10.3). Respondents with low cultural and socioeconomic levels reported increased consumption of convenience food: 28.9 and 17.5 percent, compared respectively with only 18.6 and 14.1 percent reporting such increases among those with high cultural and socioeconomic resources. Lower-resourced students were more likely to report an increase in skipping main meals: 28.9 and 30.2 percent, compared to 23.9 and 25.8 percent, respectively, for the groups of low *versus* high cultural and socioeconomic resources.

Repeating the same comparisons of the four groups – two of low cultural and socioeconomic resources and two of high resources – we consistently see data of relative worsening of health conditions for the lower-resourced groups: 10.5 and 19 percent report increased consumption of alcoholic beverages with meals, compared to 9 and 11.7 percent for the higher resourced groups; 15.8 and 15.9 percent report increased use of alcohol outside mealtimes compared to 14.4 and 14.1 percent for higher-resourced groups; 18.4 and 11.1 percent report increased smoking (tobacco or electronic cigarettes) against the only 6.4 and 5.5 percent of those with high cultural and socioeconomic resources.

Finally, the lower-resourced students were more likely to report difficulties in falling asleep, especially those among the group with low cultural capital (36.8 percent, compared to 28.7 percent of respondents with high cultural capital).

Concluding Remarks: Characterizing Profiles in the Light of Two Interpretative Axes

It should be noted that the analyses of data found no noteworthy differences relating to the nationality of the persons examined, as well as the possible diagnosis of COVID-19.

TABLE 10.3 Comparison about the frequency of several habits between pre- and post-pandemic period, by cultural and socioeconomic capital (%)

	Cultural capital		*Socioeconomic capital*	
	Low	*High*	*Low*	*High*
Consuming convenience food	28.9	18.6	17.5	14.1
Skipping one of the main meals (breakfast, lunch or dinner)	28.9	23.9	30.2	25.8
Eating main meals (breakfast, lunch or dinner) while watching TV, PC, etc.	31.6	37.2	31.7	37.5
Drinking alcoholic beverages outside meals time	15.8	14.4	15.9	14.1
Consuming alcoholic beverages during meals time	10.5	9.0	19.0	11.7
Smoking cigarettes or electronic cigarettes	18.4	6.4	11.1	5.5
Difficulty in falling asleep	36.8	28.7	33.3	34.4

Source: Authors' own elaboration.

In other words, the interactive effects of the individual's cultural and socioeconomic capital took precedence over those from any citizenship, geographic localization or COVID-19 diagnosis. Moreover, confirming the Parsonian proposal explained in the previous section, the the empirical results obtained seem to confirm that the decisions of individuals are embedded in and influenced by their cultural frame of reference.

Returning to the conceptual map of dimensions and indicators seen in Figure 10.1, the interpretative axis of distinction along destruction *versus* rebirth serves to indicate the prevalence of attitudes of optimism/pessimism towards the future in the individual's responses. A second axis of interpretation concerns the orientation towards immediate/future temporality. Working from this framework, it is

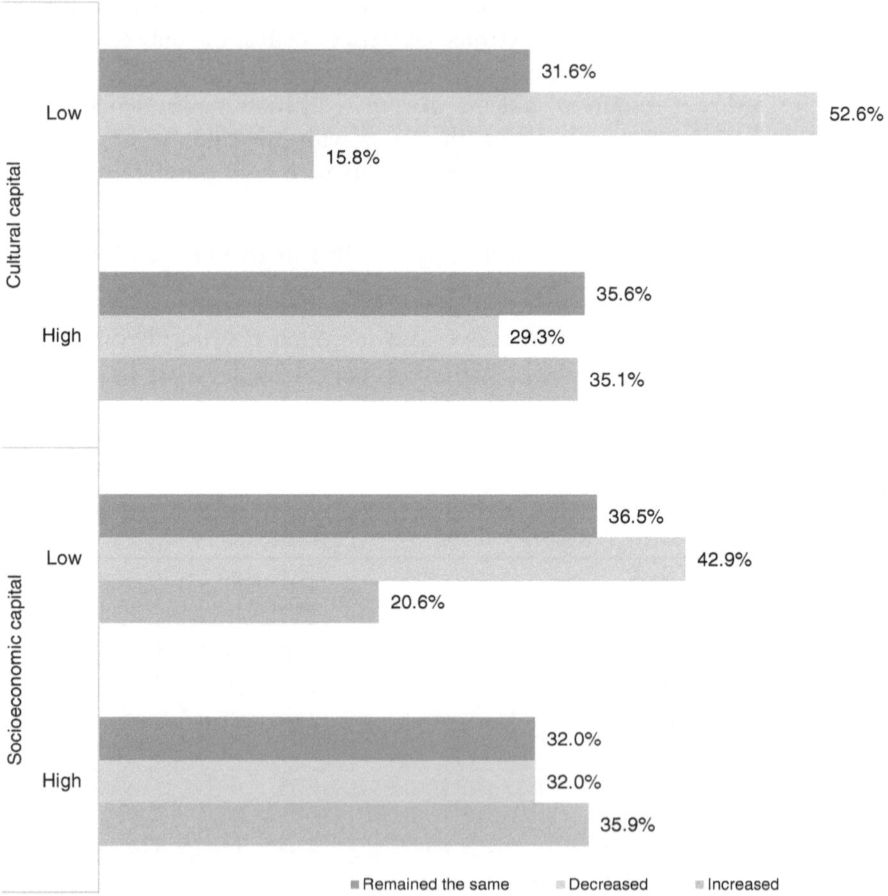

FIGURE 10.2 Comparison of the frequency of physical activity between pre- and post-pandemic period by cultural and socioeconomic capital (%).

Source: Authors' own elaboration.

possible to construct two characterizing profiles, of the cognitive-emotional dimension and dimension of intention to action, for the cases of the two groups of lesser and greater cultural and socioeconomic capital.

Low cultural and socioeconomic capital. On the destruction/rebirth axis, the profile of individuals with low cultural and socioeconomic capital is characterized by more pessimistic cognitive views and negative emotions. Individuals of this group were more likely to declare feelings of anger, boredom, depression, nervousness, powerlessness and sadness, and state that their most intense feelings are those of uncertainty about the future.

Consistent with this, on the immediate/future temporality axis, the group of lesser-resourced individuals clearly tended to express much greater inability to project into the future. They were more likely to report worries over their financial status, and beliefs that COVID-19 pandemic would lead to severe national and worldwide economic crises. Regarding both their personal and social spheres, these respondents were more likely to express anxiety over the future, again responding that in this perspective they felt frightened, angry, demoralized, depressed, nervous, powerless and sad.

Uncertainty can lead to desires for immediate relief, limited conceptions of temporality and loss of long-term perspective, all of which then translate into propensities for unproductive and contrasting actions, such as eating excessively for the immediate satisfaction of "filling up", *versus* also wanting to lose weight. Subjects of the lower-resourced profile record low values in frequency of the physical activity and, where they are active, to find the relative motivation in the desire to lose weight. At the same time, individuals of this group, in the observed emergency context, were more likely to increase consumption of convenience food and of alcoholic beverages (both during and outside mealtimes), more likely to increase smoking and to have trouble in falling asleep.

High cultural and socioeconomic capital. Along the destruction/rebirth axis, however, the profile of individuals with high cultural and socioeconomic capital was characterized by optimistic orientations to action and emotions. Individuals of this group were more likely to declare they were amused, confident, proactive and happy following the 2020 onset of the pandemic. Due to restrictions on movement, however, individuals of this same group were more likely to lament the distance from loved ones, and the lack of their typical freedom of movement.

Consistent with this, along the immediate/future temporality axis, subjects with higher resources were more likely to declare being quite satisfied concerning their future. In general, with greater access to resources and so less urgent financial pressures or problems, they were more oriented towards long-term planning. To confirm, these same individuals were more likely to maintain or increase their level of physical activity, for motivations of long-term healthy lifestyle and improved physical appearance.

Notes

* This chapter was written as part of a research programme financed with funds from the Sapienza University of Rome. It is the result of the joint work of all the authors; thus, everybody has contributed. However, Barbara Sonzogni was specifically involved in the "Introduction" and in the "Change in Physical Well-being" section, while Gabriella D'Ambrosio was involved in the "How COVID -19 Exacerbates Social Inequalities" and "During and Post-Pandemic" sections. The "Concluding Remarks" were co-written by the authors.

1 The values shown in Table 10.1 are the sums of responses "often" and "very often".

2 The values in Table 10.2 are the sums of responses "agree" and "strongly agree".

References

Adams-Prassl, Abi, Teodora Boneva, Marta Golin, and Christopher Rauh. 2020. "Inequality in the impact of the coronavirus shock: evidence from real time surveys". *Journal of Public Economics* 189: 104245.

Bambra, Clare, Ryan Riordan, John Ford, and Fiona Matthews. 2020. "The COVID-19 pandemic and health inequalities". *Journal of Epidemiology and Community Health* 74: 964–968.

Barnes, Sarah B., Deekshita Ramanarayana, and Sara Matthews. 2021. *The Lasting Effects of the COVID-19 Pandemic on Women's Work, Health and Safety*. Washington: Wilson Center.

Blundell, Richard, Monica Costa Dias, Robert Joyce, and Xiaowei Xu. 2020. "COVID-19 and Inequalities". *Fiscal Studies* 41, 2: 291–319.

Bonolis, Maurizio. 2007. *Storicità e storia della sociologia*. Milano: FrancoAngeli.

Bonolis, Maurizio, Giovanna Gianturco, and Barbara Sonzogni. 2020. "Angoscia e identità di immagine. Differenza fra guerra e pandemia". In *La società catastrofica: vita e relazioni sociali ai tempi dell'emergenza Covid-19*, edited by Carmelo Lombardo and Sergio Mauceri, 169–180. Milano: FrancoAngeli.

Carstairs, Vera, and Russell Morris. 1989. "Deprivation and mortality: an alternative to social class?". *Community Medicine* 11, 3: 210–219.

Coleman, James Samuel. 1990. *Foundation of Social Theory*. Cambridge: Harvard University Press.

Deaton, Angus, and Charles I. Jones. 2021. *COVID-19 and Global Income Inequality*. Cambridge: National Bureau of Economic Research.

Durkheim, Émile. 1914. "Le Dualisme de la nature humaine et ses conditions sociales". *Scientia* 15: 206–221.

Durkheim, Émile. 1925. *L'Éducation morale*. Paris: Alcan.

Elster, Jon. 2007. *Agir contre soi: la faiblesse de volonté*. Paris: Odile Jacob.

Fang, Peixun, Adam Kennedy, and Danielle Resnick. 2020. *Scaling up and Sustaining Social Protection under COVID-19*. Washington: International Food Policy Research Institute.

Garthwaite, Kayleigh, Ruth Patrick, Maddy Power, Anna Tarrant, and Rosalie Warnock, eds. 2022. *COVID-19 Collaborations: Researching Poverty and Low-Income Family Life during the Pandemic*. Bristol, Great Britain: Bristol University Press.

Goffman, Erving. 1961. *Encounters: Two Studies in the Sociology of Interaction*. Indianapolis: The Bobbs-Merrill Co. Inc.

Goldblatt, Peter. 1989. "Mortality by social class, 1971–85". *Population Trends* 56: 6–15.

Gunter, Barrie. 2022. *Psychological Impact of Behaviour Restrictions during the Pandemic. Lessons from COVID-19*. New York: Routledge.
Haas, John G. 2021. *COVID-19 and Psychology. People and Society in Times of Pandemic*. Wiesbaden: Springer.
International Association for the Evaluation of Educational Achievement – UNESCO. 2022. *The Impact of the COVID-19 Pandemic on Education. International Evidence from the Responses to Educational Disruption Survey (REDS)*. Paris: United Nations Educational, Scientific and Cultural Organization (UNESCO).
Kawachi, Ichiro. 2020. "Covid-19 and the 'rediscovery' of health inequities". *International Journal of Epidemiology* 49: 1415–1418.
Khan, Nazneen. 2022. *COVID-19 and Childhood Inequality*. London: Routledge.
Koehler, Claudia, George Psacharopoulos, and Loes Van der Graaf. 2022. *The Impact of Covid-19 on the Education of Disadvantaged Children and the Socio-economic Consequences Thereof*. Luxembourg: Publications Office of the European Union.
Lazarsfeld, Paul Felix. 1958. "Evidence and inference in social research". *Daedalus* 87, 4: 99–109.
Łuszczyńska, Maria, and Marvin Formosa. 2021. *Ageing and COVID-19: Making Sense of a Disrupted World*. London: Routledge.
Mangone, Emiliana. 2018. *Dalle "calamità" di Sorokin alla "rinascita"*. Milano: Franco Angeli.
Michie, Jonathan, and Maura Sheehan, eds. 2022. *The Political Economy of COVID-19: COVID-19, Inequality and Government Responses*. New York: Routledge.
Molina, George, and Eduardo Ortiz-Juarez. 2020. *Temporary Basic Income. Protecting Poor and Vulnerable People in Developing Countries*. New York: United Nations Development Programme.
Navarro, Sharon A., and Samantha L. Hernandez. 2022. *The Color of Covid-19: The Racial Inequality of Marginalized Communities*. London: Routledge.
OECD (Organization for Economic Co-operation and Development). "2020. OECD Policy Responses to Covid-19 (Covid-19). Covid-19: Protecting people and societies". Available at www.oecd.org/coronavirus/policy-responses/covid-19-protecting-people-and-societies-e5c9de1a/.
OECD (Organization for Economic Co-operation and Development). 2021a. *COVID-19 and Well-being: Life in the Pandemic*. Paris: OECD Publishing.
OECD (Organization for Economic Co-operation and Development). 2021b. *Tackling the mental health impact of the COVID-19 crisis: An Integrated, Whole-of-Society Response*. Paris: OECD Publishing.
Oxfam. 2020. *Fighting Inequality in the Time of COVID-19: The Commitment to Reducing Inequality Index 2020*. Brussels and New York: Development Finance International, Oxfam.
Papyrakis, Elissaios. 2022. *COVID-19 and International Development*. Switzerland: Springer.
Parsons, Talcott. 1951. *The Social System*. New York: Free Press of Glencoe.
Parsons, Talcott, and Robert F. Bales. 1955. *Family, Socialization and Interaction Process*. New York: Free Press of Glencoe.
Ryan, J. Michael, and Serena Nanda. 2022. *COVID-19: Social Inequalities and Human Possibilities*. London: Routledge.
Smith, Katherine, Kamaldeep Bhui, and Andrea Cipriani. 2020. "COVID-19, mental health and ethic minorities". *Evidence-Based Mental Health* 23, 3: 89–90.
Solomos, John. 2021. *Race and Ethnicity in Pandemic Times*. London: Routledge.
Sonzogni, Barbara, and Gabriella D'Ambrosio. 2022. "Enattivismo, intenzionalità, simulazione computazionale: una prospettiva di ricerca". *Sociologia e Ricerca Sociale* 128: 20–34.

Sorokin, Pitrim Aleksandrovič. 2010. *Society, Culture, and Personality: The Structure and Dynamics*. Brunswick and London: Transaction Publishers.

Sumner, Andrew, Eduardo Ortiz-Juarez, and Chris Roy. 2020. *Precarity and the Pandemic: COVID-19 and Poverty Incidence, Intensity, and Severity In Developing Countries*. Helsinki: United Nations University World Institute for Development Economics Research.

The World Bank. 2021. "2021 Year in Review in 11 Charts: The Inequality Pandemic". Available at www.worldbank.org/en/news/feature/2021/12/20/year-2021-in-review-the-inequality-pandemic.

Thomas, Melvin, Loren Henderson, and Hayward Derrick Horton. 2022. *Race, Ethnicity, and the Covid-19 Pandemic*. Cincinnati: University of Cincinnati Press.

Thomeer, Mieke Beth, Myles D. Moody, and Jenjira Yahirun. 2022. "Racial and ethnic disparities in mental health and mental health care during the COVID-19 pandemic". *Journal of Racial and Ethnic Health Disparities*, 22: 1–16.

Vargas Hill, Ruth, and Ambar Narayan. 2020. "COVID-19 and inequality: a review of the evidence on likely impact and policy options". *Centre for Disaster Protection Working Paper* 3: 1–28.

Weber, Max. 1922a. *Wirtschaft und Gesellschaft*. Tübingen: Mohr.

Weber, Max. 1922b. *Gesammelte Aufsätze zur Wissenschaftslehre*. Tübingen: Mohr.

Weill, Joakim A., Matthieu Stigler, Olivier Deschenes, and Michael R. Springborn. 2020. "Social distancing responses to COVID-19 emergency declarations strongly differentiated by income". *Proceedings of the National Academy of Sciences (PNAS)* 117: 19658–19660.

Wilkinson, Richard G. 1989. "Class mortality differentials, income distribution and trends in poverty 1921–1981". *Journal of Social Policy* 18, 3: 307–335.

11

THE DIGITAL (IN)EQUITY CRISIS DURING THE COVID-19 PANDEMIC

Narratives from the Field

Yaprak Dalat Ward and Anil Yasin Ar

This chapter presents a study with a phenomenological focus revealing how the digital inequity issue turned into a major crisis when the face-to-face education was forced into virtual teaching during the COVID-19 pandemic lockdowns as reported by the schoolteachers. The chapter concludes with critical questions to be considered for discussion.

The significance of the pandemic, together with the newly introduced online teaching modality, termed emergency remote teaching (ERT), and the existing digital inequity issue led to collecting narratives from 46 teachers during the lockdowns. The thematic and sentiment analysis of these lived experiences revealed that digital inequity was a major crisis presented in three phases: *the alarm mode, the shift mode*, and *the hot wash mode*. As a result, this research not only captured the digital inequity crisis in educational settings, exposing the impacts of social and economic inequities, but also underscored that this was not a standalone crisis but a multilayered one encompassing political, economic, and social factors.

Beyond documenting the digital inequity crisis, the chapter concludes with critical questions derived from the findings to set the tone for further academic, as well as practical, discussions. Moreover, the authors anticipate that the research findings could be beneficial regarding stakeholder engagement, such as thinking through preventative measures concerning the political, economic, and social implications of digital inequity and inviting further research to be conducted on this topic.

Introduction to the Study

Digital information and communication technologies (ICTs) have become increasingly extensive, specifically as the centerpiece of social interactions. These technologies enrich connectivity and communication (Moore et al. 2018),

DOI: 10.4324/9781003459682-13

and under social theory, increase human interactions and enable individuals to access various capitals (economic, social, or otherwise) with ease. Underlined as "the near global exposure of almost all individuals to various forms of mass media content" (Moore et al. 2018, 13), the uses of ICTs range from being employed, citizenry, free flow of information and education (to a certain extent) to organization of various state departments and governments; and, recently, the delivery of financial aid to COVID-19 victims (Ar and Abbas 2021). However, the initiatives employed, and strategies devised to ease the adoption of ICTs, have so far failed to deliver the desired outcomes. Although the intended results of these initiatives had been set for the betterment of societies, the rushed and miscalculated implementation steps resulted in unwanted consequences. One of the adverse outcomes of the mentioned missteps is "digital inequity" and its adverse progression over the years. Although many experts have indicated the existing gap in education as well as in civic life concerning the intersection of management, policy, and education perspectives, the severity of the digital divide is still not fully recognized and continues to be minimized (Olesen 2022). Despite efforts to mitigate and eradicate digital inequity, it has become more conspicuous with the COVID-19 pandemic, turning into a major crisis, as reported in this research.

In March 2020, when the COVID-19 outbreak was declared a pandemic (World Health Organization 2020), many nations implemented diverse strategies to prevent the spread of the virus, ranging from mask mandates to lockdowns. Triggered by the state of emergency, medical authorities and educational institutions acknowledged that face-to-face learning modality was futile, as it would cause a faster spread of the COVID-19 virus. Under these circumstances, as a prevention strategy, the ERT modality was introduced as the only option for uninterrupted face-to-face education for most institutions. During this time, not every individual had the same experience during the transition. While certain socioeconomic factions benefited from this shift tremendously and felt the safe environment created by the government, economically disadvantaged individuals and families were tremendously and negatively impacted by the initiatives. It is the significance of this context from which this study originated.

The research found that the digital inequity problem was amplified into a multilayered crisis encompassing political, economic, and social factors. The implications these findings hold for our society are such that, as ICTs become more integrated, society becomes increasingly interdependent. While interdependency presents numerous opportunities, those with limited access to ICTs are at a significant disadvantage in today's hyperconnected society, which can result in isolation. Ignoring individuals and families' restricted access to ICT tools and, thus, limiting these individuals' employability and citizenry, leads to a grimmer social picture. Therefore, a large-scale comprehensive, inclusive, equitable digital reform must be carried out. To make this vision a reality, decision-makers must collaborate and urgently develop policies to eliminate or minimize digital inequity by addressing individuals from all social classes and socioeconomic backgrounds. Otherwise, as the pandemic has demonstrated, taking short-term actions, ignoring the impact of digital inequity could deprive societies of opportunities to overcome future crises.

Inequity as Opposed to Inequality

Defining the terms "equality" and "equity" will enable the readers to note why authors preferred using the term "inequity" rather than "inequality." First, while "equality" and "equity" are used interchangeably in diverse contexts, experts point out significant differences. Equality is "often depicted as uniformity in rights or experiences despite differences in resources, capabilities and backgrounds" (Levy et al. 2006, 3). Moreover, these are two different words derived from the Latin root *aequus* in the following manner: "The distinction between the two has to do with whether we're taking the circumstances of the situation into consideration while making judgments about 'even' or 'just.' If we are not, we have equality; if we are, we have equity" (Berg 2022, 8). Furthermore, inequality is described as a "violation of human dignity" and "a socio-cultural order, which (for most of us) reduces our capabilities to function as human beings ... and takes many forms" (Therborn 2014, 1).

In addition, given technology's rapid development, "inequity" is the most fitting in this context, as it describes each person's distinct levels of knowledge, skills, and needs, and addresses other factors rather than just accessibility to a specific set of tangible or intangible assets. Finally, it encapsulates the required conditions and prerequisites that an individual needs to have to benefit and derive utility from the consumption or usage of any tangible or intangible items.

Moreover, digital inequity is a major defect in the education system and in the social justice field (Stewart 2000). To understand the digital divide better, it is crucial to scrutinize the significance of the term "digital self-sufficiency," conceptualized as having the essential computer hardware and affordable broadband access with a combination of skills to be able to make use of digital technologies. Based on this definition, not having the required access or device causes fractions in education and communities: "Inequitable access to electronic devices and effective internet connections contributes to opportunity, achievement, and equity gaps in education" (Moore et al. 2018). Such inequities prevent students from fully participating in a "creative, active, and innovative" learning environment, while educators struggle to deliver the state-of-the-art knowledge that is necessary (Salceanu 2020). Furthermore, lack of digital self-sufficiency not only obstructs students' ability to participate in learning activities in various learning mediums but also takes away opportunities from citizenry regarding "civic and cultural participation, employment, lifelong learning, and access to essential services" (National Digital Inclusion Alliance 2019, 1). Such disparities become a significant barrier to skill development and economic growth in most countries. Without equal access to technology, individuals from marginalized communities further experience discrimination and may be unable to thrive in the modern workforce, leading to an underdeveloped labor market and persistent income inequality. In short, as shown in this research, shifting education modalities or expecting citizens to survive or make contributions without considering such struggles can have negative consequences.

When most institutions had to abruptly adapt ERT during the lockdowns, the initial outburst stemmed from students and educators, who had varying levels of broadband access or even no access in their environments, exposing digital haves and have-nots in a stark manner. The underserved households lacked affordable and robust broadband internet services and, as a result, students and teachers alike struggled to conduct their day-to-day teaching/learning activities. During this time, causing a domino effect, the smoldering digital inequity became a major crisis which could no longer be dismissed. As a result, most institutions and societies quickly came to the realization that many teachers, students, and citizens did not have the required access, nor were they proficient in "applications and online content designed to enable and encourage self-sufficiency, participation, and collaboration" (National Digital Inclusion Alliance 2019). In addition to coordinating limited resources, inadequate communication, collaboration, and interoperability quickly turned the situation into a crisis-induced chaos (Kapucu et al. 2010).

The Differences Between Online Teaching and Emergency Remote Teaching

The significance of ERT makes it imperative to emphasize the differences between "online teaching" and "ERT" in order to understand the root cause of the problem. The ERT modality was introduced as a temporary means of sustaining uninterrupted education during the lockdowns and, therefore, should not be considered a typical online modality. Under normal circumstances traditional virtual teaching follows the principle of creating an education system that requires accessibility and a certain level of digital competencies. It leverages formal education structures and well-established pedagogical approaches to provide and deliver high-standard learning outcomes. However, ERT refers to the translation and transformation of the existing face-to-face education format into digital learning commons. The distinction is stark: "a well-planned online learning experiences are meaningfully different from courses offered online in response to a crisis or disaster … it is this careful design process that will be absent in most cases in these emergency shifts" (Hodges et al. 2020, 1).

With online education, as teachers are separated from students in time and place, they all experience "a whole new set of physical, emotional, and psychological problems that can be experienced as the technology is used extensively" (Palloff and Pratt 1999, 7). Under ideal conditions, to solve such problems, educational institutions provide training in course design preparation and digital competencies and offer technical support services.

When disasters, large-scale national events, and emergencies abruptly appear and intensify the nature of needs during abnormal conditions (Ucok-Sayrak and Brazelton 2022), and contact teaching shifts to an virtual environment, the three fundamentals of teaching – method, media, and modality – urgently need to be reconfigured and adapted.

Additionally, anecdotal evidence reveals that changing swiftly from contact teaching to remote teaching can present significant problems for both teachers and students. One challenge may be that "Online learners must be able to determine where and how to seek help and make decisions concerning the most appropriate sources for such help" (Lynch and Dembo 2004, 5). Prior to the pandemic, schools provided students with devices used in classroom settings. For students, receiving help and being motivated were expected parts of face-to-face learning. However, with ERT, help and motivation abruptly had to become secondary or nonexistent as the modality, method, and media shifted. Most teachers did not have the time to learn or adapt to the newly implemented fundamentals of online teaching. When asked to leave behind the comfort of their classrooms, together with their control and confidence, teachers felt forced to perform and exist in an unknown cyberterritory, resulting in another layer of fear, anxiety, and trauma added to the concern of the pandemic. With such a rapid transformation to ERT, asymptomatic digital gaps and systematic failures became more significant and highly problematic. With the pandemic, when most countries moved to online education, there were growing concerns about students who were socially and economically disadvantaged (UNESCO 2023). Although a set of ten key recommendations were issued to ensure that learning remained uninterrupted during the pandemic (UNESCO 2023), in numerous institutions, these recommendations became ineffective and had to be disregarded because of the existing factors contributing to digital inequity, one of which manifested itself as the absence of quality technical support. Once asked to shift, teachers felt unsupported in tackling ERT. Students were unable to have access to critical support to set up their learning environment or could not cater to the demands of the online learning experience. In short, ERT was a temporary way out which overlooked various required elements that made up quality online teaching and learning (Quality Matters 2015).

How did a Smoldering Digital Inequity Issue Turn into a Crisis?

Prior to the pandemic, despite warnings, red flags, and stark reminders of national and global data (International Telecommunication Union and UNESCO 2020), the digital inequity problem had been intentionally or inadvertently ignored, or at best avoided, perhaps due to human nature minimizing major risks: "minor risks are exaggerated, major risks which have further impacts are minimized, overlooked" (Sunstein 2005, ix). When the lockdowns forced students and teachers to cybercommunities, the divide could no longer be dismissed and, in fact, became highly visible at an alarming rate, forcing the world to pay attention to its true meaning.

The word "crisis" has differing definitions and interpretations based on personal, professional experiences, or contextual differences such as businesses, institutions, communities, and countries an individual exists: "The normal flow of life is occasionally interrupted by critical episodes, accompanied by a sense of threat and insecurity, challenging the way in which people understand the world around them" (Mladen 2019, 9). While these interruptions may have harmful consequences, their severity depends on the crisis management. Additionally, because disasters/crises are unexpected events, the possibility of responsiveness is disrupted (Quarantelli 1985).

Although crisis experts view crises as unforeseeable and unpredictable, it is possible to mitigate them by having an appropriate preparedness plan. This is due to the belief that, even though each crisis is unique due to diverse factors, they may still have similarities to various degrees. In other words, previous experiences in the crisis can inform how to tackle future crises (Pearson and Clair 1998). Even though the COVID-19 pandemic was a novel disaster, teachers could have managed the shift in education modalities effectively if the specific competencies and protocols had been mapped out in advance.

A Course Activity and the Discussions on Lived Experiences

This study's phenomenological approach is "descriptions of what people experience and how it is that they experience what they experience" (Patton 2015, 117). Through analyzing the individual experiences of 46 teachers (ages ranging from 24 to 42 and from various states in the USA), the authors were able to capture the digital inequity crisis intensified by the pandemic lockdowns.

The teachers were also students in an online graduate program at a university in the USA and the data were curated from a course activity. For this research only the spring 2020, fall 2020, and spring 2021 semesters were included, since this period symbolized the forced lockdowns and adaptation of ERT. For the course activity, teachers were asked to map their experiences and interactions by means of reflections and discussions. The course provided learning objectives ranging from understanding underserved populations to inequalities and inequities in schools and societies. Due to the topics, the focus was transformative learning, challenging the learners to "assess their value system and worldview and be [sic] subsequently changed by the experience" (Quinnan 1997, 42) by means of core elements including individual experience, deep learning, critical reflections, and dialogues. The students shared their lived experiences, perceptions, and feelings related to these inequalities in real-world settings, engaging in critical reflections, discussions, and interacting with each other in the form of dialogues (Taylor 1998).

The course materials included open educational resources, current research articles, and materials available for public use, and were continuously revised based on political, economic, and social events. A quality assurance benchmark for online teaching was employed (Quality Matters 2015), promoting cognitive, social, and instructor presence with three interactions as part of adult learning: learner-learner, learner-content, and learner-instructor.

The narrative derived from a discussion activity with the following objectives: 1) understand the meaning of *digital inequity*; 2) analyze the socioeconomic impact of digital inequity in education; 3) evaluate the terms "problem/issue," "crisis," and "crisis management." After a critical reflection phase, students discussed their experiences using the following guiding questions: 1) Prior to the pandemic, what was your institution's strategic approach to digital inequities? 2) During ERT, how did your institution manage the digital inequity issue? 3) How did you feel about ERT? 4) How do you and your institution keep up with technology? 5) How did your institution cope with digital literacy?

Prior to reporting their experiences on digital inequity as part of a discussion activity, the teachers were required to read the following materials to be able to reflect and challenge their deeply rooted assumptions which included: "Section I. Understanding (In)equity in Technology"; "Section II. Understanding Issues, Crises, and Crisis Management"; and "Section III. Understanding Lived Experience and Interactions." Introducing such fundamental knowledge allowed teachers to accurately interpret and report their experiences and surroundings.

Section I: Understanding (In)equity in Technology

Due to their limited knowledge on digital self-sufficiency, it was fundamental to start with the definitions, including digital literacy, digital self-sufficiency, digital divide, digital equity, and digital inclusion, to be able to make reliable observations. The following materials were covered and discussed so the students could make observations and reflect on their experiences.

1 ***Digital Equity.*** Understand digital equity defined as "a unified voice for home broadband access, public broadband access, personal devices and local technology training and support programs" (National Digital Inclusion Alliance 2019, 1).
2 ***Technology, Growth, Inequality.*** Outline and exemplify technology, growth, and inequality based on the following reading materials: "Tackling the inequality pandemic: is there a cure?" (Qureshi 2020) and "Technology, growth, and inequality: changing dynamics in the digital era" (Qureshi 2020, 1).
3 ***Effects of Digital Learning in Economically Disadvantaged Contexts.*** Analyze and evaluate the effects of digital learning in underserved contexts based on the following reading: "The state of broadband: tackling digital inequalities – a decade for action" (International Telecommunication Union and UNESCO 2020).
4 ***The Next-Normal.*** Collaborate and create *the next-normal* blueprint to promote digital equity in schools by reading the following report: "The next normal: the recovery will be digital – digitizing at speed and scale" (McKinsey & Company 2020).

Section II: Understanding Problems/Issues, Crisis, and Crisis Management

Recall the differences between a problem/an issue, a crisis, distinct types of crises, and understand crisis management. The following materials were covered and discussed.

1. ***Disaster vs. Crisis.*** Understand the difference between disaster and crisis to be able to interpret the context of COVID-19 and crisis management by reading "That is disaster? The need for clarification in definition and conceptualization in research" (Quarantelli 1985).
2. ***Problem, Issue or Crisis?*** Recognize the difference by reviewing "Issue or problem? managing the difference and averting crises"(Jaques 2007b).
3. ***Crisis Management.*** Interpret and evaluate crisis management based on "Issue management and crisis management: an integrated, non-linear, relational construct"(Jaques 2007a).
4. ***Crisis Leadership.*** Understand crisis and crisis leadership by reading Parts I and 2 of a book entitled *Crisis Leadership: How to Lead in Times of Crisis, Threat and Uncertainty* (Johnson 2017). In addition, read "How to lead in a time of crisis" (Johnson 2017).

Section III: Understanding Lived Experiences and Interactions

This section helped the teachers make sense of their observations, insights, feelings, and interactions. A virtual session first presented what sense-making entailed with the following questions and instructions for reporting: "What consists of a *lived experience* as opposed to a secondhand experience?" "How do we experience the world?" "How do we make sense of the context we work in?" (Patton 2015). Then, the following question was tackled: "What makes a qualitative data qualitative?" (Patton 2015). Teachers grasped the description of qualitative research, particularly *phenomenological inquiry*, and collection of data (perception, feelings, description, interactions, observations), together with examples to capture their experiences effectively. Prior to capturing their lived experiences, the teachers were asked to take mental or written notes – because "consciousness" was fundamental. Explanation and discussions allowed the teachers to understand the meaning of lived experiences as part of phenomenological inquiry as they read certain sections of *Researching Lived Experience: Human Science for an Action Sensitive Pedagogy* (Van Manen 2016). Finally, the meaning of raw data was covered, together with how raw data transformed into findings, including *themes, patterns, concepts, insights*, and *understandings* (see Patton 2015).

The readings and learner-learner interactions served as a framework for teachers to be able to "convert a complex goal choice into concrete actions ... have [sic] vocabulary to deal with a particular situation ... expert-driven, meaning they come from a credible source" (Duncan et al. 2021, 99). This framework enabled the teachers to interpret their context in a trustworthy manner and be able to reflect and, eventually, interact with each other.

Following their reflections on experiences, feelings, and interactions, the teachers interacted on a social platform, Yellowdig, which was compatible with such discussions, as it promoted both cognitive and social presence and aimed to "build active, social, and experiential learning communities for online, hybrid, and in-person programs" (Yellowdig Co., n.d., 1). These posts and responses made up the textual data. The identities of the teachers were deleted. The researchers also went beyond the formal discussion posts and responses: "It is not just the responses to the intended questions that need to be analyzed, but rather the conversations that took place" (Guest et al. 2012, 23).

During the three semesters, a total of 76 teachers were enrolled in the same courses. All narratives were filtered based on one criterion – the texts had to reflect the "first-hand lived experiences," which meant capturing a visual representation or record of their experiences and interactions during the pandemic and the lockdowns. Eleven texts were disregarded, as they could not be defined as first-hand experiences. Additionally, 19 teachers dropped the courses due to excuses related to the pandemic, which narrowed the reliable data down to 46 narratives. Eventually, the data included 14 narratives from the spring 2020 course, 17 narratives from the fall 2020 course, and 15 narratives from the spring 2021 course.

What Did the Narratives Reveal?

First, all teachers noted that their reading materials and initiative-taking discussions with guiding questions enabled them to scrutinize their assumptions and assess their surroundings more accurately, eliminating bias. They were able to make more sense of how things worked or did not work at their institutions and communities. They also reported that they were able to describe their experiences truthfully. Second, related to the course, the deep learnings, critical reflections, and dialogues helped them widen their perspectives so they could effectively decipher the complexity of the digital inequity issue.

The sociodemographic characteristics of the 46 teachers indicated that 18 lived in rural or smaller towns and taught in public schools scattered around the USA, and 27 lived in larger cities or commuted to cities from smaller towns and taught in public schools. The majority of the teachers identified themselves as white, two as African American, and seven as Hispanic. Females made the 68 percent of the teachers and males the 32 percent. Regarding the students they taught, most were socioeconomically disadvantaged, ranging from middle- to mostly low-income families and came from single-family homes.

With a specialty in linguistics, one researcher looked into *text segmentation, keywords-in-context following the mainstream conduct in literature* (Guest et al. 2012) and, for reliability, the other researcher, with a background in business management, completed *sentiments analysis* (Liu 2012), looking into "natural language utterances" regarding positive, negative, and neutral emotions, attitudes, opinions towards ERT, and digital inequity. Following the individual analysis, *member checking* (Creswell and Guetterman 2019) resulted in the validation of the findings for reliability.

An initial review of the narratives displayed negative emotions and revealed words/phrases such as "heightened anxiety," "frustration," "fear," "anger," "isolation," and "worry." All narratives indicated the "adversely affected players" of the situation and included the administrators themselves, their learners, parents, guardians, and the community members with whom they interacted. Keywords and phrases such as "victim," "suffering," "mentally drained," "an alarming stage," "felt the shift," "waking up," "cannot stop criticizing," "what can be done as an after action," and "totally helpless," or similar words/phrases, were used repeatedly for "the affected groups."

Based on a second-level analysis, the keywords/phrases identified, digital inequity was beyond being an issue. The word "crisis" appeared in all texts, many indicating that this was "beyond an issue" as "became evident with lockdowns." There were repetitious phrases, similar lexicons related to feeling "deserted" and phrases such as "felt alone," "being dumped," and "being abandoned." Added to the heightened fear of the pandemic, it became apparent that switching to ERT adversely affected all players in one way or another. It was reported that the administrators all "felt shocked" and "unprepared," as they had no plans to manage such an "unexpected and unprecedented crisis." All 46 teachers revealed that they felt ill-equipped, as they were "forced to leave their comfort zones" of their classrooms. They felt "thrown into cyberspace with limited digital skills." Their students ranged from "haves and have-nots," the have nots being "in the majority." It was also reported that most parents and/or guardians were not able to help. Many were working one or two jobs or looking for employment. Everyone felt their "livelihood" was threatened. Moreover, they experienced other social inequalities in their communities. The consensus was that this was a major crisis, which resulted in three phases including *the alarm mode, the shift mode*, and *the hot wash mode*.

The Alarm Mode

According to the narratives, when lockdowns were enforced, massive gaps and weaknesses in institutional structures, regarding inequities at all levels, started to surface. Although most institutions had been aware of the digital inequity issue, it was observed that administrators were caught off guard, as there was no crisis or emergency management plan of this scope in place. All narratives revealed that the crisis was "unprecedented." According to the perspectives, technology was advancing at an uncontrollable pace, resulting in "powerlessness" and "slowing down to catch up." While certain institutions were swift and provided internet-enabled devices and at times created hot spots, most failed to provide "quality technical support" and/or to "enable and encourage self-sufficiency, participation, and collaboration." Moreover, because teaching and learning became an urgent priority, other issues were downplayed. Most underserved students complained and suffered, as they did not have the required connections or help at home. In a way, both teachers and students were left to "survive on their own." In addition, parents or grandparents could not provide the much-needed help. Most parents had to work and could not afford to pay attention to their children. Teachers, who had to leave their old way of teaching, felt helpless in creating cybercommunities. With two exceptions, most teachers reported that they felt "abandoned" and that ERT was "dumped onto them, their students." According to the experiences, only a few privileged students who were not disadvantaged were able to receive help and, thus, manage their digital environment. Otherwise, it became impossible to control this environment. It was also reported that communication ceased to exist or, if it did exist, it was mostly by random and included inconsistent messages which were "not helpful."

In addition to the heightened 'fear of contracting the disease," most teachers reported that the more they felt "extremely helpless," the more "more panic" set in. The teachers revealed that they were "pushed into managing the situation themselves." The domino effect of the dual sided fear triggered "immense pressure" and "terror." On the one hand, as reported, teachers were asked to manage their teaching with "whatever they had in hand," and, on the other hand, they were treated like "a piece of furniture rather than a human being." They had "no right to become ill." Most considered themselves novices concerning technology. Those who were experienced reported shortfalls in teaching online. The narratives also reported the complaints from parents concerning ERT. which resulted in online learning receiving an "undeserved negative reputation." This was no longer a problem, but an enormous crisis which could not be halted. The crisis required urgent action and crisis management was nothing more than a temporary-fix approach.

The Shift Mode

During the loosened lockdown restrictions, according to the narratives, when most institutions were forced to go back to face-to-face learning, the "shift" proved to be "poor." The digital equity became secondary. Problems such as "socioeconomic inequalities," "lack of health insurance coverage," as well as "student and teacher absences," continued to surface. During this period, "digital connectivity remained a barrier;" and educational and socioeconomic inequalities continued to persist. While the entire world felt the domino effects of the pandemic, the groups that suffered the most were those who were disadvantaged economically. In a way, the inequality issues which had been a pressing issue and had been minimized was felt even more during the pandemic lockdowns: "The stagnation of total investments in education observed in recent decades ... has contributed both to the rise in inequality and to the slowdown in the rate of average income" (Piketty and Couper 2021, 9).

The Hot Wash Mode

As reported by the teachers, once the crisis was over and students returned to their face-to-face classroom, despite policy interventions and recommendations, "the crisis continued to negatively affect students' lives," particularly those who were economically underserved and socially disadvantaged. While the institutions "tried to adapt" to the "next normal," the digital inequity crisis required "urgent solutions both short-term and long term." It became apparent that, first, there was a pressing need for "digital coaches" to provide the much-needed support and training and development for the teachers and administrators to become self-sufficient, which would have a multiplier effect in that teachers could become more competent in serving their students. Second, "understanding the root cause of the crisis was pivotal," because digital inequity was not a standalone educational issue but rather a complex problem involving political, economic, social factors, and the solution required accountability and a large-scale comprehensive reform. Third, to establish a new and more equitable normal, visionary leaders, sustainable structural systems, and policy interventions were essential. The urgency for "strategic conversations beyond education" was fundamental. This was not a time for waiting around for other disasters to further amplify the crisis and cripple the education system. This was, and has been, a time to focus on human dignity and devise strategies to mitigate impact of future disasters.

The authors would like to note that these findings are limited to the experiences and interactions of 46 teachers during the COVID-19 pandemic lockdowns, providing a single country and single language setting, and cannot be generalized to all cases and institutions.

Conclusion

During the global lockdowns, "over 100 countries implemented nationwide closures, impacting over half of the world's student population" (UNESCO 2020, 1). While an increasing number of students were not able to go to school because of poverty, others did so, as certain schools favored the wealthy and disqualified the vulnerable children and youth. The digital inequity issue was exposed and became a crisis encompassing political, economic, and social factors.

To bring about a large-scale comprehensive digital reform, crisis management dictates devotion, and cross-functional commitment, involving interdisciplinary decision-makers to get urgently to the root cause of the crisis as a starting point. The Broadband Commission for Sustainable Development acknowledges "the critical roles of digital connectivity, capacity and content in transforming education and lifelong learning systems" (The Broadband Commission 2022). However, the same report states that many countries are behind regarding building the required infrastructure and establishing policies. While the commission makes "recommendations" for "connecting schools to the

Internet and digitalizing education to enable a more inclusive and sustainable approach to learning" (The Broadband Commission 2019, 1), they remain recommendations. The solution rests with all stakeholders acting beyond "recommendations" and acting now.

A critical issue is to investigate, and at the same time to invest in, technology which moves at an unimaginable speed with new developments. Even if 60 percent of the youth are educated, they would still need to develop lifelong learning skills (The Broadband Commission 2022). Additionally, if they manage to get jobs, continuous upskilling would be essential in the workforce (Waddil 2021). In a world where artificial intelligence and virtual reality are the new rulers, not having connectivity, devices, skills, training cannot be an option. If anything, the pandemic has shown us that digital self-sufficiency must be today's agenda, not a future plan, and hasty policy interventions must be prioritized: "Is rising inequality an inevitable consequence of today's technology-driven economic transformations – and globalization? The answer is no. Policies have been slow to respond to the challenges of change. With better, more responsive policies, more inclusive economic outcomes are possible" (Qureshi 2020, 1).

In concluding this study, the authors think these findings could be an impetus for further research, such as exploring one of the domino effects of the pandemic particularly affecting health workers and teachers: "hundreds of thousands of students without full-time, certified teachers ... districts without enough bus drivers to transport kids or enough paraprofessionals to support teachers and students" (Florida Education Association 2022, 1). The significance of this problem could also lead to exploring the depreciation of certain professions so that necessary steps could be taken to prevent or mitigate the possible shocks to the education or health systems. Additional recommended research would be exploring multi-country setting sentiments with multilingual research teams.

Critical Questions for Discussion

This research exposed a key problem in schools and societies which turned into a major crisis during the pandemic. Critical questions emerge from the findings (listed below). While the climax of the pandemic has given way to new normalcy, all educators and community leaders are invited to reflect on some of these questions and discuss the implications related to economic, social, and political factors:

- Is digital inequity a problem or a crisis?
- What are the two-three takeaways from this digital inequity crisis?
- How does digital inequity affect citizenry?
- Is digital inequity a standalone problem? If yes, why? If not, why not?
- Can the problem of digital inequity be fixed? If yes, how? If not, why not?
- What is the root cause of digital inequity?
- Based on the definition of *digital self-sufficiency*, what are the long-term effects of digital inequity in communities?

References

Ar, Anil Yasin, and Asad Abbas. 2021. "Public-private ICT-based collaboration initiative during the COVID-19 pandemic: the case of Ehsaas Emergency Cash program in Pakistan". *Brazilian Archives of Biology and Technology* 64: e21200616. https://doi.org/10.1590/1678-4324-2021200616.

Berg, Jill Harrison. 2022. *Uprooting Instructional Inequity: The Power of Inquiry-Based Professional Learning*. ASCD.

The Broadband Commission. 2019. "The state of broadband as a foundation for sustainable Development". www.broadbandcommission.org/publications/the-state-of-broadband-2019.

The Broadband Commission. 2022. "Universal, inclusive and affordable connectivity for the digital transformation of education". *Broadband Commission*. www.broadbandcommission.org/publication/tes-open-statement/#.

Creswell, John W., and Timothy C. Guetterman. 2019. *Educational Research: Planning, Conducting, and Evaluating Quantitative and Qualitative Research*. 6th edition. London and Upper Saddle River, NE: Pearson Education, Inc.

Duncan, Sophie, Melanie Kim, and Dilip Soman. 2021. "A guide to guidelines". In *The Behaviorally Informed Organization*, edited by Dilip Soman and Catherine Yeung, 96–110. Toronto, Buffalo and London: University of Toronto Press.

Florida Education Association. 2022. "Teacher and staff shortage". https://feaweb.org/issues-action/teacher-and-staff-shortage/.

Guest, Greg, Kathleen MacQueen, and Emily E. Namey. 2012. *Applied Thematic Analysis*. 1st edition. Thousand Oaks, CA: Sage Publications, Inc.

Hodges, Charles, Stephanie Moore, Barb Lockee, Torrey Trust, and Aaron Bond. 2020. "The difference between emergency remote teaching and online learning". *EDUCAUSE Review*. https://er.educause.edu/articles/2020/3/the-difference-between-emergency-remote-teaching-and-online-learning.

International Telecommunication Union and UNESCO. 2020. "The state of broadband: tackling digital inequalities: a decade for action". www.broadbandcommission.org/event/annual-fall-meeting-2020/.

Jamieson, Lynn. 2013. "Personal relationships, intimacy and the self in a mediated and global digital age." In *Digital Sociology*, edited by Kate Orton-Johnson and Nick Prior, 13–33. London: Palgrave Macmillan UK. https://doi.org/10.1057/9781137297792_2.

Jaques, Tony. 2007a. "Issue management and crisis management: an integrated, non-linear, relational construct". *Public Relations Review* 33, 2: 147–157. https://doi.org/10.1016/j.pubrev.2007.02.001.

Jaques, Tony. 2007b. "Issue or problem? Managing the difference and averting crises". *Journal of Business Strategy* 28, 6: 25–28. https://doi.org/10.1108/02756660710835888.

Johnson, Tim. 2017. *Crisis Leadership: How to Lead in Times of Crisis, Threat and Uncertainty*. London and New York: Bloomsbury Business.

Kapucu, Naim, Tolga Arslan, and Fatih Demiroz. 2010. "Collaborative emergency management and national emergency management network". *Disaster Prevention and Management: An International Journal* 19, 4: 452–468. https://doi.org/10.1108/09653561011070376.

Levy, Jonathan I., Susan M. Chemerynski, and Jessica L. Tuchmann. 2006. "Incorporating concepts of inequality and inequity into health benefits analysis". *International Journal for Equity in Health* 5, 1: 2. https://doi.org/10.1186/1475-9276-5-2.

Liu, Bing. 2012. "Sentiment analysis and opinion mining". Synthesis Lectures on Human Language Technologies. Cham: Springer International Publishing. https://doi.org/10.1007/978-3-031-02145-9.

Lynch, Richard, and Myron Dembo. 2004. "The relationship between self-regulation and online learning in a blended learning context." *The International Review of Research in Open and Distributed Learning* 5, 2. https://doi.org/10.19173/irrodl.v5i2.189.

McKinsey & Company. 2020. "The next normal: the recovery will be digital – digitizing at speed and scale". www.mckinsey.com/~/media/mckinsey/business%20functions/mckinsey%20digital/our%20insights/how%20six%20companies%20are%20using%20technology%20and%20data%20to%20transform%20themselves/the-next-normal-the-recovery-will-be-digital.pdf.

Mladen, Pecujlija. 2019. *Crisis Management: Introducing Companies Organizational Reactivity and Flexibility*. Business Issues, Competition and Entrepreneurship. New York: Nova Science Publishers, Inc.

Moore, Reale, Dan Vitale, and Nycole Stawinoga. 2018. "The digital divide and educational equity". R1698. ACT Research & Center for Equity in Learning. www.act.org/content/dam/act/unsecured/documents/R1698-digital-divide-2018-08.pdf.

National Digital Inclusion Alliance. 2019. "Definitions: digital equity and digital inclusion". www.digitalinclusion.org/definitions/.

Olesen, Thomas. 2022. "Whistleblowing in a time of digital (in)visibility: towards a sociology of 'grey areas'". *Information, Communication & Society* 25, 2: 295–310. https://doi.org/10.1080/1369118X.2020.1787484.

Palloff, Rena M., and Keith Pratt. 1999. *Building Learning Communities in Cyberspace: Effective Strategies for the Online Classroom*. 1st edition. The Jossey-Bass Higher and Adult Education Series. San Francisco: Jossey-Bass Publishers.

Patton, Michael Quinn. 2015. *Qualitative Research & Evaluation Methods: Integrating Theory and Practice*. 4th edition. Thousand Oaks, CA: SAGE Publications, Inc.

Pearson, Christine M., and Judith A.Clair. 1998. "Reframing crisis management". *The Academy of Management Review* 23, 1: 59. https://doi.org/10.2307/259099.

Piketty, Thomas, and Kristin Couper. 2021. *Time for Socialism: Dispatches from a World on Fire, 2016–2021*. New Haven: Yale University Press.

Quality Matters. 2015. "Course design rubric standards". www.qualitymatters.org/qa-resources/rubric-standards/higher-ed-rubric.

Quarantelli, Enrico L. 1985. "That is disaster? The need for clarification in definition and conceptualization in research". In *Disasters and Mental Health: Selected Contemporary Perspectives*, edited by Barbara J. Sowder, 41–73. US Department of Health and Human Services Public Health Service.

Quinnan, Timothy William. 1997. *Adult Students "at-Risk": Culture Bias in Higher Education*. Critical Studies in Education and Culture Series. Westport, CN: Bergin & Garvey.

Qureshi, Zia. 2020. "Tackling the inequality pandemic: is there a cure?" Global Economy and Development Brookings Institution, 17 November. www.brookings.edu/research/tackling-the-inequality-pandemic-is-there-a-cure/.

Salceanu, Claudia. 2020. "Higher education challenges during COVID-19 pandemic: a case study". *Revista Universitara de Sociologie* 16, 1: 104–114.

Stewart, Angus. 2000. "Social inclusion: an introduction." In *Social Inclusion: Possibilities and Tensions*, edited by Peter Askonas and Angus Stewart. Basingstoke: Palgrave Macmillan.

Sunstein, Cass R. 2005. *Laws of Fear: Beyond the Precautionary Principle*. Cambridge, UK: Cambridge University Press.

Taylor, Edward W. 1998. "The theory and practice of transformative learning: a critical review". Information Series 374. Office of Educational Research and Training for Improvement, Ohio State University. https://files.eric.ed.gov/fulltext/ED423422.pdf.
Therborn, Göran. 2014. *The Killing Fields of Inequality*. Cambridge: Polity Press.
Ucok-Sayrak, Ozum, and Nichole Brazelton. 2022. "Regarding the question of presence in online education: a performative pedagogical perspective". *Educational Philosophy and Theory* 54, 2: 131–144. https://doi.org/10.1080/00131857.2021.1880389.
UNESCO (United Nations Educational, Scientific and Cultural Organization). 2023. "COVID-19: 10 recommendations to ensure that learning remains uninterrupted". *UNESCO*. www.unesco.org/en/articles/covid-19-10-recommendations-plan-distance-learning-solutions.
UNESCO (United Nations Educational, Scientific and Cultural Organization). 2020. "COVID-19 educational disruption and response", Education Sector Issue Notes, 7.1. UNESCO.
Van Manen, Max. 2016. *Researching Lived Experience: Human Science for an Action Sensitive Pedagogy*, 2nd edition. London and New York: Routledge.
Waddil, Deborah. 2021. "4 strategies for upskilling and reskilling your workforce". https://hbr.org/sponsored/2021/12/4-strategies-for-upskilling-and-reskilling-your-workforce.
World Health Organization (WHO). 2020. "Coronavirus disease 2019 (COVID-19) Situation Report", 96. *World Health Organization*. www.who.int/docs/default-source/coronaviruse/situation-reports/20200425-sitrep-96-covid-19.pdf?sfvrsn=a33836bb_2.
Yellowdig Co. n.d. "Yellowdig", 1. www.yellowdig.co.

12

GENERATION Z AND CIVIC ENGAGEMENT IN A PRE- AND POST-VACCINE WORLD

Stephanie Garrone-Shufran, Kirstie Lynn Dobbs and Laura M. Hsu

Introduction

In this chapter, research from sociology, political science, education, and other social science disciplines will be woven together to describe the need for a social reform movement in education that mobilizes young people in all communities to become engaged and informed citizens of a thriving democracy in the aftermath of the COVID-19 pandemic. We argue that education reform targeting skill building in civics education is, in itself, a social movement given its ability to reverse radically the direction of deepening polarization within the United States and abroad. Tackling polarization through building young people's civic skills leads to the increased promotion of social equity while protecting democratic freedoms currently under threat as a result of global democratic backsliding. In *Teaching Democracy: Unity and Diversity in Public Life*, Walter C. Parker (2003, 20) argued that "the central citizenship question of our time" is "[h]ow can we live together justly, in ways that are mutually satisfying, and which leave our differences, both individual and group, intact and our multiple identities recognized?" Nearly 20 years and one global pandemic later, the United States is still searching for the answer to that question.

Generation Z

Generation Z, the generation of people born between 1997 and 2012, comprise nearly 21 percent of the United States' population (Duffin 2022). In this chapter, this population will be referred to as "Gen Z" or "Gen Zers". This generation is the most racially and ethnically diverse generation in United States history, as nearly 50 percent of 6- to 21-year-olds identify as Hispanic, Black, Asian, or Other, a noticeable increase over previous generations (Parker and Igielnik

DOI: 10.4324/9781003459682-14

2020). As the most diverse generation in United States history, Gen Zers show more awareness and concern about racial inequality (Seemiller and Grace 2019).

As digital natives, "Gen Zers have grown up with massive interconnectivity to peers and strangers alike through access to social media, global news, and research, resulting in a high awareness of what is occurring around the world" (Sladek 2021). Research indicates that 98 percent of Gen Zers own a smartphone (Young 2017), and, whether on a phone or computer, Gen Zers spend eight hours or more a day online (Todorov 2022). Being a "digital citizen" may include both consuming and producing content and disseminating information via various social media types and outlets (Levinson 2014, 3). With this type of interconnectedness, information spreads rapidly (Sladek 2021). One study of Gen Z immigrants to the United States found that they use social media to share information on politics, including voting and protesting opportunities, with other members of their cultural or linguistic group (Wilf et al. 2022, 22). "The online world offers somewhere for them to claim the agency they may not get in traditional civic spaces like their schools, universities or workplaces" (Carnegie 2022).

Civic Engagement of Gen Z

Gen Z's activism is beginning at a younger age, spurred by role models such as Malala Yousafzai, Greta Thunberg, and the students at Marjory Stoneman Douglas High School in Parkland, Florida (Rue 2018, 9). The fact that so much of Gen Z's activism is concentrated online – via Tik Tok, Instagram, and other social media platforms – allowed similar efforts to continue throughout the COVID-19 pandemic when in-person methods were curtailed for much of the world (Pleyers 2020, 303). The politicization of COVID-19 in the United States was driven by (then) President Donald Trump, a tactic which served to widen the divide that already existed among Americans regarding the government (Carothers and O'Donoghue 2020). In June 2020, the murder of George Floyd and the resurgence of the Black Lives Matter movement sparked a new wave of protests, and "social media became a portal of unfiltered user-generated content on the brutalisation of Black citizens" (Mungroo 2021). Distrust of government, especially in lower-income communities and communities of color, is the result of decades of interaction with "the routine brutalities of the criminal justice system or the paternalism and complexity of welfare and Medicaid" (Schmitt 2020). However, a poll conducted by Civiqs, a nonpartisan online survey firm, showed that a year and a half after Floyd's murder, there was declining support among Americans for the Black Lives Matter movement (Bellamy 2021). In tandem, resistance to including Critical Race Theory in schools (Ray and Gibbons 2021) reinforces institutional oppression and perpetuates lack of knowledge about oppressive structures – the awareness of which belies many social justice movements.

Pleyers (2020, 308) wrote that "[t]he COVID-19 outbreak is a battlefield for alternative futures". Focusing only on loss and deficits among youth negates the fact that living through adversity can build new skills and new ways of thinking (Center on Reinventing Public Education 2021, 12). Gen Z needs equitable access to civic empowerment opportunities. Schools do not seem to be taking on this responsibility, as systems focus their attention on gaining back pandemic losses in reading and math; however, educational settings provide opportunities for youth to connect their unique personal stories to their place in the broader community. This connection is especially important in a post-pandemic world after youth experienced extreme periods of isolation and social marginalization. Through civic engagement, young people – especially youth of color – can challenge injustices, address social problems, and develop important cognitive and socioemotional skills (Wray-Lake and Abrams, 2020, 12).

However, the definition of civic engagement is changing with the rise of social media. In fact, many young people view social media as their choice form of participation, especially for expressing their political voice and raising awareness about issues important to them (Dobbs et al. 2022, 19). In a series of qualitative interviews with members of Gen Z, many young interviewees remarked that they started to "tune in" to politics a lot more during the pandemic because of the volume of information they saw on social media. When asked how Gen Z was going to impact the future, one youth stated: "We care in a different way than older generations do... we will post something on social media and we believe that we did our job, whereas older generations are more willing to go out and have these conversations in person (Aiden Joseph Burke, interview, 9 June 2022).

Although many Gen Zers are ineligible to vote due to age restrictions, nearly half of them think voting is important (Rue 2018, 9). Members of Gen Z are less likely to identify with party labels and may cast votes based on issues and ideology (Norwood 2020). In previous years, youth turnout for elections has not been a match for older generations. However, youth voter turnout (ages 18 to 29) surged from 45 percent in 2016 to 53 percent in 2020 (Center for Information and Research on Civic Learning and Engagement 2020). Additionally, the percentages of young people who donated money to a political campaign (29 percent) or volunteered for one (18 percent) in 2020 were about three times higher than in 2016 (Center for Information and Research on Civic Learning and Engagement 2020). Perhaps more critically, Gen Z cast their votes in some of the key battleground states. In 2021, Georgia's runoff elections showed a major increase in youth voter turnout as well, notable in that runoff elections tend to have lower turnout than presidential races (Lee 2020).

In summer 2022, 42 interviews were conducted with members of Gen Z ages 14 to 25 to learn more about the impact of the pandemic on Gen Z's political identity. In their interviews, many Gen Zers praised their generation as being more politicized than previous generations and as being more likely to engage in politics. One student remarked, "I think more people are going to get into politics at a much younger age" (John Liddy, interview, 23 June 2022). Another stated, "[Gen Zers] are much more on the political side given everything we have seen throughout the pandemic" (Kiley Martel, interview, 7 June 2022). Especially when it comes to their involvement in recent social movements related to racism, gun violence, and gender and sexual equality, Gen Z believes in themselves as political agents. The COVID-19 pandemic may have a "persistent negative effect on confidence in political institutions and leaders" (Aksoy et al. 2020, 1) which, in turn, could influence Gen Z to continue this more hands-on participation in civic matters, such as protests and boycotts.

Despite Gen Zers expressing and demonstrating increased engagement in politics, many young people are aware of the dangers of misinformation and disinformation and its connection with social media. Gen Zers often consume news and other information on social media where misinformation and disinformation can abound (Watson 2022b). A survey conducted in February 2022 found that Gen Zers most frequently obtain their news from social media, with 50 percent reporting that they used social networks as their news source daily and close to 60 percent saying that they never read newspapers (Watson 2022a). One young Gen Zer remarked, "There is a lot of fake news, I don't really know what to believe so it's tough to find sources to become politically involved because you don't really know who you can trust" (John Liddy, interview, 23 June 2022). Many youth noted that fake news is more prevalent on Instagram and Facebook – yet they are still more likely to use these platforms for political engagement. Thus, a civics education focusing on skill building related to not only political expression through digital technology, but also improving digital media literacy, is central to developing youth into effectively engaged citizens.

The access to technology in general – and social media in particular – might increase feelings of isolation and loneliness in young people; this hyper-connectedness can also fuel "a steady drum-beat of negative news stories, a fear of missing out, and shame in falling short of a social media-worthy standard" (Annie E. Casey Foundation 2021). Gen Z is the most depressed generation: just 45 percent rated their mental health as "very good" or "excellent", the lowest percentage of any surveyed generation (Annie E. Casey Foundation 2021). In addition to technological access, various factors related to the COVID-19 pandemic have likely resulted in these mental health concerns, including the loss of family income, the death of a loved one, and the isolation of remote learning and school closures (Annie E. Casey Foundation 2021).

The COVID-19 pandemic, democratic back-sliding across the globe, and the rise of social media have mobilized this generation to promote radical social and political transformation in society. Yet, Gen Z is not necessarily unique in the trend of being radically politicized; youth are often at the forefront of social movements that lead to radical social and political change, such as the Student Non-Violent Coordinating Committee in the 1960s in the United States, *Otpor!* in Ukraine and *Pora* in Serbia in the early 2000s, as well as the February 20 movement in Morocco and the April 6 Youth Movement during the Arab Spring protests. However, young people's tendency towards radicalization is not always positive. For example, many modern-day terrorist organizations like the Taliban and the Islamic State in Syria (ISIS) are effective manipulators of youth by indoctrinating them with misinformation and disinformation. To promote youth socialization for the greater good and impede the chances of their activism being used against societal progress, countries must prioritize civics education.

Inequitable Access: The "Civic Empowerment Gap"

Levinson (2012, 46) called the unequal distribution of "civic and political knowledge, skill, efficacy, sense of membership, and participation" in Generation Z the "civic empowerment gap". Part of the decline in America's civic health can be traced back to the increase in the number of civic deserts in which individuals live. The term "civic desert", coined by Kawashima-Ginsberg and Sullivan (2017), refers to "places characterized by a dearth of opportunities for civic and political learning and engagement, and without institutions that typically provide opportunities like youth programming, culture and arts organizations and religious congregation". Atwell et al. (2017, 8), building upon the ideas of Putnam's (2000) *Bowling Alone: The Collapse and Revival of American Community*, wrote that, when civic health "is absent, we see disengagement, polarization, and alienation that threaten our political system, which depends heavily on public participation. Severe disparities in who participates also threaten the social fabric". Kawashima-Ginsberg and Sullivan (2017) found that youth living in civic deserts were less likely to vote in the 2016 presidential election compared to those who had access to more civic resources (regardless of rural, suburban, or urban location). The idea that the loss of connection to the community is damaging for individuals in the United States had been described earlier by Klinenberg (2002) in *Heat Wave: A Social Autopsy of Disaster in Chicago* and Jacobs (2004) in *Dark Age Ahead.*

The other component of the civics empowerment gap is the "civics opportunity gap," evidenced in the score differences on the National Assessment of Educational Progress (NAEP) civics test between white students and students of color. The NAEP civics test has been administered to eighth-grade students every four years since 1998. For the first time, scores on the test declined in 2022 with average scores falling by two points (The Nation's Report Card 2022). In 2022, 22 percent of students performed at or above the NAEP *Proficient* level, as compared to 24 percent of students in 2018 (The Nation's Report Card 2022). While achievement dropped across all subgroups, on average, Black students still scored 25 points lower and Hispanic students 19 points lower than their white peers (The Nation's Report Card 2022).

As of 2018, 31 states required that high school students take a half-year of civics, nine states and Washington, DC, required a full year, and ten states did not require any civics (Shapiro & Brown 2018). On the 2022 NAEP civics survey, 49 percent of eighth-grade students reported having a class mainly focused on civics or government that year, 32 percent stated that they had taken a class that included some information on those topics, and 8 percent reported that they had not learned anything about those topics (The Nation's Report Card 2022). Students who reported taking courses that included content on civics or government and those whose teacher had primary responsibility for teaching those topics had higher scores (The Nation's Report Card 2022).

Content knowledge in civics is not standardized at the national level. The National Council for the Social Studies published *National Curriculum Standards for Social Studies* in 2010. However, there has been no large-scale adoption of this document in the United States. In 2013, a companion text called the *College, Career & Civic Life C3 Framework,* naming specific ideas and principles of civics that students must know at the ends of second, fifth, eighth, and twelfth grades, and "the virtues – such as honesty, mutual respect, cooperation, and attentiveness to multiple perspectives – that citizens should use when they interact with each other on public matters", was released (National Council for the Social Studies 2013). To confuse the matter even further, in 2021, Educating for American Democracy, an initiative led by university faculty and funded by the United States Department of Education, released *The Roadmap to Educating for American Democracy*, an "advisory document" that "identifies high-priority history and civics content essential to robust and authentic civic participation" – elements the organization believes to be missing from the *C3 Framework* (Educating for American Democracy 2021).

The implementation of a civics curriculum itself is deeply politicized. In his critique of the *Roadmap*, Butcher (2021) echoed the concerns that many conservatives have about "progressive" approaches to civics, namely that civics education should be the responsibility of the state and local government. Additionally, some conservatives believe that progressive approaches such as "action civics" encourage students with little knowledge of government to become involved in political matters (Winingham and Butcher 2021). In the post-COVID-19 era, two bipartisan bills aimed at improving outcomes for civics education – the Educating for Democracy Act of 2020 and the Civics Learning Act of 2021 – were introduced in Congress and have failed to move forward. The text of the Civics Learning Act of 2021 includes the arguments that the lack of civics education in the country has "helped to foster a political climate that is deeply partisan and divided" and that the polarization of the nation "has created an environment in which people are less likely to be well-informed on the current state of affairs and to participate in the political process" (Civics Learning Act of 2021, H.R. 400, 117th Congress). Affective polarization, the measure of how much more negative a person feels about the opposing party than one's own, has increased in the United States since the year 2020 (Boxell et al. 2020, 3).

Although most teachers agree that students need to learn personal responsibility through civics, teachers' beliefs on approaches to civics education differ between conservatives' emphasis on historical facts and dates and a liberal approach that includes a more critical view with a focus on social justice issues (Anderson et al. 1997, 348). Classrooms are thought to be the ideal place to engage in political discussions, due to the diversity of perspectives present (Hess and McAvoy 2015, 6), yet teachers are often quick to curtail any "emotional, heated, or controversial" discussions among students in the current political climate, despite feeling that discussing these very types of issues is an important practice (DiGiacomo et al. 2021, 270). Thus, it is no surprise that Gen Z is "no more prepared to discuss race, bias, or privilege than earlier students" (Rue 2018, 7).

The America Gen Z Will Inherit

The persistent gap in civic empowerment arguably leads to de facto disenfranchisement of citizens living in underresourced areas, thereby exacerbating existing racial, social, and economic stratification. The Census shows the United States is becoming increasingly more diverse (Jensen et al. 2021), and the wealth gap continues to increase amidst the fallout of the pandemic (Semega and Kollar 2022, 10). Globally, simulations on the long-term effect of COVID-19 on educational outcomes predict that close to 11 million students from primary to secondary education may drop out due to the income shock, and school closures will result in a loss of between 0.3 and 0.9 years of quality education for students (Azevedo et al. 2021, 23). Students in the secondary grades at the onset of the pandemic, 14 to 17 years old, as well as students from marginalized groups, who have been facing inequities in their access to quality education well before 2020, will feel these effects most deeply (Azevedo et al. 2021, 19). In fourth grade, for both math and reading, students in the bottom 25th percentile were more negatively impacted compared with students at the top of their class, and Black and Hispanic students, who started out behind white and Asian peers, experienced sharper declines than those groups in fourth-grade math (Mervosh and Wu 2022). These cumulative learning and economic losses will result in a cycle of decreasing access to quality education, which will eventually lead to a decrease in young people obtaining the civic skills gained from a high-quality education.

The widening disparity in academics was one manifestation of the pandemic, but recovery needs to address more than academic gaps. The pandemic also deepened a mental health crisis among youth. The average weekly number of emergency department visits for adolescent suicide attempts increased by 39 percent between 2019 and 2021 (Yard et al. 2021, 889). With regard to the sociopolitical sphere, particularly for people of color, George Floyd's murder, magnified xenophobia and racism during Trump's presidency, and the increased visibility in white nationalist groups led to a widening distrust of government (Fording and Schram 2020, 59; Wu et al. 2022, 193). The solutions for civic re-engagement must include raising critical social consciousness about race, class, and other identities; strengthening social-emotional skills; educating students how to be critical consumers of information in a digital world; and making students aware of allies in their community to counteract oppression that they and their families experience.

Youth Voice – A Civic Engagement Opportunity

The authors argue that an effective civics curriculum includes skill building that is constructed upon three major pillars: 1) coping with mental health challenges; 2) digital media literacy; and 3) cognitive skills (including writing, reading, and critical thinking). Figure 12.1. represents our theoretical framework for "how to" build a civics curriculum in a post-pandemic world. This figure draws from our experiences creating Youth Voice, an interdisciplinary and transdisciplinary civic engagement program that promotes well-being, individuality, community building, and social justice for middle schoolers, high school students, and college students.

The Youth Voice program supports the empowerment of middle school students by sharpening their tools for enacting advocacy in their communities. As a result of this summer program, participants are able to use their written and oral communication skills, participate in open-minded engagement with others, and express their voice using a variety of mediums (including art, music, and social media). Through Youth Voice, young people improve their ability to identify false information online, which empowers them to be in control of their own ideologies and enhances their ability to form evidence-based opinions.

Currently, a focus on skill building related to digital media literacy is notably lacking in the K-12 school system in the United States. The Youth Voice middle

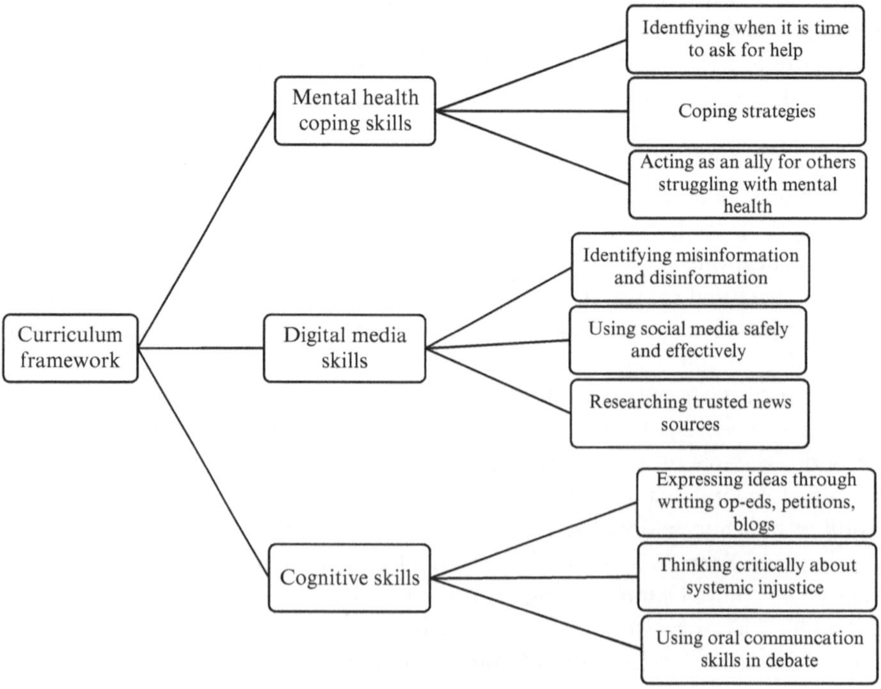

FIGURE 12.1 The Youth Voice Curriculum Framework.

school participants took a pre-survey on the first day of the Youth Voice program and a post-survey on the final day. The survey consisted of 24 questions related to creating, sharing, reading, and posting content online, creating online communities around common interests, confidence levels in discerning truthful information online, and tendency to participate in advocacy activities when raising awareness around issues they cared about. In this survey that 57 middle school students aged nine to 14 completed in 2021 and 2022, only 14 percent indicated that they talked *often* in their classrooms about how to identify fake news, while 38 percent of students reported *a few times*, 25 percent marked *once*, and 23 percent recorded *never*. Thus, almost half the participants had very little engagement (if any) with learning the tools for identifying fake news during their academic school year.

On the other hand, the middle school students did report higher levels of learning about trustworthy news sources, with 55 percent reporting they talked about news sources they can trust *a few times*, and 14 percent reporting they discussed this with their teachers *often*. Still, about 31 percent of the students reported they *never* discussed news sources they can trust, or they discussed it only *once*. This signals that some discussion on the media is taking place in the classroom, but direct conversations about misinformation and disinformation are notably lacking among this sample of students: "The students most underserved by our nation's schools are similarly underserved in the realm of access to quality materials for evaluating digital sources" (Breakstone et al. 2021b, 21). There is evidence that direct instruction in fact-checking strategies can increase college students' use of these strategies when reading information online (Breakstone et al. 2021a, 4). More research is needed to determine the impact of weaving this content into civics education with middle and high school students as well.

Structurally, to support the capacity building in the three pillars of a civics curriculum, the program must also be situated within a dense network of local community support. Education Reimagined developed a visual framework for community-centered learning called the "ecosystem of learning" (Education Reimagined, n.d. 2021). The ecosystem of learning represents a radical reform in education that decenters the traditional school building and classrooms as the locations where most student learning takes place. Ecosystems are comprised of three general spaces for learner engagement: home bases (advisors/mentors at academic institutions), learning hubs (libraries, YMCAs, museums, religious institutions, theaters, etc.), and field sites (places of internships, field projects, jobs, service learning).

The Youth Voice program is designed to support an ecosystem of learning where local and national organizations contribute to the learning of each youth participant in the program. This chapter posits that the learning ecosystem is better equipped to build upon the relational dimension of civic empowerment, given its propensity to build social networks. The Youth Voice ecosystem is displayed in Figure 12.2. This ecosystem has two main home bases: the Early College Program and Merrimack College in North Andover, Massachusetts,

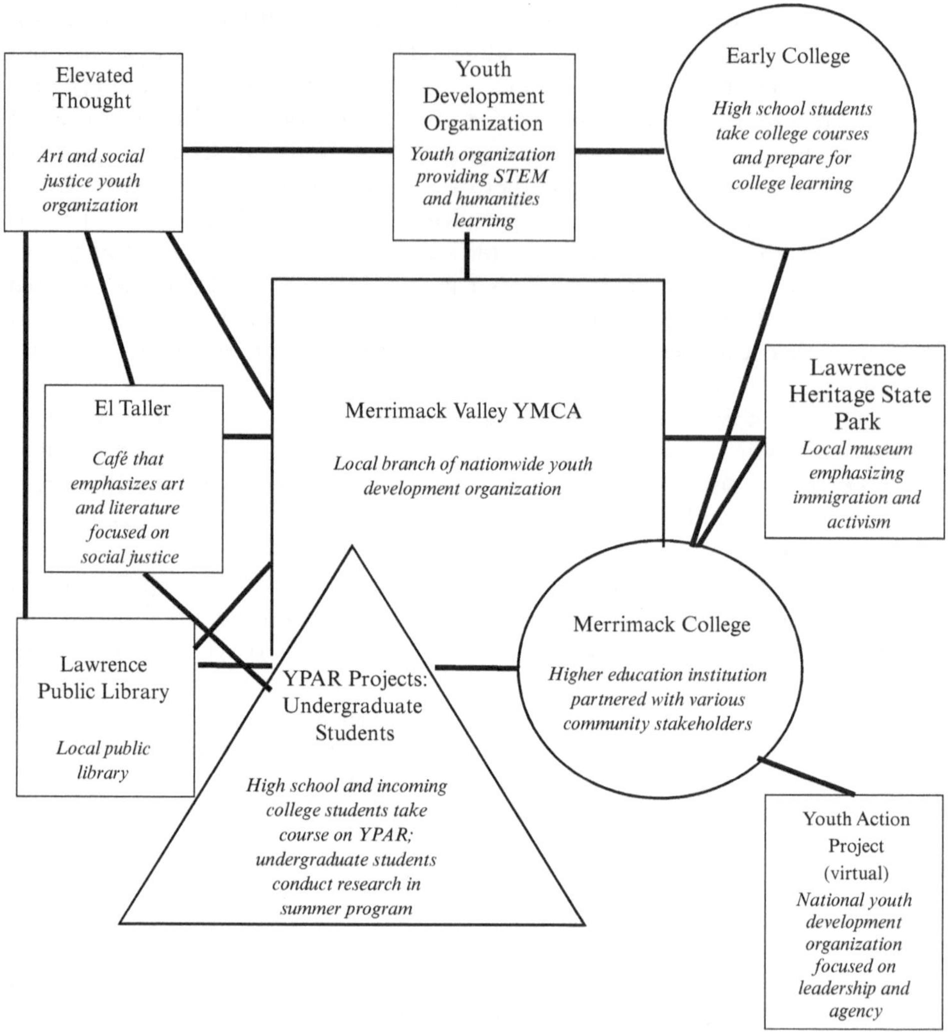

FIGURE 12.2 The Ecosystem of Youth Voice.

which is adjacent to the town of Lawrence, where Youth Voice is implemented. Three Merrimack faculty (one in political science, one in education, and one in human development), along with four Merrimack College undergraduates and three high school students, enrolled in an Early College program, have been involved, with the undergraduates and Early College students trained by the faculty to be primary facilitators in a program for youth in middle school. Several learning hubs include local organizations: Youth Development Organization, Elevated Thought, El Taller Cafe and Bookstore, the Lawrence Public Library, The Lawrence History State Park Museum, and the Merrimack Valley

YMCA. The YMCA serves as the center of the ecosystem because the program is housed through this organization, and youth are recruited through YMCA programming. One virtual learning hub, the Youth Action Project (YAP), is a youth development organization focused on leadership. YAP conducted a virtual workshop with the Youth Voice participants on building a public narrative and how to tell stories about their passions and calls for leadership. The one field site represented in this ecosystem is for the Early College students to conduct field research through their engagement with Youth Voice. For these participants, the Youth Voice program is their field site, where they engage in participant observation, survey data collection, and focus group interviews.

Various consultants were also present during the program. For example, a specialist in mental health and clinical counseling discussed mental health and strategies for self-care. Two local politicians also visited Youth Voice to speak about their path and call for leadership. The youth, in turn, communicated to the politicians' needs of the community, and, in 2021, the participants wrote testimonials that were sent directly to the offices of both representatives. Additionally, local youth activists visited Youth Voice to talk about why they engage in activism and how they connect their identity to the work that they are doing. In 2021, a podcast episode was recorded with a biology professor from Merrimack College, during which the youth participants asked questions related to COVID-19 and fears around vaccines.

During the summer of 2022, we conducted focus group interviews with the middle school participants. Many of the respondents mentioned elements of the ecosystem as their favorite part of the program. For example, many middle school participants expressed that working with the Merrimack undergraduate facilitators, the Early College students, and each other was their favorite part of the program. There were also several mentions of how they enjoyed connecting with a local youth activist who gave a presentation on T-shirt activism. When a state representative spoke to the students about proposed policy changes for curtailing gun violence, a middle school youth participant stated: "Youth Voice helped me learn about what's going on in Lawrence, like gun violence. I didn't know gun violence was a big issue, but now I am starting to listen to more people talking about it and how we can stop it."

A participant also remarked how the visits with the state representatives helped them "understand the politics side of their city" and that the state representative's "energy was bouncing off everyone in the room; he was enlightening and uplifting". Another participant recalled how talking to the state representatives was the most helpful activity in helping him think through how he could enact positive change in his school and community. He said, the representative "was talking about the community and how he wanted to be a state representative to work on issues, like immigration, that people in Lawrence face every day". Through the state representative visits, it became clearer for the middle schoolers how the government and politics fit into the equation of trying to influence change.

Another participant stated that "Youth Voice helped me with looking at Lawrence differently ... we need to make more opportunities for people to give back to the community, like when it comes to tackling homelessness." Participants also noted that Youth Voice helped them recognize issues they did not see before and helped them envision how they can try to influence change. They were taught how to collaborate with several youth social justice organizations in the area, which might account for their increased likelihood to engage with community groups to enact positive change.

The facilitators witnessed the students engage enthusiastically with Lawrence's history of worker mobilization to fight injustices surrounding labor exploitation by large corporations. Early in the program, the students took a trip to the Lawrence Heritage Visitor Center, where they learned about the Bread and Roses Strikes of 1912. These strikes were led by a diverse population of immigrants, including young children, to level the power dynamic between the wealthy mill owners and the factory workers. The theme of strikes and resistance to exploitation by large businesses resonated with the students and came up frequently during our discussions of cancel culture – notably regarding the Amazon strikes. In sum, the program appears to motivate the youth regarding specific policies and issue areas given their interactions with the community; they want to become civically engaged when they know who they can target and try to influence.

Conclusion

There is a critical need for civics education as threats to democracies and campaigns of misinformation and disinformation continue to grow. A pandemic of ignorance, white supremacy, mental health crises, and isolation persists. Counteraction of these forces with education (especially in underserved areas) around digital literacy and citizenship, social emotional learning, and communities of care is needed, particularly among youth. Ecosystems of learning – which involve dynamic interactions among community members, schools, and local and national organizations that support the cognitive, social, emotional, and political development of its members – are needed, and models of success exist. Devoting resources to such ecosystems is vital for the health and humanity of all.

References

Aksoy, Cevat G., Barry Eichengreen, and Orkun Saka. 2020. *The Political Scar of Epidemics*. SRC Discussion Paper 97. London: Systemic Risk Centre. www.systemicrisk.ac.uk/sites/default/files/2020-08/dp-97.pdf.

Anderson, Christopher, Patricia G. Avery, Patricia V. Pederson, Elizabeth S. Smith, and John L. Sullivan. 1997. "Divergent perspectives on citizenship education". *American Educational Research Journal* 34, 2: 333–364. https://doi.org/10.3102/00028312034002333.

Annie E. Casey Foundation. 2021. "Generation Z and mental health". www.aecf.org/blog/generation-z-and-mental-health.

Atwell, Matthew N., John Bridgeland, and Peter Levine. 2017. "Civic deserts: America's civic health challenge". *National Conference on Citizenship*. www.ncoc.org/wp-content/uploads/2017/10/2017CHIUpdate-FINAL-small.pdf.

Azevedo, Joao Pedro, Amer Hasan, Diana Goldemberg, Koen Geven, and Syedah Aroob Iqbal. 2021. "Simulating the potential impacts of COVID-19 school closures on schooling and learning outcomes: a set of global estimates". *The World Bank Research Observer* 36, 1: 1–40. https://doi.org/10.1093/wbro/lkab003.

Bellamy, Claretta. 2021. "Support for Black Lives Matter movement is declining, according to new poll". *NBC News*, November 16. www.nbcnews.com/news/nbcblk/support-black-lives-matter-movement-declining-according-new-poll-rcna5746.

Boxell, Levi, Jacob Conway, James N. Druckman, and Matthew Gentzkow. 2021. "Affective polarization did not increase during the COVID-19 pandemic", August. https://web.stanford.edu/~gentzkow/research/VirusAffect.pdf.

Breakstone, Joel, Mark Smith, Priscilla Connors, Teresa Ortega, Darby Kerr, and Sam Wineburg. 2021a. "Lateral reading: college students learn to critically evaluate internet sources in an online course". *Harvard Kennedy School Misinformation Review* 2, 1. https://misinforeview.hks.harvard.edu/article/lateral-reading-college-students-learn-to-critically-evaluate-internet-sources-in-an-online-course.

Breakstone, Joel, Mark Smith, Sam Wineburg, Amie Rapaport, Jill Carleton, Marshall Garland, and Anna Rosefsky Saavedra. 2021b. "Students' civic online reasoning: a national portrait". *Educational Researcher*, April 14: 1–40. http://dx.doi.org/10.2139/ssrn.3816075.

Butcher, Jonathan. 2021. "Improving civics education means preserving America's character". *The Heritage Foundation*, March 11. www.heritage.org/education/report/improving-civics-education-means-preserving-americas-character.

Carnegie, Megan. 2022. "Gen Z: how young people are changing activism". *British Broadcasting Corporation*, August 8. www.bbc.com/worklife/article/20220803-gen-z-how-young-people-are-changing-activism.

Carothers, Thomas, and Andrew O'Donoghue. 2020. "Polarization and the pandemic". *Carnegie Endowment for International Peace*, April 28. https://carnegieendowment.org/2020/04/28/polarization-and-pandemic-pub-81638.

Center on Reinventing Public Education. 2021. "How has the pandemic affected students' social emotional well-being? A review of the evidence to date". August 2021. https://crpe.org/wp-content/uploads/SEL-report-2021-final-8-10.pdf.

Center for Information and Research on Civic Learning and Engagement. 2020. "Election week 2020: young people increase turnout, lead Biden to victory". *Tufts University*, November 25. https://circle.tufts.edu/latest-research/election-week-2020.

DiGiacomo, Daniela Kruel, Erica Hodgin, Joseph Kahne, and Sara Trapp. 2021. "Civic education in a politically polarized era". *Peabody Journal of Education* 96, 2: 1–14. https://doi.org/10.1080/0161956X.2021.1942705.

Dobbs, Kirstie Lynn, Laura M. Hsu, Stephanie Garrone-Shufran, Nicholas Barber, Fatoumata Kourouma, Yarielis Perez-Castillo, and Samantha Rich. 2022. "Centering youth voices: an interdisciplinary and transdisciplinary approach to civic engagement". *Issues in Interdisciplinary Studies* 40, 2: 11–38.

Duffin, Erin. 2022. "Population distribution in the United States in 2021, by generation". *Statista*, September 30. www.statista.com/statistics/296974/us-population-share-by-generation.

Educating for American Democracy. 2021. "How is the road map different from C3?" www.educatingforamericandemocracy.org/the-roadmap.

Education Reimagined. n.d. "An ecosystem approach to unleashing learner-centered transformation". https://education-reimagined.org/ecosystem-approach.

Education Reimagined. 2021. "Learning out loud: why we must invent community-based ecosystems of learning", May 26. https://education-reimagined.org/learning-out-loud-why-we-must-invent-community-based-ecosystems-of-learning.

Fording, Richard C., and Sanford F. Schram. 2020. *Hard White: The Mainstreaming of Racism in American Politics*. New York: Oxford University Press.

Hess, Diana E., and Paula McAvoy. 2015. *The Political Classroom: Evidence and Ethics in Democratic Education*. New York: Routledge.

Jacobs, Jane. 2004. *Dark Age Ahead*. New York: Random House.

Jensen, Eric, Nicholas Jones, Megan Rabe, Beverly Pratt, Lauren Medina, Kimberly Orozco, and Lindsay Spell. 2021. "The chance that two people chosen at random are of different Race or ethnicity groups has increased since 2010". *United States Census Bureau*, August 12. www.census.gov/library/stories/2021/08/2020-united-states-population-more-racially-ethnically-diverse-than-2010.html.

Kawashima-Ginsberg, Kei and Felicia Sullivan. 2017. "Study: 60 percent of rural millennials lack access to a political life". *The Conversation*, March 26. https://theconversation.com/study-60-percent-of-rural-millennials-lack-access-to-a-political-life-74513.

Klinenberg, Eric. 2002. *Heat Wave: A Social Autopsy of Disaster in Chicago*. Chicago: University of Chicago Press.

Lee, Michelle Ye Hee. 2020. "Youth voter turnout in Georgia runoffs shows signs of sustained enthusiasm post-November". *The Washington Post*, December 30. www.washingtonpost.com/politics/georgia-runoff-youth-vote/2020/12/30/8104720c-4605-11eb-b0e4-0f182923a025_story.html.

Levinson, Meira. 2012. *No Citizen Left Behind*. Cambridge, MA: Harvard University Press.

Levinson, Meira. 2014. "Citizenship and civic education". In *Encyclopedia of Educational Theory and Philosophy*, edited by Denis C. Phillips. http://nrs.harvard.edu/urn-3:HUL.InstRepos:12701475.

Mervosh, Sarah, and Ashley Wu. 2022. "Math scores fell in nearly every state, and reading dipped on national exam". *New York Times*, October 24. www.nytimes.com/2022/10/24/us/math-reading-scores-pandemic.html.

Mungroo, Pam. 2021. "Passive or active? Generation Z and the social marketing of Black Lives Matter". *Cambridge Social Innovation Blog*, August 18. https://socialinnovation.blog.jbs.cam.ac.uk/2021/08/18/passive-or-active-generation-z-and-the-social-marketing-of-black-lives-matter.

National Council for the Social Studies. 2013. "College, career & civic life C3 framework for social studies state standards". www.socialstudies.org/system/files/2022/c3-framework-for-social-studies-rev0617.2.pdf.

The Nation's Report Card. 2022. "NAEP report card: civics". https://www.nationsreportcard.gov/civics.

Norwood, Candace. 2020. "How new Gen Z voters could shape the election". *PBS News Hour*, October 31. www.pbs.org/newshour/politics/how-new-gen-z-voters-could-shape-the-election.

Parker, Walter C. 2003. *Teaching Democracy: Unity and Diversity in Public Life*. New York: Teachers College Press.

Parker, Kim, and Ruth Igielnik. 2020. "On the cusp of adulthood and facing an uncertain future: what we know about Gen Z so far". *Pew Research Center*, May 14. www.pewresearch.org/social-trends/2020/05/14/on-the-cusp-of-adulthood-and-facing-an-uncertain-future-what-we-know-about-gen-z-so-far-2.

Pleyers, Geoffrey. 2020. "The pandemic is a battlefield: social movements in the COVID-19 lockdown". *Journal of Civil Society* 16, 4: 295–312. https://doi.org/10.1080/17448689.2020.1794398.

Putnam, R. D. 2000. *Bowling Alone: The Collapse and Revival of American Community*. New York: Simon & Schuster.

Ray, Rashawn, and Alexandra Gibbons. 2021. "Why are states banning critical race theory?" *Brookings*, November. www.brookings.edu/articles/why-are-states-banning-critical-race-theory/

Rue, Penny. 2018. "Make way, millennials, here comes Gen Z". *About Campus* 23, 3: 5–12. https://doi.org/10.1177/1086482218804251.

Schmitt, Mark. 2020. "In the wake of Its COVID-19 failure, how do we restore trust in government?" *New America Weekly*, April 23. www.newamerica.org/weekly/wake-its-covid-19-failure-how-do-we-restore-trust-government.

Seemiller, Corey, and Meghan Grace. 2019. *Generation Z: A Century in the Making*. New York: Routledge.

Semega, Jessica, and Melissa Kollar. 2022. "Increase in income inequality driven by real declines in income at the bottom". *United States Census Bureau*, September 13. www.census.gov/library/stories/2022/09/income-inequality-increased.html#:~:text=The%20ratio%20of%20the%2090th,a%204.9%25%20increase%20from%202020.

Shapiro, Sarah, and Catherine Brown. 2018. "The state of civics education". *Center for American Progress*, February 21. www.americanprogress.org/article/state-civics-education.

Sladek, Anna. 2021. "Gen Z: The youth vote and the 2020 election". *XYZ University*, January 14. www.xyzuniversity.com/gen-z-youth-vote-2020-election.

Todorov, Georgi. 2022. "Top Generation Z marketing statistics, facts and trends". *Thrive My Way*, October 17. https://thrivemyway.com/gen-z-marketing-stats.

Watson, Amy. 2022a. "Gen Z news consumption sources in the US 2022". *Statista*, October. www.statista.com/statistics/1124119/gen-z-news-consumption-us.

Watson, Amy. 2022b. "Trust in selected news sources in the US 2022". *Statista*, February. www.statista.com/statistics/1251903/trust-news-sources-us.

Wilf, Sarah, Elena Maker Castro, Kedar Garzón Gupta, and Laura Wray-Lake. 2022. "Shifting culture and minds: immigrant-origin youth building critical consciousness on social media". *Youth and Society* 55, 8: 1–26. https://doi.org/10.1177/0044118X221103890.

Winingham, Hance, and Jonathan Butcher. 2021. "Why action civics is more action than civics: K-12 students aren't ready to be activists". *The Heritage Foundation*, February 8. www.heritage.org/education/commentary/why-action-civics-more-action-civics-k-12-students-arent-ready-be-activists.

Wray-Lake, Laura, and Laura S. Abrams. 2020. "Pathways to civic engagement among urban youth of color". *Monographs of the Society for Research in Child Development* 85, 2: 1–54. https://doi.org/10.1111/mono.12415.

Wu, Cary, Rima Wilkes, and David C. Wilson. 2022. "Race & political trust: justice as a unifying influence on political trust". *Daedalus* 151, 4: 177–199. https://doi.org/10.1162/daed_a_01950.

Yard, Ellen, Lakshmi Radhakrishnan, Michael F. Ballesteros, Michael Sheppard, Abigail Gates, Zachary Stein, Kathleen Hartnett, *et al.*2021. "Emergency department visits for suspected suicide attempts among persons aged 12–25 years before and during the COVID-19 pandemic – United States, January 2019–May 2021". *Morbidity and Mortality Weekly Report* 70: 888–894. http://dx.doi.org/10.15585/mmwr.mm7024e1, www.cdc.gov/mmwr/volumes/70/wr/mm7024e1.htm.

Young, Katie. 2017. "98% of Gen Z own a smartphone". *GWI*, 17 October. https://blog.gwi.com/chart-of-the-day/98-percent-of-gen-z-own-a-smartphone.

PART III

Pandemic, Social Movements and Democracy

13

HOW DID THE PANDEMIC SHAPE THE DYNAMICS OF TWO CIVIC COMMUNITIES?

Unraveling Complementarities and Divergences Within Spain's Civic Culture

Rubén Díez García and Ariel Sribman Mittelman

Introduction

The COVID-19 pandemic in Spain has taken place in a context of intense political dispute and partisan polarization, both in terms of the action of the different levels of government and the behavior of citizens (González 2017; Simón 2020, 2021). These political hostilities – which also permeate the daily, or affective, sphere – are not exclusive to the Spanish case, and are closely related to conflicts around identity that have been afflicting many democratic societies in recent decades (Fukuyama 2019). In fact, as shown by Boxell et al. (2021), affective polarization grew dramatically in the US through the period 1980–2020, and it grew less dramatically, but still consistently, during the same period in Organisation for Economic Co-operation and Development (OECD) countries such as Switzerland, France, Denmark, Canada, and New Zealand.

In the case of Spain, the trend has been less consistent and presents substantial oscillations through time. Torcal and Comellas (2022, 10) show that "this phenomenon is election specific and responds to the dynamics of party competition", identifying peaks in 1993, 2008, and 2015, and chasms in 2000–2004 and 2011. As for the current situation, however, Spain is among the countries with the greatest affective polarization, which has increased considerably in recent years and, probably, during the pandemic (Miller 2020; Torcal 2020). In this chapter, we approach the concept of civic culture and the behavior of citizens and civil society during the first phases of the pandemic. In those early phases (spring 2022), Spain was one of the countries with a more extremely restrictive lockdown, which in turn had serious social implications (Martínez-Garcia et al. 2022). Those social implications include the polarization of beliefs based on political ideology (Bernacer et al. 2021).

DOI: 10.4324/9781003459682-16

In particular, we address two complementary ways of understanding this type of civic awareness in the hardest moments of confinement and the state of alarm. The central hypothesis is twofold: i) there are two dimensions to this system of values that crystallize in two ideal types of civic community,[1] which we will call "Rousseaunian" and "Montescan"; and ii), even when dealing with communities that are often divided and polarized, they are complementary and maintain features in common – just as the citizenry revealed through action guidelines and forms of behavior that accentuated their responsibility, solidarity, and social recognition towards health personnel and public order forces.

Similarly, we suggest that some of the features or attributes that make it possible to delimit both ideal types of civic community have their roots in the evolution of networks of groups and organizations of civil society and social movements in Spain. The presence and visibility of both communities over time inform about the most relevant public consensuses and controversies in the country and are proof that, within the framework of democratic societies, the tension between social organization and change can be balanced based on the potential of a shared system of civil values and beliefs – civic culture (Díez García 2019).

Finally, we will show that the pandemic triggered two different stages in terms of civic culture. The first stage blurred the dividing lines between the "Rousseaunian" and the "Montescan" communities. However, a few weeks into the confinement established by the central government, it led to a rearticulation of preexisting positions within Spain's polarized sociopolitical context and opened the field for those positions to manifest their differences on how to address this threat. It unleashed attributions of cross-liabilities between communities that already had different ideals and material interests before the pandemic but found reprehensible preferences in its expressions of the other communities (and their political representatives').

Theory and (Pre-) Pandemic Politics

The COVID-19 pandemic highlighted the socially constructed definition of the risks we cope with (Douglas & Wildavsky 1982; Dake 1992). Disregarding whether their origin is (as in this case) of a medical or biological nature, and its potential connection with environmental issues (Arias-Maldonado 2022), this chapter deals with the fact that society defines, interprets, and elaborates the medical or biological facts to face the above-mentioned risks, and different parts of each society can do so in different, even strongly opposed, ways – as happened in Spain with the COVID pandemic. Public debates around the management of the pandemic are a clear example of the collective definitions that we face in our global society around scientific (epidemiological) controversies, political and national security measures, public health strategies, or patterns of collective behavior by citizens. These collective definitions, and how we act based on them, have a direct effect on biological reality itself – in its indissoluble interdependence with social reality; that is, on the number of infected and deceased by the outbreak.

Although there is no optimal and fully adequate theoretical perspective on risk to confront a socionatural global threat of both a premodern and a modern nature, such as this pandemic (Arias-Maldonado 2020), social risks are (following Beck (1992)) a consequence of the very process of modernization that seeks to control them. In complex societies, risks are not easily assessable or controllable through the scientific-technical logic that generate, or feeds, them in their interrelationship with the economic and political institutions of the globalized world. Political institutions are incapable of responding, with the consequent increase in distrust towards institutional (or formal) politics, and new conflicts and forms of politicization of social life emerge outside of formal politics – the *subpolitical* sphere. Thus, the definition of these risks and their social perception and acceptability became the subject of important public debates, scientific controversies, and conflicts, through the public policy process (Laraña 2001; Wynne 2004).

In every democratic society, other conflicts also arise that affect different and multiple spheres of social and political life. In Spain, the events that, since the Transition to democracy (1975–1978),[2] have given rise to the emergence of strong controversies and public debates around the event or situation that motivates them are notorious. Examples of this are the public debates and controversies around terrorism and the ways to deal with it, or the separatist process of independence in Catalonia and the pardoning of its leaders convicted of sedition; also, on issues as disparate as the relationship between men and women, gender politics, and sexual identity; education and the language to be used in certain contexts; or citizens' relationship with the environment and living conditions. This last aspect has become especially relevant during the pandemic, given that our lifestyles directly affect the number of infections.

The existence of diverse opinions and preferences within a society, as well as the possibility of expressing them openly and having them represented in the public institutions, is usually considered a positive feature of liberal democracies (Fukuyama 2022). However, Sartori (1987) establishes a relevant difference between two forms of materialization of diversity – *dissensus* and conflict. The former is a positive asset in a society and constitutes the foundations of peaceful diversity; and the latter can be understood as a negative feature, that is, as "warlike behavior" (Sartori 1987, 92). In this sense, we interpret affective polarization as grounds for conflict, not as a manifestation of diversity in its positive aspect. Unlike pluralism as a "belief in the value of diversity" (Sartori 1987, 92), polarization does not lead to deliberation; it does not promote an exchange of arguments that enriches the decision-making processes and their outcomes. On the other hand, it creates divisions within the society – which, in turn, constitute a serious threat to democracy.

In moments of great uncertainty and of threat to democracy and daily life, conflict does not prevent actions of collective expression that allow numerous and diverse individuals to identify with their political community – for example, the approval of the constitutional pact during the Transition, or the rejection of the 1981 coup d'état; the feelings of indignation and contempt towards the murders of the terrorist organization ETA in the mid-1990s and the jihadist terrorist attacks in 2004; or the corruption and collusion between politicians and plutocratic groups hatching in 2011. Episodes like these have the capacity to generate a broad consensus within civil society regarding their scope and meaning, but they regularly lead to a logic of conflict and give rise to polarization dynamics.

These forms of expression reveal the existence of circumstances that motivate a collective definition of the situation, shared by multiple actors. In these cases, citizens recognize themselves as part of the same community and subordinate their material and ideal interests in ritual forms of collective expression, which translate into mobilizations or ostensible democratic exercises of citizen participation – transversal in nature. The relevance of these events not only marks citizens biographically and generationally due to their relationship with modernization processes, but is also related to the development of a system of democratic or civic beliefs and values in Spain (Díez García and Laraña 2017).

These dynamics are promoted and disseminated by intermediate groups of civil society that act as agencies of *social reflexivity* by introducing public controversies and persuading citizens about a certain *state of affairs*. On the one hand, within the framework of this value system, changes are faced with resistance, since in such conflicts emotional aspects linked to the identities of people and their behaviors emerge. On the other hand, the situations that give rise to a widely shared definition by a plurality of actors are scarce, since particular and competing interests often emerge, manifested in the dissemination of rival discourses around the causes and the actions to be developed to face them. An analogous process seems to have taken place during the pandemic.

Although we do not have data to confirm the level of irradiation and the intensity with which these political disputes move between the institutional and media level, on the one hand, and the level of everyday life (the *subpolitical* sphere) on the other, we can find in our interactions examples of the growing tension and *politicization* of social life to which such controversies give rise – discussions and intolerant attitudes on networks, between friends, family, and colleagues in social gatherings and instant messaging groups. During this pandemic, different actors have resorted to demagogic and binary discursive structures that are related to these dynamics, which point to an increase in polarization.[3]

The expression of this type of conflict around material and ideal interests is compatible with the maintenance of coexistence and democratic life, thanks to value and regulatory systems that drain the expression of such conflicts through civil channels (Alexander 2006; Díez García and Alexander 2021). Civic culture implies a form of conscience, which is manifested in the behavior of people and in their social relationships, from which citizens perceive themselves and builds their identity as such, as well as their relationships with others under principles of responsibility, respect, tolerance, and recognition of the other – of their values, goals, projects, and life opportunities. It is a system of beliefs and values linked to the ideas of the Enlightenment and the liberal-humanist tradition that is spreading in modern societies, observable in our social relations, that crystallizes in democratic institutions and produces a social order whose main actor is the citizen as a subject of rights and duties within a political community (Díez García and Laraña 2017).

The emergence and development of civic culture is a process promoted by civil society organizations and social movements since the transition to democracy. Such a process is described by some scholars as a startling paradox between the construction of a weak civil society and a strong democracy (Encarnación 2003). That is, Franco's regime's prohibition of associationism would have built on a national tradition of "great weakness when it comes to organizing themselves [the Spaniards] into units or groups that will together form a stable social pattern capable of withstanding the tensions and struggles normally generated within the boundaries of any nation" (Amodia 1977, 203). These dynamics would persist at least until the end of the 20th century, with the World Values Survey presenting Spain throughout that period as "one of the least-prone nations to generate the kind of associational life attached to vibrant and robust civil societies" (Encarnación 2003, 48).

Remarkable changes in this area could begin to be perceived, however, during the 1990s. In the mid-1990s there was a widespread mobilization that breathed vitality into international solidarity movements, as well as into the affiliation and participation in NGOs (Díez García and Laraña 2017). In that decade the victims' organizations played a decisive role in the development of a civic culture, since citizens overcame their fear of the organized violence of the nationalist terrorism of ETA.[4] In the next two decades, in the 21st century, these changes were linked to the emergence of crises, and therefore they were temporary. The first occurred in 2008, with the economic crisis; the second, in 2020, with the pandemic: "Spanish civil society has gained impetus with shocks like the 2008 economic crisis or the COVID-19 pandemic, but it still lacks the capacity to sustain this momentum and achieve transformation in the long term" (Rey-García and Royo 2022, 6).

An Ad Hoc Methodology for the Pandemic

Regardless, what is relevant for this study is that the coronavirus pandemic did trigger a reaction by Spanish civil society. So what *was* that reaction? In other words, how did the two phenomena that emerged as reactions of the civil society to the pandemic crisis – the impetus towards solidarity and unity, versus the tendency towards polarization – act and interact?

We argue that the former is currently compromised by dynamics that promote discourses and actions that favor polarization and identity conflict. Such dynamics are related to at least two phenomena that have intensified in recent decades. One is the colonization of civil society actors by political parties and related media groups, and the resulting loss of autonomy (these media groups act as sounding boards of discursive positions around highly controversial issues). The other phenomenon is the display of world-views that revolve around hermetic and segmented collective identities, which makes it difficult to recognize other civic groups as part of the political community.

To address our hypothesis, we conducted the CiudCovid2020 pilot survey and carried out ten qualitative interviews.[5] This pilot survey presents particularities that make the sample of 793 people between 18 and 85 years old (43.4 percent men, 56.6 percent women) a case study, given the sampling strategy and the exceptional nature of the confinement.[6] It is not, therefore, a representative sample, although the margins of error on which it works are assimilable to some common panel studies among social and market research institutes that handle samples of a comparable size. Likewise, no stratification or weighting criteria were established, with the aim of making the sample resemble the population with respect to certain parameters.

The aim, instead, was to create a sample with a substantial representation of citizens linked to political and union organizations, networks, initiatives, and associations of civil society. If we refer to some survey series from the Centro de Investigaciones Sociológicas, the frequency with which Spanish citizens are linked to this type of organization and civil society networks is considerably lower than that found in this pilot study.[7] In the sample, which takes the 2010s as a reference, nearly two out of ten people have been, or continue to be, affiliated with a union or party, or have been, or are, registered party supporters. In addition, half of the respondents, 49.7 percent, affirm that over the last ten years they have been affiliated with, participated in, collaborated with, or supported an association, group, or citizen movement of civil society.

The questionnaire was spread across three ("ideal types") nodes, each of them representative of citizen networks, associations, and social movements that have functioned as agencies of social reflexivity, promoting civic culture (Díez García and Laraña 2017).

The first node is represented by associations oriented to the defense of interests and specific groups, social intervention and inclusion, entrepreneurship or social economics – that is, broadly speaking, NGOs and foundations of Spain's Third Sector.[8] Considering the dual nature – expressive and instrumental – of these associations, among the people linked to them we can find some who share close relationships with the second node (which we discuss next), but also with the third node, according to their interests and ways of working or the situations and public debates that are generated.

The second node is made up of organizations and networks of social movements of an alternative nature, focused on social justice, which have a long history. This ideal type is epitomized by the agenda implemented by certain activists and groups in the framework of action (initially transversal and reformist) generated by the irruption of the *indignados* (15M) movement in May

2011. Far from of the character originally shown by the movement, that agenda displaced and excluded the key elements displayed during its birth – dialogue, inclusivity, respect, and tolerance. These dynamics can be explained by the co-optation and institutionalization of the afore-mentioned agenda at the level of formal (institutional) politics and the classic dispute within the political order by new parties such as Podemos.

At the institutional level, such parties embody – inspired by Latin American populism –confrontation with the principles of liberal democracy in favor of an agonistic model (Mouffe 2000) that "bulldozes" it by building a new hegemony. The connection between those parties – and their leaders – with Latin American populism is threefold: many such leaders built their careers on studying the Pink Tide, populist governments, leaders, and political projects; they based their political theory on philosophers such as Ernesto Laclau, who wrote positively about populism; and they wrote positively about populism themselves (Seguín 2017, 290–291).

The third node is represented by the associations that for decades have been defending the civil rights of numerous citizens in the Basque Country and Catalonia. This node has its origins in the fight against terrorism in the Basque Country at the end of the 20th century, and promoted demonstrations against the negotiation between the Socialist government and ETA between 2004 and 2007 (Argomaniz 2019). After a long period of latency, it gained visibility and power of persuasion through two large mobilizations – one held in Barcelona in October 2017 against the independence process in Catalonia; the other, in June 2021, in Madrid, against pardoning Catalonian pro-independence leaders sentenced to prison by Spain's Supreme Court in October 2019.

Submerged networks of academics, intellectuals, and associations with a plurality of material and ideal interests have played (indeed, still play) a prominent role in this node. In recent years, associations from this node have been acting in defense of the common language, Spanish, in regions with co-official languages. The origin of new parties in public life since the 2000s is located in Unión, Progreso y Democracia (2007), Ciudadanos, and VOX (2013), the last of which gave birth to a nativist populism (Turnbull-Dugarte et al. 2020) whose agenda confronts the principles and values of political liberalism. Such principles and values are essential to define a concept for many years present in the core of this node – "civic constitutionalism".

The Civic-Normative and Civic-Communitarian Dimensions

The criteria for the design and selection of the variables to operationalize the dimensions of civic culture that appears in Table 13.1 and Figure 13.1 is based on previous works on its emergence and development in Spain (Díez García y Laraña 2017). In particular, we considered the importance citizenship attaches to six civic attitudes. The difficulty of operationalizing this concept does not preclude us from highlighting some central features in this type of value system

TABLE 13.1 Factorial analysis results

Items included in the analysis	*Factor 1*	*Factor 2*
To obey laws and regulations	**0,805**	0,075
To respect people with other opinions	**0,793**	0,053
To be a responsible person	**0,654**	0,377
To vote in elections	0,335	**0,529**
To help people who are worse off than yourself	0,173	**0,764**
To be active in social or political associations	–0,037	**0,830**
Explained variance by factor (percentage)	40,1	19,1
Total explained variance (percentage)	40,1	59,2
Source: Pilot Survey 2020. Own elaboration.		

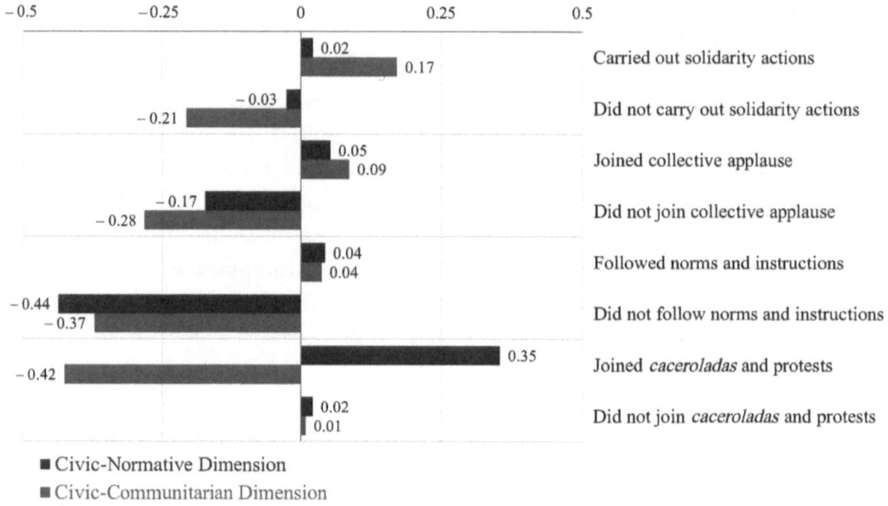

FIGURE 13.1 Differences in the "Civic-Normative" and the "Civic-Communitarian" Dimensions. Source: Pilot Survey 2020. Own elaboration.

that allows an approach via aggregate data. Some of these traits can be operationalized through the importance that people give to these civic attitudes and behaviors guided by that type of civic consciousness. Previous analyses of time series on these attitudes show how strong they are in Spain, with levels comparable to those of countries with a long democratic tradition (Fernández and Díez García 2018).

Applying factor analysis to these variables allows us to extract two factors that reflect the two expected underlying dimensions. A communitarian (or Rousseaunian) dimension considers democracy as a principle of legitimacy and fosters the expression of citizen will, and the second node of activist networks, collectives and organizations of the alternative movements, and for social justice, has gravitated on this dimension. The liberal dimension (of a Montescan character) refers to the rule of law in general, specifically as a guarantee of equality and liberties[9] – that is, it represents the limits set upon public power by the law, in order to protect basic individual rights and freedoms, and it crystallizes in the networks and associations of civic constitutionalism, linked to the third node (Díez García and Laraña 2017, 430).

In other words, following Ortega y Gasset's (1963) distinction between democracy and liberalism, the former can be understood as the question about how many hands hold the public power, regardless of the limits of that power, whereas the latter can be understood as the question about the limits of public power, regardless of how many hands hold it. In this sense, the communitarian dimension focuses on the democratic element (that is, on the materialization of the will of the majority), whereas the liberal dimension (focusing on the liberal element) prioritizes the protection of basic individual rights and liberties according to the rule of law – that is, the restraint of public power.

The first factor highlights three key features in the delimitation of a value and institutional system of civic nature – "civil", if we follow Jeffrey Alexander (2006): (i) compliance with laws and regulations, (ii) respect for the different ideas of other people, and (iii) responsibility as a criterion or guide for citizen action (Table 13.1). These features inform a dimension that we define as "civic-normative", which is oriented towards a form of civic consciousness centered on the individual as a subject of rights and duties; on personal autonomy and pluralism guaranteed by the existence of stable normative frameworks. Additionally, in accordance with a perspective that emphasizes the formal aspects of democracy, a fourth feature acquires presence in this dimension: the exercise of the vote.

The second factor, on the other hand, emphasizes three essential features of civic culture for the expression of civil solidarity: (i) an active citizenry that is aware of the importance of participating in intermediate groups of civil society; (ii) solidarity towards those people in a worse situation; and (iii) voting as an expression of citizen will. These features inform a dimension that we define as "civic-communitarian", which is oriented towards a form of civic consciousness centered on participation and the civil incorporation of new groups (Alexander 2006). Consistent with this commitment of citizens in matters that concern them, a fourth feature appears in this dimension: personal responsibility for shaping one's own life in the community.

Having identified these dimensions, we have verified the existence – or not – of their differences, based on the behavior of citizens during the weeks of strictest confinement and of state of alarm in 2020 in relation to: (i) collaboration in networks of support for people or families who have gone through a difficult economic situation or assimilable solidarity actions (54 percent);[10] (ii) participation in the daily applause at 8.00pm in recognition of the work of healthcare professionals (76 percent); (iii) compliance with rules and instructions (time slots and type of activities allowed to be carried out, or use of a face mask, 91 percent); and (iv) participation in *caceroladas* [11] to protest against the management of the pandemic (10 percent).[12]

The results show that, in the "civic-normative" dimension, significant statistical differences appear between those who claimed to participate in the health applause and follow the rules and instructions, and those who did not, as well as between those who participated in *caceroladas* and protests, compared to those who did not. No differences were observed between those who claimed to carry out solidarity actions and those who did not. This dimension reaches its highest scores among those who participated in the health applause, perceived themselves as people who followed the rules and instructions, and those who participated in the protests.

In the "civic-community" dimension, the same trend is observed for the case of the first two variables, but with an additional factor. Significant differences are also observed between the people who stated that they carried out solidarity actions and those who did not, with higher scores reached among the former. However, the trend is reversed among those who participated in *caceroladas*, since the scores for those who did not participate in them for this dimension turn negative.

Concluding Remarks

This pilot study suggests that during the pandemic two civic communities coexisted, which had already been playing a leading role in the development of civic culture in Spain. The application of factor analysis to the sample, prepared on the basis of this premise, shows the existence of two dimensions of this civic consciousness: one of a normative nature, oriented towards the individual and pluralism; and one of a communitarian nature, focused on participation and solidarity. These connect with two networks or nodes of civil society and social movements that have been cohabiting and involved in important conflicts since the transition to democracy. However, their foundations are complementary, and are essential in the defense and maintenance of the modern democratic order, civil incorporation, and change.

During the first weeks of confinement, citizens and civil society exhibited the complementarity and balance of both civic communities in their commitment and sense of belonging to the broader political community in the fight against the spread of the virus. They did so through a responsible attitude, in following the rules and indications of mobility and public health, the organization of networks and solidarity actions, and the massive, daily applause for the healthcare professionals that took place since 14 March 2020.

The highest scores of the civic-communitarian dimension are linked to solidary people who participated in the applause, notwithstanding the fact that these people may also present positive scores in the civic-normative dimension if we compare these scores with those who did not participate in the applause. Likewise, both dimensions present higher and equivalent scores among people who stated that they followed the rules, compared to those who indicated that they did not, with significantly negative scores. The course of events, however, evidenced the conflict that the situation would lead to in an already polarized context. This became visible in early May 2020, when residents began to celebrate *caceroladas* and protests in the Madrid neighborhood of Núñez de Balboa, spreading quickly to other neighborhoods and cities. People who participated in them show very high scores in the civic-normative dimension, becoming negative in the civic-community dimension.

This gap is related to two conflicting interpretations of the origin of *caceroladas*. On the one hand, there is the interpretation that motivated its promoters, who attributed responsibility for the management of the pandemic and its serious consequences to the central government. They charged the government with its lack of foresight and late reaction, the strict confinement measures, and the state of alarm (which meant a de facto suppression of individual rights) and the procedure followed to legally sanction it.

On the other, there is an interpretation that described the promoters as disloyal to the government and/or individualistic and unsupportive people focused solely on their own economic and political interests, holding them responsible for a possible increase in infections. Successively, after summer 2020, groups and neighborhood associations called to protest the selective confinements and the restrictions on mobility established by the government of the Community of Madrid in the municipalities and health areas with the highest incidence. These neighborhood groups, which had described the promoters of the *caceroladas* in May as irresponsible and unsupportive, promoted mobilizations in September against the measures of the regional government, considering them arbitrary, discriminatory, and segregationist, since such restrictions were concentrated in "poor neighborhoods".

This type of dynamics exemplifies how the pandemic unleashed attributions of cross-liabilities between communities with different material interests and ideals, which has continued over time, and that political parties and related media groups have been monopolizing for partisan purposes, deepening the growing infiltration of its structures in civil society and in public debates. This is a phenomenon that already existed – the "partitocracy" (González, 2017) – and both the *indignados* (15M) in its beginnings and various civic associations denounced it long ago (Díez García and Laraña 2017). However, it has acquired greater strength with the appearance of new political formations, the independence process in Catalonia, and the calls for mobilization of political parties whose objective is to align audiences and potential voters with their organization and interests. The most serious consequence of these dynamics of polarization is that they dilute and discredit the very principle of responsibility of rulers and citizens, and political accountability – that is, our civic culture and the civil institutions that sustain democracy, and enable us as a society to face crises of this magnitude.

Notes

1 The expression "civic community" was suggested to us by Josep Lobera.
2 There is no consensus on the starting and finishing date of the Transition. As a reference, we will consider here the period between the death of Francisco Franco in late 1975 and the passing of the democratic Constitution in late 1978.
3 The first controversy over the government's possible lack of foresight and the potential measures to be adopted focused on the suitability (or otherwise) of supporting the 8-M feminist demonstration and the holding of public events during the first weekend of March 2020, including a VOX rally. Likewise, the exaltation or criticism of public figures with a prominent role in the management of the pandemic accounts for this type of discursive structure, inspired and disseminated by political organizations and their related groups in the media and in civil society, which invites citizens to align themselves with – and display – a certain collective identity of a binary type.
4 According to Laraña and Díez García, until 2010, the leading issue of mass mobilizations was the defense of civil rights, which motivated 70 percent of them; the majority against terrorism and the role played by political parties and government on this issue. The rest were motivated by pacifism, gay marriage, and LGBT rights, education, family, environmental protection, social (and global) justice, labor rights, and conflicts between the Autonomous Communities (the Spanish Regions) and the State.
5 The sample consisted of professionals and researchers in the fields of virology, biology, applied economics, politics, the third sector and cooperatives, nursing, business, or law – members or sympathizers, mostly, of organizations and networks of civil society, or political parties.
6 The collection of information took place between 26 May and 4 June 2020. The sampling error, for a confidence level of 95.5 percent, and under the assumption of simple random sampling, is ±3.48 percent. The sample has two important biases: a territorial bias, given that the Community of Madrid represents 58 percent of the sample and Catalonia 15 percent; as well as a predominance of people with undergraduate and graduate studies, close to 80 percent. The questionnaire was distributed through two instant messaging applications, and through Twitter, LinkedIn, and Instagram, primarily contacting people employed and/or affiliated with civil society organizations, and/or activists, and among academic and university networks, who spread it in turn in their networks and primary and secondary social groups in a snowball sampling.
7 Membership of associations (30 percent, 2019); membership of, and/or participation in, in the present or the past, a political party (8.1 percent, 2017), and in a trade union or business association (17.7 percent, 2017).
8 Among others, Cruz Roja (Spanish Red Cross), Caritas, food banks, EAPN, and refugee aid organizations, development cooperation, or support for children and sick people at a national and international level.
9 "Rule of law" has two different translations in Spanish: "Estado de Derecho" and "imperio de la ley". Although they are closely connected, there are nuances that differentiate one from the other. In this case, the first use (*rule of law in general*) corresponds to "Estado de Derecho", whereas the second (*rule of law as guarantee of equality and liberties*) corresponds to "imperio de la ley".
10 The percentage of affirmative answers in the survey is shown in parentheses.
11 Protests with pots and pans.
12 To calculate these differences, we have taken the factorial scores of $\overline{x} = 0$ and $s = 1$, obtained in both dimensions, and have applied a contrast of means in them – *Student's t* test – in the dichotomous variables that operationalize these behaviors.

Acknowledgments

This work has been supported by the Spanish State Research Agency (grant number PID2019–104078GB-I00/AEI/10.13039/501100011033).

References

Alexander, Jeffrey C. 2006. *The Civil Sphere*. New York: Oxford University Press.

Amodia, José. 1977. *Franco's Political Legacy: From Dictatorship to Façade Democracy*. London: Allen Lane.

Argomaniz, Javier. 2019. "Civil action against ETA terrorism in Basque country". In *Civil Action and the Dynamics of Violence*, edited by Deborah Avant, Marie Berry, Erica Chenoweth, Rachel Epstein, Cullen Hendrix, Oliver Kaplan, and Timothy Sisk, 229–255. Oxford: Oxford University Press.

Arias-Maldonado, Manuel. 2020. "COVID-19 as a global risk: confronting the ambivalences of a socionatural threat." *Societies* 10: 92. https://doi:10.3390/soc10040092.

Arias-Maldonado, Manuel. 2022. "What's in a pandemic? COVID-19 and the anthropocene." *Environmental Values*, 32, 1: 45–63. https://doi.org/10.3197/096327122X16452897197793.

Beck, Ulrich. 1992. *Risk Society: Towards a New Modernity*. London: Sage.

Bernacer Javier, Javier García-Manglano, Eduardo Camina, and Francisco Güell. 2021. "Polarization of beliefs as a consequence of the COVID-19 pandemic: the case of Spain". *PLoS ONE* 16, 7: e0254511. https://doi.org/10.1371/journal.pone.0254511.

Boxell, Levi, Matthew Gentzkow, and Jesse Shapiro. 2021. "Cross-country trends in affective polarization". *NBER Working Paper* 26669, January 2020, revised November 2021, *JEL* D72. www.nber.org/papers/w26669.

Dake, Karl. 1992. "Myths of nature: culture and the social construction of risk". *Journal of Social Issues*, 48, 4: 21–37.

Díez García, Rubén. 2019. "Sociedad civil y movimientos sociales: entre el cambio y la organización social". *Revista Española de Sociología*, 28, 1. https://doi.org/10.22325/fes/res.2018.55.

Díez García, Rubén, and Jeffrey C. Alexander. 2021. "En defensa de la democracia liberal: la superposición del binomio 'acción-reacción' y la politización de la vida social como amenazas a la democracia". *Política y Sociedad*, 58, 2. https://doi.org/10.5209/poso.74514.

Díez García, Rubén, and Enrique Laraña. 2017. *Democracia, dignidad y movimientos sociales: El surgimiento de la cultura cívica y la irrupción de los indignados en la vida pública*. Madrid: Centro de Investigaciones Sociológicas.

Douglas, Mary, and Aaron Wildavsky. 1982. *Risk and Culture: An Essay on the Selection of Technological and Environmental Dangers*. Berkeley: University of California Press.

Encarnación, Omar G. 2003. *The Myth of Civil Society: Social Capital and Democratic Consolidation in Spain and Brazil*. New York: Palgrave Macmillan.

Fernández, Juan J., and Rubén Díez García. 2018. "Cambio de valores y cultura cívica en España, 1981–2014." *Informe España 2018*. Universidad Pontificia Comillas. https://blogs.comillas.edu/informeespana/wp-content/uploads/sites/93/2019/05/IE2018Parte-2%C2%AA.pdf.

Fukuyama, Francis. 2019. *Identity: Contemporary Identity Politics and the Struggle for Recognition*. London: Profile Books.

Fukuyama, Francis. 2022. *Liberalism and Its Discontents*. New York: Farrar, Straus and Giroux.

González, Juan Jesús. 2017. "Crisis de la democracia de partidos y segunda transición". *Revista de Derecho Político*, 100. https://doi.org/10.5944/rdp.100.2017.20712.

Laraña, Enrique. 2001. "Reflexivity, risk and collective action over waste management: a constructive proposal". *Current Sociology*, 49, 1: 23–48. https://doi.org/10.1177/0011392101049001003.

Martínez-Garcia, Marina, Emilio Sansano-Sansano, Andrea Castillo-Hornero, Rubén Femenia, Kristof Roomp, and Nuria Oliver. 2022. "Social isolation during the COVID-19 pandemic in Spain: a population study." *Scientific Reports*, 12: 12543. https://doi.org/10.1038/s41598-022-16628-y.

Miller, Luis. 2020. "Polarización en España: más divididos por ideología e identidad que por políticas públicas." *Esade EcPol*, October. www.esade.edu/ecpol/wp-content/uploads/2020/11/EsadeEcPol-insight-polarizacion-espana.pdf.

Mouffe, Chantal. 2000. *The Democratic Paradox*. London: Verso.

Ortega y Gasset, José. 1963. "V. Ideas de los castillos: liberalismo y democracia". In *Obras Completas*, vol. 2, *El Espectador (1916–1934)*, 6th edition. Madrid: Revista de Occidente.

Rey-García, Marta, and Sebastián Royo. 2022. *Strengthening Civil Society in Spain: A Post-COVID-19 Agenda*. Cambridge, MA: Belfer Center for Science and International Affairs.

Sartori, Giovanni. 1987. *The Theory of Democracy Revisited*. London: Chatham House.

Seguín, Bécquer. 2017. "Podemos and the ideals of populist proceduralism". *Arizona Journal of Hispanic Cultural Studies* 21: 287–309.

Simón, Pablo. 2020. "The multiple Spanish elections of April and May 2019: the impact of territorial and left-right polarisation". *South European Society and Politics*. https://doi.org/10.1080/13608746.2020.1756612.

Simón, Pablo. 2021. "Two-bloc logic, polarisation and coalition government: the November 2019 general election in Spain". *South European Society and Politics*. https://doi.org/10.1080/13608746.2020.1857085.

Torcal, Mariano. 2020. "Enfrentados y enfadados, una realidad preocupante" *Agenda Pública*. http://agendapublica.elpais.com/enfrentados-y-enfadados-una-realidad-preocupante. May 31.

Torcal, Mariano, and Josep M. Comellas. 2022. "Affective polarisation in times of political instability and conflict. Spain from a comparative perspective". *South European Society and Politics*. https://doi:10.1080/13608746.2022.2044236.

Turnbull-Dugarte, Stuart, José Rama, and Andrés Santana. 2020. "The Baskerville's dog suddenly started barking: voting for VOX in the 2019 Spanish general elections". *Political Research Exchange* 2, 1. https://doi:10.1080/2474736X.2020.1781543.

Wynne, Brian E. 2004. "May the sheep safely graze? A reflexive view of the expert-lay knowledge divide". In *Risk, environment and modernity: towards a new ecology*, edited by Scott Lash, Bronislaw Szerszynski, and Brian Wynne. London: Sage. https://doi.org/10.4135/9781446221983.

14

MORAL PANIC, SPANISH RROMA,[1] AND POLITICAL CONTESTATION DURING THE COVID-19 HEALTH CRISIS

Antonio Montañés Jiménez and Demetrio Gómez Ávila

In this chapter, we document and investigate the diffusion of news, political statements, and social media hoaxes that scapegoated and blamed Spanish Rroma – also known as Gitanos – for spreading the COVID-19 virus in Spain. The chapter combines sociological insights with discourse analysis and evidences the role of mass media[2] and prejudiced social media users in reproducing negative views on minorities during health crisis episodes. It shows that the COVID-19 pandemic stands not only as a medical and epidemiological phenomenon but also one in which racial, moral, and ethnic hierarchies were reinforced and contested.

The chapter is co-authored by a non-Rroma academic and a leading Rroma activist. We have examined the production of news and online messages on social media platforms from a period spanning from the first lockdown (March 2020) to the end of the first state of alarm (June 2020) in Spain. Our analysis relies and builds on secondary data and empirical material previously gathered and elaborated by Spanish and international Rroma NGOs, associations, and activists. By examining and utilizing sources crafted by Rroma civil society and associational fabric, we acknowledge the Rroma as key knowledge producers in the study of their own social experience.[3]

During COVID-19 pandemic times, in which everyone was potentially a victim of the virus and a suspect of carrying it, the idea of a good citizen was redefined. Good citizens stayed at home, cleaned their hands, wore face masks, and kept to social distancing. Good citizens followed health and lockdown guidelines and, above all, shared a joint responsibility and a willingness to make individual sacrifices for the long-term good of society. Those perceived to fail to comply with those emerging standards of good citizenship and social ethics were deemed a danger to society.

DOI: 10.4324/9781003459682-17

Drawing on Cohen's seminal work on moral panic, Cârstocea (2002) has recently argued that this sociological concept is well placed to understand the construction of Rroma communities as a threat during COVID-19 pandemic times. Moral panic episodes involve an overreaction driven by widespread fear or concern based on a perception that some "evil" group might endanger society's core values and well-being. By labeling the behavior of a group as deviant and a social problem, those fearing a threat to prevailing and moral social or cultural values often call for actions to re-establish order. Also, by using fearful rhetoric and hostile language, they seek to generate animosity towards the "deviant group." Following that line of inquiry, here we contend that epidemic anxieties led to scattered episodes of moral panic involving Spanish Rroma during the pandemic. As we will show below, Spanish Rroma were the subject of moral framing and exaggeratedly portrayed as a public health hazard deserving of reproach, control, and policing during the pandemic. Episodes of moral panic concerning the Rroma are recurrent in Spain; therefore, we argue that the extraordinary circumstances surrounding the coronavirus health crisis acted just as one of the frequent catalysts that trigger ordinary anti-Rroma sentiment to manifest. The COVID-19 pandemic thus reveals a far more dangerous and problematic scenario: the persistence of structural ethnic-based hierarchies and unequal power in crafting and enforcing narratives about who to blame in times of crisis, uncertainty, and despair.

We identified three master narratives (the virus spread rapidly among Rroma families and places where Rroma live; Rroma are a reckless group that fails to follow COVID-19 health guidelines and regulations; Rroma benefited from State subsidies during the pandemic to a greater extent than other groups in Spanish society) that questioned that the Rroma belonged to the emerging pandemic moral community. Inter-group power dynamics, double standards, and prejudices shaped blame-attributing practices and moral judgments for alleged lack of regulation compliance. When non-Rroma broke the rules, they were usually judged as individuals and therefore depicted as extreme individualists. However, it was the collective irresponsibility of Gitanos as an ethnic group that was emphasized when Rroma individuals did so (Gay y Blasco 2023). Also, while it is true that other social groups in Spain, such as young people or antivax groups, were consistently reported to breach health guidelines recklessly, and portrayed negatively in the media and social media platforms too, in the case of Rroma communities, accusations of improper behavior reinforced and built upon well-entrenched stereotypes portraying them as problematic, dangerous, and undesirable (Gay y Blasco 2016; Cortés 2021; Gómez Ávila and Saéz 2021). The existence of previously established general negative views about Rroma communities led to the proliferation and, to some extent, the normalization of abusive language against Rroma, especially in places where hate speech is difficult to track, control, or prosecute, such as social media.

The chapter is divided into three sections. First, we introduce a broad historical and comparative perspective on how scapegoating practices often re-emerge during pandemic times. Next, we investigate the use of moral framings and hate speech against Spanish Rroma during the pandemic, focusing on the channels of diffusion and identifying the various narratives that structure the construction of argumentative repertoires against Rroma. Finally, we look at the dynamics of suffering, exclusion, and contestation shaping the collective pandemic experience of Rroma during the pandemic.

Minorities, Pandemics, and Scapegoating: A Historically Repeating Pattern

Pandemics are disease outbreaks that rapidly spread across countries or continents, infecting a large number of people within a short period of time. Throughout human history, there have been several recorded pandemics of diseases, such as smallpox, the Black Death, and the 1918 influenza pandemic. More recent pandemics include HIV/AIDS, tuberculosis, and the recent COVID-19 virus spread. Extraordinary threats to global public health, pandemics disrupt social life and frequently cause massive economic crises. Indeed, the COVID-19 pandemic has become synonymous with death, worldwide lockdowns, and social collapse.

The COVID-19 virus can spread from an infected person's mouth or nose in small liquid particles when they cough, sneeze, speak, sing, or breathe. The pandemic prompted fear of others and their potentially infected bodies; consequently, physical contact and social closeness were deemed unsafe. Pressure to comply with health guidelines and protective measures was enormous. Different agents, including the State, communities, and individuals, enforced social control using varying strategies, from punitive actions to moral reprobation. Consonantly, distrust became a salient element in defining the new modes of sociability in pandemic times. Are people interacting with you carrying the virus? Are they strictly following prevention measures to avoid contagion? In other words, who can we trust?

Racialized and ethnic minorities often get affected disproportionately in pandemics (Clissold et al. 2020; Khunti et al. 2020; Resnick et al. 2020; Saeed et al. 2020). Black people, Asian people, and Latinx minorities were seriously affected by COVID-19 and experienced a disproportionate number of deaths in the US (Zakrzewski, 2020; Truman et al. 2022). In the UK, death rates for most ethnic minorities were also higher than for white ethnic groups (Barr et al. 2020; ONS 2020).

Social and not biological factors account for the higher prevalence of infections among vulnerable groups (Maqbool 2020; Reuters 2020; Ross 2020; Zakrzewski 2020). Minorities are frequently at greater risk of infection due to several socioeconomic factors, inequalities in access to health care or housing arrangements (Saeed et al. 2020). Also, working-class people and minorities are often disproportionately represented in some high-risk jobs such as childcare, elder care, food service, and transport. During the COVID-19 pandemic, most of these occupations were deemed "essential work" and therefore had to be continued to avoid further collapse.

The historical record shows that poor, vulnerable, and otherized people are usually scapegoated during pandemics and health emergencies (Nelkin and Gilman 1988; Clamp 2020; Resnick et al. 2020; Cârstocea 2022), fracturing societies when social cohesion is most needed (Montañés Jimenez and Gómez Ávila 2022). Pandemic-related discrimination against minorities ranges from the experience of being called names or insulted, to being threatened or harassed, and includes those instances in which people act afraid of minorities because they hold unsubstantiated assumptions about them carrying contagion.

During the Black Death in the 14th century, Jews in Europe suffered harassment because they were believed to spread the disease intentionally by poisoning wells, rivers, and springs (Markel 1999; Clamp 2020). In 1900, Chinese people were unfairly vilified for a plague outbreak in San Francisco's Chinatown. Following panic surrounding a local smallpox outbreak, the Chinese Exclusion Act of 1882 was created, not only preventing Chinese immigration but also forcing the vaccination of Chinese residents without epidemiological rationale (Parmet 2007; Resnick et al. 2020). Jews, Persian merchants, Armenians, and "Gypsies" were blamed for spreading cholera at the beginning of the 20th century, the last being expelled from Italian cities (Cohn 2018, 259). More recently, in the 1980s, Haitians were blamed for carrying HIV/AIDS to the USA (Farmer 2004; Lu 2021), and the spread of the Ebola virus led to a rise in anti-African racism in European communities in 2014 (Prati and Pietrantoni 2016). Similarly, during the US swine flu epidemics, Mexicans and immigrants from South America were accused of spreading the disease (Schoch-Spana et al. 2010).

Unfortunately, the COVID-19 pandemic proved to be no exception to such a general trend, and discrimination toward minorities continued. According to the World Health Organization, COVID-19 is caused by the emergence of a new coronavirus called SARS-CoV-2, first identified on 31 December 2019, following a report of a cluster of "viral pneumonia" cases in Wuhan, the People's Republic of China (World Health Organization, 2021). The Chinese community was the first national minority globally scapegoated and stigmatized. Since China was the country where the first case was reported, the concept "Chinese virus" gained traction in popular conversations and right-wing rhetoric. Metonymic thinking associated with infection, region, and culture, and images that exoticized and ridiculed Chinese dietary practices, circulated extensively on social media. The subtext was clear: Chinese people lack proper notions of cuisine and Chinese dietary practices based on eating "dirty" things that should not be eaten – such as bats – are unhygienic. Therefore, the rapid rise of the virus was perceived by many, especially in Western countries, as the consequence of Chinese people's allegedly "polluted" feeding habits.

The Asian American community experienced a striking rise in hate incidents since the onset of COVID-19, especially following former USA President Trump's repeated use of the term "Chinese virus" on Twitter and in his public appearances to refer to the COVID-19 virus (Gusterson 2020). Police records in the UK revealed a 300 percent increase in reported incidents towards British

Chinese people at the beginning of 2020 compared with 2019. Incidents ranged from banning Chinese-born citizens from shops and restaurants to declining trade for local Chinese businesses (Amnesty International 2020b) and even the unprovoked physical assault of Asian British and Asian American citizens (Campbell 2020).

Moreover, in a study recently published in the *American Journal of Public Health,* researchers measured the prevalence of COVID-19 – related discrimination in all major racial and ethnic groups in the US (Strassle et al. 2022). Using data from the "COVID-19's Unequal Racial Burden (CURB)" survey, researchers found that minorities reported experiencing more COVID-19-related discrimination than white adults. The groups who reported the highest number of discriminatory acts were Asian, American Indian, and Alaska Native people. Individuals identifying as Latinx, Pacific Islander, or Hawaiian also experienced more significant discrimination (Strassle et al. 2022). Scapegoating practices were not limited to the Western world. In India, Muslims were targeted and blamed for spreading the virus amid accusations that an Islamic missionary organization was responsible for the outbreak of COVID-19 in the country (Ellis-Petersen and Rahman 2020).

Hate Speech and Scapegoating Narratives Blaming Spanish Rroma for the Spread of the COVID-19 Virus

From the pandemic's beginning, European Romanies were subjected to practices of securitization (Surová 2022) and received discriminatory institutional treatment. In the name of security, human rights were violated (European Roma Rights Centre 2020), and surveillance and policing of Roma communities by states and police forces were increasing across Europe. In Slovakia, Greece, and Portugal, states enacted extreme measures targeting Romani neighborhoods, including lockdowns and sanitary fences (FRA 2020). Reports from Bulgaria, Romania, and Slovakia indicated that governments imposed precautionary measures not applied to other groups or the general population, including militarised quarantines, selectively targeting Roma settlements (Amnesty International 2020a; FRA 2020). The Bulgarian government imposed particularly harmful measures, including roadblocks and police checkpoints in several Romani neighborhoods despite no evidence of positive COVID-19 test results there (Matache and Bhabha 2020). Also, in Bulgaria, a plane sprayed 3,000 liters of disinfectant on Roma houses and neighborhood streets (FRA 2020). In France, Rroma and Travellers were singled out as "unconfinable" diehards, closely followed by public officials during the lockdown, and sedentary people suspected them of carrying and propagating the virus (Loiseau and Rémy 2022, 252).

Anti-Rroma rhetoric pervaded discourses in Western and Eastern European politics as well as media reports during the pandemic. Local politicians in Bulgaria, Hungary, Romania, and Slovakia utilized media reports of mass returns of Roma migrant workers from countries with a high prevalence of COVID-19 to foment fears about its spread (FRA 2020). In Moldova, a local mayor alarmed by a funeral decided to place a town in self-isolation, despite having limited legal scope to do so, and issued a lengthy statement in which he associated Rroma culture, disrespect for rules, and the risk of the virus spreading (Cârstocea 2022). In Slovakia, the mayor of Rimavská Sobota published an open letter to the prime minister calling for the lockdown of Roma settlements to prevent the spread of the virus (FRA 2020). In Romania, media sources spread hatred toward Romani neighborhoods by portraying them as sources of infection (Matache and Bhabha 2020). In Serbia, TV coverage portrayed Roma waste collectors as virus carriers (Cârstocea 2022). Actions sometimes followed rhetoric. Cases of harassment, property damage, physical assault, and violent attacks against Roma were reported and documented by media and civil society in North Macedonia, the Czech Republic, and Ukraine (OSCE 2020). Police abuse toward the Rroma was also documented and denounced by NGOs in Albania (Cârstocea 2022).

In Spain, Spanish Rroma were targeted, suspected, and suffered from abuse as well as institutional racism. Over the course of the pandemic, pro-Rroma NGO Fundación Secretariado (FSG 2021, 2022) reported an increase in online hate speech, fake news, biased and derogatory mass media features, as well as police and neighbor harassment against Rroma. The situation reached the point at which the Spanish Council for the Elimination of Racial and Ethnic Discrimination expressed their concern regarding the sudden spike in the number of discrimination cases detected against Rroma. Two months into the pandemic, the Servicio de Asistencia y Orientación a Víctimas de Discriminación Racial o Étnica (Welfare and Counselling Office for Victims of Racial and Ethnic Discrimination from the Spanish Government) declared that 46 out of 53 cases of discrimination during the pandemic involved Rroma people (Consejo para la Eliminación de la Discriminación Racial o Étnica 2020).

In some regions of Spain, WhatsApp audios called Spanish people to avoid flea markets – where Rroma have a strong presence as vendors – as they might catch the virus from Rroma (FSG 2021, 14). Some other audio recordings circulated, calling for protests against Rroma communities and even calling for them to be attacked (Kethane 2020):

> Let us catch them all and take them to prison … and let us have them there, inside the walls, let them sing and dance locked up like in a concentration camp until they all die … They are infecting everyone … Let's see if all those sons of the great whore, little ones, children, grandparents, and their fucking mother die.
>
> *(Kethane 2020)*

Although old historical patterns regarding scapegoating practices do remerge in contemporary societies, something perhaps novel to this current COVID-19 pandemic is that social media played a significant part in rapidly diffusing racism. USA-based companies such as Twitter, Facebook, YouTube, and Microsoft recently signed a code of conduct to fight discrimination and hate speech. However, the efficacy of social media in preventing hate speech from spreading during the pandemic can be easily called into question. Rroma activists and organizations have denounced social media as a haven for hate speech and fake news. A recent report based on a study concerned with online hate speech against the Rroma in Albania, Ukraine, Turkey and Serbia concluded that:

> online commentary variously accuses Roma of involvement in petty theft and organized crime, welfare abuse and fraud, and being work-shy and undeserving beneficiaries of affirmative action programs. While the tone varies from sarcasm and contempt to fuming full-on race hate, there can be little doubt concerning the corrosive, cumulative impact of online hate speech which disparages and dehumanizes Romani people.
>
> *(Ćuk and Rorke 2023, 7)*

In our own monitoring of the development of hate speech and abuse against Rroma in Spain, we found that social media is a fast and easy-to-use vehicle for spreading anti-Rroma sentiment. Below we show a few instances from public Facebook pages reacting to news of Rroma allegedly breaching the COVID-19 protocols:

> I wished Gitanos would kill each other and none of them would survive; they are just misfits.
>
> *(Facebook user, 27/03/2020)*

> Gitanos are trash; they are always so troublesome!
>
> *(Facebook user, 12/04/2020)*

> They are always the same sort of people creating problems, sons of a fucking bitch!
>
> *(Facebook user, 13/04/2020)*

> Everyone in the neighborhood thinks like us, but they are afraid to speak up. I am fed up with "do-gooders." We all know Gitanos live off the State and sell drugs. Why would you defend them? I take no pity on them. They are poor because they want to be poor. They are used to it. For us seeing Gitano kids barefooted and malnourished is shocking, but for them, it just is normal; they live like that.
>
> *(Facebook user, 15/05/2020)*

Thus, although social media indeed became one of the most important sources of communication for eliminating feelings of loneliness and isolation during quarantine and periods of physical distancing, its use had a dangerous, abusive side, one that disproportionally affected the Rroma.

When analyzing mass media and online material produced by Rroma and pro-Rroma organizations in Spain, we identified several master narratives underlying the generation of discourses blaming and scapegoating the Rroma for spreading the virus.

The first narrative emerged when the virus was breaking out, and it asserts that it spread rapidly among Rroma families and places where Rroma live. Telling examples of the prominence of this frame include when local newspapers and anonymous WhatsApp audios reported that in Haro (La Rioja) and Vitoria (Basque Country), Rroma had brought the COVID-19 virus to these regions (Kethane 2020). In the same vein, the mayor of Santoña in Cantabria informed local newspapers that Rroma families had brought the virus to the town after attending a funeral and declared that, since most people infected in town were Rroma, local authorities must keep a watchful eye on this community (Navarro 2020). A Rroma family in Karrantza (Basque Country) complained to the police that some of their neighbors threatened them because they were perceived to be virus spreaders (Kethane 2020). In the above-mentioned town of Haro, police were deployed to watch the homes of the quarantined families and, in Seville, a prominent leader of civil society who works for the city council demanded the urgent deployment of the army in a deprived Rroma neighborhood upon arguing, "we must prevent that a single minority keep doing as they please" (Tubio 2020). Here, Rroma association with dirtiness and pollution in Spanish cultural consciousness is re-elaborated and used to connect Rroma with disease (FSG 2021, 9).

The second narrative emerged following the enforcement of lockdowns and social distancing to contain the spread of the virus. It contends that Rroma are a reckless group that fail to follow COVID-19 health guidelines and regulations. The key to understanding the negative impact of this frame lies in the overexposure Rroma are subjected to when it comes to reporting negative incidents. During the first weeks of the pandemic, mass media reported 21 cases of Rroma breaching lockdown regulations in instances in which the ethnicity of the perpetrators added nothing to the understanding of the news (FSG 2021,13). Additionally, news coverage often recreates the image of Rroma as an irresponsible group. An extreme case that shows how deeply ingrained stereotypes about Rroma guided the representations of Rroma during the pandemic was found in a video that reported that Rroma people have purposely infected others in a public hospital (FSG 2021, 25).

In Andalucía, some conservative local media outlets portrayed Rroma as religious fanatics by reporting that some Rroma believers breached lockdown regulations and observed evangelical religious services outdoors in the streets when ceremonies were forbidden by the government (Montañés Jiménez and Carmona 2023; Montañés Jimenez and Gómez Ávila 2024). Subsequently, a video of a Rroma family celebrating an open-air ceremony circulated widely among WhatsApp users. Notably, reports failed to mention that most Rroma churches followed government guidelines. The Iglesia Evangélica de Filadelfia, the national Evangelical Gitano Church, reproved this isolated act of a small church (Montañés Jiménez and Carmona 2023).

The third narrative emerged when the Spanish government approved emergency economic aid to people affected by the rampant lockdown-driven financial crisis and the massive escalation of unemployment rates. It asserts that Rroma benefit from state subsidies to a greater extent than other groups in Spanish society. The notion that Rroma are privileged by the state predicates on preconceptions shared by many Spanish people about Rroma being free riders favoured by the Spanish state that exploit and take advantage of social welfare schemes and resources. For instance, a fake piece of information claiming Rroma families were awarded 3,000 euros during the pandemic was spread as a malicious hoax (FSG 2021, 13).

The three narratives mentioned above come together to advance a line of thinking that portrays Rroma as a social threat, a social group whose allegedly reckless and immoral behavior is not punished, but rewarded by, the Spanish state.

The dynamics of exclusion, mobilization, and contestation among Rroma during the COVID-19 pandemic

We have discussed how minorities are repeatedly scapegoated during health crisis episodes and how Rroma communities were on the receiving end of moral panic-driven stigmatizing narratives and discriminatory actions, and now we shift our analytical lens to include Rroma voices and their experiences of marginalization, and to recount their political mobilization.

Statistics on the number of Spanish Rroma infected by the COVID-19 virus are not available, since ethnicity is not a variable collected in official datasets in Spain. However, key determining social health factors during the pandemic, such as housing, occupation, and income levels, placed Rroma communities in an extremely vulnerable position (Gay y Blasco and Rodriguez Camacho 2020). When members of Rroma families were infected during the pandemic, the scenario that followed for most of them was far from ideal. As a result of a shortage of affordable private accommodation and limited public housing stock in large Spanish cities, Rroma often live in overcrowded homes (Gay y Blasco and Rodriguez Camacho 2020) that sometimes include three or even four generations of family members and adult married sons, spouses, and children. This residential pattern made the avoidance of contagion to family members through self-isolation unlikely.

Social risk for Rroma during the pandemic extended to their finances. Rroma communities entered the global health crisis from an exceptionally disadvantaged position: already before the health crisis, Rroma suffered from extreme marginality (Gay y Blasco and Fotta 2023) and were affected by high unemployment rates and job insecurity. Many Rroma families' primary source of income comes from selling goods in street flea markets and scrap collecting. Given that the national lockdown halted these economic activities to contain the virus's rapid spread, the economic impact of pandemic-related lockdowns on the Rroma community was immediate and overwhelming (FSG 2021; Gay y Blasco and Rodriguez Camacho 2020). Importantly, given that the Rroma often engage in diverse forms of precarious work, they faced difficulties claiming support and benefits available to workers in the formal labor market (FRA 2020). Sadly, some Rroma families inhabiting deprived informal settlements – such as La Cañada Real in Madrid, today one of the largest informal settlements of Europe – faced enormous difficulties paying their electricity bill, medicines, and even feeding their children.

In our project, we interviewed several Rroma families. One of the most outrageous family accounts we found in "Las 3000 Viviendas," a set of highly marginalized neighborhoods in Sevilla, a city located in the south of Spain. The area is well known for being a segregated area that gives shelter to some of the most deprived residents of Sevilla, including hundreds of Spanish Roma families. The family account was revealed by family members Antonia, Rosi, Diego, and Juana:[4]

ANTONIA: Once, in the midst of lockdown restrictions, my six-year-old daughter and I went to the local supermarket to use some food vouchers an NGO gave us to provide my family with basic foodstuffs. The coupons were crucial to our economic survival. You know, because of the lockdown and the pandemic, I could not sell things in the street as I usually do. My husband sometimes makes some money scavenging stuff, but he was not permitted to do so during the lockdown. When we were queuing in the supermarket to check out our groceries, a private guard who had been following me around accused me of stealing! On top of this, some local police who happened to be making their daily rounds near the store heard the hustle and joined in. Can you believe they interrogated me openly before everyone? Some neighbors of mine were there and saw the whole thing! My little girl broke down in tears, as she thought they would take me to jail. They left when they verified with the NGO that my vouchers were real and that I had not shoplifted anything. Worst of all, no one apologized to me afterward

ROSI: During the lockdowns, you know, schools were forced to transition to online teaching. My dear little Jesus fell behind in his lessons because, unfortunately, we do not have the money to buy a laptop or purchase electronic devices. When the lockdown was lifted, thank God my little Jesus's primary school bought some tablets for students. One day, I was cooking lunch when a teacher rang home to ask me about a tablet's whereabouts. It seems some teacher noticed my little Jesus's tablet was missing from the school. To my surprise, before I could get in touch with my little Jesus to ask him about it, another teacher on the school bus accused and frisked him before his whole class. It turned out Jesus's tablet was hidden in his low-drawer desk at school. Do you think they apologized to my 11-year-old Jesus? Of course, they did not!

DIEGO: We are having a tough time with the pandemic. It's a dramatic situation. We have no savings, and government aid is taking too long to reach us. We are always treated like dogs; we are not even human to them. They would kill us like the Nazis did if they could.

JUANA: A guy took a picture of a Gitano man in our neighborhood. The poor thing looked very sick; it was apparent he had come down with COVID. The image spread quickly on WhatsApp. People said nasty things about Gitanos. Many assumed we did not comply with the rules and got infected because of it. Yesterday I went to buy some groceries and ran into a neighbor. She shouted at me, "Gitana, go home!" This is just unbelievable; I tested negative and wore my face mask just like everyone else. I do not know what to do; I wish they would leave me alone!

The above family account illustrates the punitive dimension of some encounters between Gitanos and their neighbors in Spain during the crisis across social spaces, ranging from schools to food markets and social media. Of course, not every Gitano family encountered discrimination to the same extent, and the negative consequences of punitive encounters varied across Gitano individuals. However, it is worth noting again that these statements and stories are not isolated cases prompted by the fear of the virus. Rroma's collective experience is historically defined by severe discrimination and exclusion.

Grassroots organizations quickly took action to help improve the living conditions of the Rroma. In Spain and other European countries, they collected information and data to assess the impact of the pandemic and the social and economic measures to mitigate its effects on Rroma families (FRA 2020; FSG 2020). Also, some Rroma NGOs organized campaigns to inform the Rroma about state resources available to them (Kamira 2020) and provide children in Rroma neighborhoods with digital devices to help them complete their school year, as well as face masks and other hygiene materials. In partnership with the Spanish government, various Rroma organizations launched awareness-raising campaigns and distributed leaflets to engage the Rroma in vaccination schemes (Union Romani 2021).

During the COVID-19 pandemic, Rroma activists in Spain were highly concerned about the possibility of racism spiraling out of control. In the face of adversity, Rroma organizations and activists organized to fight the spread of hoaxes and hate speech. Also, they made a massive effort to report hate speech crimes during the pandemic and pushed for more effective implementation of anti-hate speech regulations (Fakali 2020).

In the early 2000s, the European Union urged state members to establish national legal frameworks to protect the Rroma population against discrimination and hate speech. However, the development of such legal apparatus in Spain is long overdue.[5]

The current political term at the time of writing (2019–2023) has borne witness to an unprecedented occurrence: this is the first time in the history of democratic Spanish politics that three Members of Parliament (MPs) (Ismael Cortés, Beatriz Carrillo, and Sara Giménez) identify as Rroma. Previously, only one individual of Romani origin, Juan de Dios Ramírez Heredia, had held a representative position – from 1977 to 1986 – in the Spanish Parliament.

In a joint effort, Spanish Rroma politicians are organizing to address the historical injustice done to Roma and amend an outdated Spanish legal system, seeking to introduce novel laws paving the way for a more comprehensive framework to protect the Rroma. On 14 December 2020, Rroma MPs led an ongoing initiative to create a comprehensive nationwide legal framework focused on anti-Gypsyism that aims to provide an effective apparatus to protect the Rroma against hate and discriminatory actions comprehensively (Montañés Jimenez and Gómez Ávila 2022). They seek to create a "national pact" focused on anti-Gypsyism that provides an effective apparatus to protect Rroma against discriminatory actions (Montañés Jimenez and Gómez Ávila 2022). In Spanish politics, a national pact is a long-term agreement between Congress-represented parties providing a general framework for addressing priority issues. National pacts must be complied with regardless of the political party in office. In addition, in July 2022, the Spanish government adopted the much-anticipated Ley de Igualdad de Trato y no Discriminación, a progressive Spanish law on equal treatment and nondiscrimination that introduced anti-Gypsyism as a crime in the Spanish national criminal code and imposed sanctions on discriminatory behaviors and offenses toward minorities (Montañes Jimenez and Gómez Ávila 2022).

Against the backdrop of a global pandemic that made visible the structural injustices the Rroma face in their everyday life, the juxtaposition of Rroma family testimonies and Rroma grassroots movements, organizations, and political representatives' actions exemplifies the dynamics of exclusion and contestation shaping the Rroma collective experience during the pandemic.

Conclusive remarks

As we have shown, the historical record painfully reveals that pandemics usually exacerbate preexisting resentment against racial/ethnic minorities and marginalized communities. As was the case with other minorities, during the COVID-19 pandemic, the Rroma, in Spain and beyond, were categorized as dangerous outsiders, ones that do not share the same notions of what is proper or right and failed to comply with lockdowns or behave like "good citizens." The generalized use of double standards, and the call for action to control the Rroma by politicians, newspapers, and media users can be interpreted as moral panic episodes predicated on previously widespread negative social perceptions. Fortunately, moral frameworks against Rroma failed to lead to generalized violence against them in Spain. However, these moral frameworks inform hate speech and normalize anti-Rroma discourses. As such, they must be interpreted as manifestations of anti-Gypsyism.

We have identified the primary narratives that guide the reproduction of negative views towards Spanish Rroma during the pandemic and shown how they remake and reinforce previously deep-seated conceptualizations of Rroma as problematic and undesirable. We have also traced four main diffusion channels through which this moral framework against Rroma is constructed and displayed: WhatsApp audios, mass media news, social media videos and users' comments, and politicians' statements.

Paradoxically, and in a sinister twist of events, those blamed for spreading the virus were, in turn, one of the groups most affected by the pandemic. The evidence collected by scholars, NGOs, and Rroma organizations shows that the pandemic affected Rroma disproportionally, particularly those living in socially excluded and marginalized settings. Spanish Rroma families' distressing accounts during the pandemic, such as the one we quoted at length in this chapter, illuminate some dark aspects of our society's social and moral crisis during the COVID-19 pandemic. Importantly, an account of Rroma's experiences in Spain must include stories of resilience and political contestation. Dynamics of suffering, exclusion, and contestation are not novel in the landscape of Spanish Romani politics. However, in this instance, Rroma grassroots mobilization overlapped with ongoing efforts to introduce new legal apparatuses and create more effective nationwide legal frameworks to protect the Rroma in Spain, adding synergy to their historical struggle for social justice and recognition.

Notes

1 Romani activists are increasingly using the term "Rroma" to describe themselves. This spelling is based on the Rromani alphabet, which was standardized in 1990 at the Fourth World Romani Congress in Poland.

2 Muyor and Segura (2021) recently published an in-depth analysis (available in Spanish) of the negative coverage by the Spanish press on Rroma during the pandemic, reaching similar conclusions to ours.

3 To gain a more comprehensive view of the dynamic processes of contestation and production of counter-narratives from the Rroma that followed the circulation of negative narratives about them during the pandemic, we recommend reading this piece with other works featuring Rroma's voices and experiences. Instances of such works include the book Romani Chronicles of COVID-19: Marginal Lives at a Time of Global Health Crisis, edited by Paloma Gay y Blasco and Martin Fotta (2023, available in English) and the report "Hate Speech against Rroma and the COVID-19 Crisis", commissioned by the Fundación Secretariado, 29–39 (available in Spanish; FSG 2021).

4 The names of the Rroma people interviewed for this project are pseudonyms.

5 In Spain, hate speech is recognized as a crime by Article 510 in the national criminal code. Whereas the EU defines hate speech as criminal verbal abuse against minorities and vulnerable individuals, Spain has strikingly taken a 'universalist approach,' meaning that everyone, not only minorities, can benefit from Article 510. This interpretation of the law is twisted, and it has been widely criticized by many European organizations and experts because it has been utilized to protect from political and social criticism individuals and institutions in a position of power, such as the Spanish police and the monarchy.

References

Amnesty International. 2020a. "Open letter to the European Commission: quarantines of Roma settlements in Bulgaria and Slovakia require urgent attention". Brussels: Amnesty International. www.amnesty.org/en/documents/ior60/2347/2020/en/.

Amnesty International. 2020b. "Responses to COVID-19 and states' human rights obligations: preliminary observations". www.amnestyusa.org/press-releases/responses-to-covid-19-and-states-human-rights-obligations-preliminary-observations/.

Barr, Caleainn, Niko Kommenda, Niamh McIntyre, and Antonio Voce. 2020. "Ethnic minorities dying of Covid-19 at higher rate, analysis shows". *The Guardian*. April 22. www. theguardian.com/ world/ 2020/ Apr/ 22/racial-inequality-in-Britain-found-a -risk-factor-for-covid-19.

Campbell, Lucy. 2020. "Chinese in UK report 'shocking' levels of racism after coronavirus outbreak". *The Guardian*, February 9. www.theguardian.com/uk-news/2020/feb/09/chinese-in-uk-report-shocking-levels-of-racism-after-coronavirus-outbreak.

Cârstocea, Andreea. 2022. "Going viral: the moral panic constructing the Roma as a hreat to Ppublic health during the first wave of the Covid-19 pandemic". *Journal on Ethnopolitics and Minority Issues in Europe* 21, 2: 57–80.

Cârstocea, Raul. 2022. "War against the poor: social violence against Roma in Eastern Europe during COVID-19 at the intersection of class and race". *Journal on Ethnopolitics and Minority Issues in Europe* 21, 2: 81–109.

Clamp, Rachel. 2020. "Coronavirus and the Black Death: the spread of misinformation and xenophobia shows we haven't learned from our past". *The Conversation*, March 5.

Clissold, Elliot, Davina Nylander, Cameron Watson, and Antonio Ventriglio. 2020. "Pandemics and prejudice". *International Journal of Social Psychiatry* 66, 5: 421–423.

Council of Europe. 2011. *ECRI General Policy Recommendation* 13, Combating Anti-Gypsyism and Discrimination Against Roma. Strasbourg. Accessed January 2023. www.coe.int/en/web/european-commission-against-racism-andintolerance/recommendation-no.13.

Cohen, Stanley. 1972. *Folk Devils and Moral Panics: The Creation of the Mods and Rockers*. New York: St. Martin's Press.

Cohn, Samuel K. 2018. *Epidemics: Hate and Compassion from the Plague of Athens to AIDS*. Oxford: Oxford University Press.

Consejo para la Eliminación de la Discriminación Racial o Étnica. 2020. "Informe del servicio de asistencia y orientación a víctimas de discriminación racial o étnica". Gobierno de España. Accessed January 2023. https://asistenciavictimasdiscriminacion.org/wp-content/uploads/2020/06/Informe-Servicio-de-Asistencia-COVID-19.pdf.

Cortés, Ismael. 2021. "Hate speech, symbolic violence, and racial discrimination. Antigypsyism: what responses for the next decade?" *Social Sciences* 10: 360.

Ellis-Petersen, Hannah, and Shaikh Azizur Rahman. 2020. "Coronavirus conspiracy theories targeting Muslims spread in India". *The Guardian*, April 13. www.theguardian.com/world/2020/apr/13/coronavirus-conspiracy-theories-targeting-muslims-spread-in-india.

Ćuk, Milena, and Bernard Rorke. 2023. *Challenging Digital Antigypsyism*. Brussels: European Roma Rights Centre.

European Roma Rights Centre. 2020. "Roma rights in the time of Covid", September 9. *European Roma Rights Centre*. www.errc.org/reports–submissions/roma-right s-in-the-time-of-covid.

Fakali. 2020. "Fakali, Antigitanismo y Covid-19: Informe del impacto del antigitanismo en la sociedad del coronavirus". Accessed January 2023. https://fakali.org/wp-content/uploads/2020/12/Informe-FAKALI-Antigitanismo-Covid-19.pdf.

Farmer, Paul. 2004. "An anthropology of structural violence". *Current Anthropology* 45, 3: 305–325.

FRA/The European Union Agency for Fundamental Rights. 2020. *Coronavirus Pandemic in the EU – Impact on Roma and Travellers*, bulletin 5. The European Union Agency for Fundamental Rights.

FSG/Fundación Secretariado Gitano. 2021. *Discursos de odio Rroma y crisis de la COVID-19: análisis sobre el origen, difusión e impacto en las personas mediante el estudio de casos*. Madrid: Fundación Secretariado Gitano.

FSG/Fundación Secretariado Gitano. 2022. *Impacto de la crisis del Covid-19 sobre la población gitana*. Madrid: Fundación Secretariado Gitano.

Gay y Blasco, Paloma. 2016. "'It's the best place for them': normalizing Roma segregation in Madrid'". *Social Anthropology* 24, 4: 446–461.

Gay y Blasco, Paloma. 2023. "Introduction to the Spanish chronicles: from ordinary crisis to pandemic emergency". In *Romani Chronicles of COVID-19: Testimonies of Harm and Resilience*, edited by Paloma Gay y Blasco and Martin Fotta. Oxford: Berghahn Books.

Gay y Blasco, Paloma, and Martin Fotta, eds. 2023. *Romani Chronicles of COVID-19: Marginal Lives at a Time of Global Health Crisis*. Oxford: Berghahn Books.

Gay y Blasco, Paloma, and Maria Félix Rodriguez Camacho. 2020. "COVID-19 and its impact on the Roma community: the case of Spain", *Somathosphere*, March. http://somatosphere.net/forumpost/covid-19-roma-community-spain/.

Gómez Ávila, Demetrio, and Javier Saéz. 2021. "La crisis de la COVID-19, los discursos de odio antigitano y el impacto en las personas". In *Discriminación y Comunidad Rroma: Informe Anual FSG 2021*, 193–197. Madrid: Fundación Secretariado Gitano.

Gusterson, Hugh. 2020. "What's wrong with 'the Chinese virus'". *Sapiens Magazine*, March 3. www.sapiens.org/culture/coronavirus-name/.

Kamira. 2020. "Mapa de recursos sociales en España en el estado de alarma". https://federacionkamira.com/mapa-de-recursos-sociales-en-espana-en-el-estado-de-alarma/.

Khetane. 2020. "El Antigitanismo en la España del Coronavirus, Crónica de la BBC". *Plataforma Kethane*. https://plataformakhetane.org/index.php/2020/05/20/el-antigitanismo-en-la-espana-del-coronavirus-cronica-de-la-bbc/.

Khunti, Kamlesh, Awadhesh Kumar Singh, Manish Pareek, and Wasim Hanif. 2020. "Is ethnicity linked to the incidence or outcomes of covid-19?" *BMJ* 369.

Liu, Ying, Brian Karl Finch, Savannah G. Brenneke, Kyla Thomas, and Phuong Thao D. Le. 2020. "Perceived discrimination and mental distress amid the COVID-19 pandemic: evidence from the Understanding America Study". *American Journal of Preventative Medicine* 59, 4: 481–492.

Loiseau, Gaëlla, and Agnès Rémy. 2022. "Gypsies and travellers confined already?" In *Anthropology of a Pandemic*, edited by Monique Selim, 251–260. Association Française des Anthropologues.

Lu, Joanne. 2021. "Why pandemics give birth to hate: from bubonic plague to COVID-19". *NPR*, March 26.

Maqbool, Aleem. 2020. "Coronavirus: why has the virus hit African Americans so hard?" *BBC News*, April 11. www.bbc.co.uk/news/world-us-canada-52245690.

Markel, H. 1999. *Quarantine! East European Jewish Immigrants and the New York City epidemics of 1892*. Baltimore: Johns Hopkins University Press.

Matache, Margareta, and Jacqueline Bhabha. 2020. "Anti-Roma racism is spiraling during COVID-19 pandemic". *Health and Human Rights* 22, 1: 379–382.

Montañés Jimenez, Antonio, with Gory Carmona. 2023. "COVID-19 is a trial from God: gitanos, pentecostal imaginaries and compliance". In *Romani Chronicles of*

COVID-19: Testimonies of Harm and Resilience, edited by Paloma Gay y Blasco and Martin Fotta, 80–92. Oxford: Berghahn Books.

Montañés Jimenez, Antonio, and Demetrio Gómez Ávila. 2022. "In Spain, scapegoating spikes during the pandemic'. *Sapiens Magazine*, 22 September. www.sapiens.org/culture/roma-pandemic-prejudice/.

Montañés Jimenez, Antonio, and Demetrio Gómez Ávila. 2024 "Bridging academia and Romani activism in the age of COVID-19". In *Gypsy, Roma and Traveller Research in the Age of COVID-19: Ethics, Methods and Engagement*, edited by Martin Fotta and Paloma Gay y Blasco. Bristol: Bristol University Press.

Muyor, Jesús, and Antonio J. Segura. 2021. "COVID-19 y comunidad gitana: enfoques en la prensa española". *Revista de Ciencias Sociales (Ve)* 27, 1: 34–52.

Navarro, Juan. 2020. "Los bulos xenófobos infectan la lucha de Santoña contra el coronavirus". *El País*. March 31. https://elpais.com/espana/2020-03-31/los-bulos-xenofobos-infectan-la-lucha-de-santona-contra-el-coronavirus.html.

Nelkin, Dorothy, and Sander L. Gilman. 1988. "Placing blame for the devastating disease". *Social Research* 55, 3: 361–378.

OSCE Office for Democratic Institutions and Human Rights. 2020. "OSCE human dimension commitments and state responses to the Covid-19 pandemic". *OSCE Office for Democratic Institutions and Human Rights (ODIHR)*. www.osce.org/odihr/human-rights-states-of-emergency-covid19.

ONS- Office for National Statistics. 2020. "Why have Black and South Asian people been hit hardest by COVID-19?" *UK Government*, December 14. www.ons.gov.uk/peoplepopulationandcommunity/healthandsocialcare/conditionsanddiseases/articles/whyhaveblackandsouthasianpeoplebeenhithardestbycovid19/2020-12-14.

Parmet, Wendy E. 2007. "Legal power and legal rights –isolation and quarantine in the case of drug-resistant tuberculosis". *New England Journal of Medicine* 357, 5: 433–435.

Prati, Gabriele, and Luca Pietrantoni. 2016. "Knowledge, risk perceptions, and xenophobic attitudes: Evidence from Italy during the ebola outbreak". *Risk Analysis* 36, 10: 2000–2010.

Resnick, Andrew, Sandro Galea, and Sivashanker Karthik. 2020. "Covid-19: the painful price of ignoring health inequities". *BMJ Opinion*, March 31.

Reuters. 2020. "False claim: African skin resists the coronavirus", March 10. www.reuters.com/article/uk-factcheck-coronavirus-ethnicity/false-claim-african-skin-resists-the-coronavirus-idUSKBN20X27G.

Ross, Janell. 2020. "Coronavirus outbreak revives dangerous race myths and pseudoscience". *NBC News*, March 19. www.nbcnews.com/news/nbcblk/coronavirus-outbreak-revives-dangerous-race-myths-pseudoscience-n1162326.

Saeed, Fahimeh, Ronak Mihan, S. Zeinab Mousavi, Renate L.E.P. Reniers, Fatemeh Sadat Bateni, Rosa Alikhani, and S. Bentolhoda Mousavil. 2020. "A narrative review of stigma related to infectious disease outbreaks: what can be learned in the face of the COVID-19 pandemic?" *Front Psychiatry* 11: 565919.

Schoch-Spana, Monica, Bouri Nidhi, Rambhia, Kunal J and Ann Norwood. 2010. "Stigma, health disparities, and the 2009 H1N1 influenza pandemic: how to protect Latino farmworkers in future health emergencies". *Biosecur Bioterror*. 8: 243–254.

Strassle, Paula D., Anita L. Stewart, Stephanie M. Quintero, Jackie Bonilla, Alia Alhomsi, Verónica Santana-Ufret, Ana I. Maldonado, Allana T. Forde, and Anna María Nápoles. 2022. "COVID-19-related discrimination among racial/ethnic minorities and other marginalised communities in the United States". *American Journal of Public Health* 112, 3: 453–466.

Surová, Svetluša. 2022. "Securitization and militarized quarantine of Roma settlements during the first wave of COVID-19 pandemic in Slovakia". *Citizenship Studies* 26, 8: 1032–1062.

Tubio, Silvia. 2020. "El Comisionado para el Polígono Sur pide que entre el Ejército en las Tres Mil Viviendas". *Periódico ABC de Sevilla*, March 19. https://sevilla.abc.es/sevilla/sevi-comisionado-para-poligono-pide-entre-ejercito-tres-viviendas-202003191920_noticia.html.

Truman, Benedict I., Man-Huei Chang, and Ramal Moonesinghe. 2022. "Provisional COVID-19 age-adjusted death rates, by race and ethnicity – United States, 2020–2021". *MMWR Morbidity and Mortality Weekly Report* 71: 601–605.

Union Romani. 2021. "'Yo me vacuno. Te digo por qué …': campaña de vacunación frente a la COVID-19 dirigida a la población gitana". *Union Romani*. https://unionromani.org/2021/06/16/yo-me-vacuno-te-digo-por-que/.

World Health Organization. 2021. "Coronavirus disease (COVID-19)". *WHO*, September 13. www.who.int/emergencies/diseases/novel-coronavirus-2019/question-and-answers-hub/q-a-detail/coronavirus-disease-covid-19.

Zakrzewski, Sonia. 2020. "No, 'racial genetics' aren't affecting COVID-19 deaths". *Sapiens Magazine*, June 11. www.sapiens.org/biology/covid-race-genetics/.

15

THE ANTI-VAXXER ATTITUDE AS A SOCIALLY ROOTED THOUGHT-STYLE

Fiorenzo Parziale and Maria Carmela Catone

Vaccination Hesitation and Institutional Distrust: The Terms of the Question

Hesitation towards COVID-19 vaccines is a multifaceted and context-dependent phenomenon that is being investigated through different approaches and perspectives.

This chapter focuses on the social roots of aversion to the COVID-19 vaccination, taking into account the moral panic resulting from the vaccine hesitancy felt by a not insignificant part of population during the pandemic. More specifically, we take into consideration not only this hesitancy, but also explicit aversion towards vaccines, attempting to overcome the typical common-sense notion according to which the anti-vaxxer attitude seems to be a mere reflection of impatience with the limits of freedom, mainly stemming from hyper-socialization to radical neoliberal individualism.

According to recent studies, hesitancy towards the vaccine may be caused by several factors (Gobo & Sena 2019), mainly associated with distrust in health institutions and more generally in the knowledge of experts (Pellizzoni 2020). Indeed, what usually characterizes the population of "No Vax" is the absence of a sufficient degree of trust in science which sometimes is reflected in the difficulty to distinguish the benefits of scientific progress from subordination to the mechanisms of capitalist accumulation by the big pharmaceutical corporations. These studies can also be read in the light of the broader analysis of the relationship between vaccine aversion and the level of institutional trust. This association has also been found in other past epidemiological situations, such as in the case of the Ebola outbreak (Vinck et al. 2019). Focusing on the COVID-19 outbreak, according to the findings of the research carried out by Kerr et al. 2021), people who were the most afraid of COVID and distrustful of institutions were the least likely to use

DOI: 10.4324/9781003459682-18

vaccines at that time. In the same direction is the investigation by Soares et al. (2021), which found that lower trust and the worse perceptions of the government and the measures implemented were associated with delay or rejection of the COVID-19 vaccine.

Moreover, results from various research projects found that vaccine behavior was associated with specific social characteristics and that certain groups are more likely to be hesitant towards the new COVID-19 vaccines; in particular, people with little education and a low income (Lin et al. 2020; Aw et al. 2021; Kessels et al. 2021; Vulpe and Rughiniş 2021). Among these are women, especially if they are in a condition of financial distress (Morales et al. 2022), and members of ethnic minorities, especially if they have suffered health discrimination (Reno et al. 2021).

Starting from these reflections, in which refusal of the COVID-19 vaccine is explored through a plurality of factors in which social and cultural issues converge, this work investigates whether vaccination hesitancy, and a fortiori open opposition to the COVID-19 vaccination, can be conceived as a way through which subordinate groups express their discomfort with the current institutional order.

The choice of this approach is also suggested by the extensive fast-growing literature on the subject, according to which among the most disadvantaged there is a growing reactionary orientation that seems to question the entire project of modernity as well as an aversion to everything that originates from global governance (Appadurai 2017; Fraser 2017).

This perspective allowed us to understand in what terms the phenomenon of vaccination hesitancy can be traced back to institutional distrust, and also to consider which component more clearly expresses a typically anti-vaccination attitude. With reference to the latter, the label "No Vax" can be used to evoke the radical opposition to the directions conveyed by the institutions mainly engaged in the dissemination of scientific discourse (the Ministry of Health and the Institutes of Public Health, etc.), according to which the outbreak of the pandemic determined the need for a vaccine for the good of all.

The analytical path traced here is developed in the theoretical framework outlined in the next section. Next, we present empirical research aimed at investigating the aversion towards the COVID-19 vaccines in a sample of Italian upper-secondary students. The methodology used is described in the third section; the presentation of the results and the final discussion on the explanation of the social roots of vaccination hesitancy are developed in the last two sections.

Social Insecurity and Opposition to Modern Rationalization

The aim of our investigation is developed from a theoretical framework in which different perspectives converge. On one hand, concerning the relationship between science, irrationality and social risk, we can benefit from the use of Weberian analysis of modern rationalization. In particular, Weber (1919) argued that the progressive dominance of science can produce a meaning vacuum filled by other, even markedly irrational, systems of beliefs. In the last few dacades, other sociologists such as Beck (1986) and Giddens (1990) already pointed out how, paradoxically, the increasing dependence of human existence on technical and scientific development led to a crisis of confidence in expert knowledge and science.

Starting from this perspective, the theoretical framework we adopted is enriched by the thought of Mannheim (1929) according to which different social classes express different worldviews. In this regard, he showed how such interpretations reveal the more general style of thinking of the social groups involved in the political and economic clash. In particular, analyzing the relationship between cognitive style, social status and modern rationalization, Mannheim (1952) noted how an irrational style of thinking, developed in reaction to modern social organization, could be found in the popular strata, particularly rooted in local traditions, reassuring them as to the condition of social marginality induced by modern rationalization.

With respect to the aim of our study, vaccination hesitation could thus be conceived as a particular manifestation of this more general tendency, thus linking social insecurity, cognitive style and relationship with the modern institutional order.

In this respect, the development of Mannheim's analysis by Bernstein (1964, 1971, 1975) is significant. The British sociologist traced the cognitive styles of different social groups back to real linguistic, and thus communicative, codes. More specifically, Bernstein identified a connection between a person's social condition and the linguistic code through which they express themselves and consequently conceive reality; he noted that social classes take shape not only around specific political-economic power relations, but also through the different ways in which they employ language to express their material conditions. In particular, Bernstein distinguished between the "restricted code" and the" elaborated code".

The former is only employed by the members of the working class as it is based on lexically flexible and syntactically condensed language; it is adequate to cope with the anxiety generated by the high level of social insecurity that usually characterizes the subordinate classes and it does not favor use and full understanding of abstract discourse, such as the use of generalizing thinking. Moreover, the restricted code can be considered the most commonly employed mode of expression in a family context linked to precarious material conditions, and therefore a source of anxiety, where the circulation of communication focused on family problems is more prevalent than on public interest issues.

Instead, the elaborated code is employed by the upper and middle classes, as it is based on the use of abstract symbols, promoters of generalizing thinking and it relates to the self-governing capacity of those who live in advantaged social conditions. Consequently, the upper and middle classes tend to build a family communication oriented towards participation and trust in the public sphere.

In our research, as in the following sections will illustrate, we investigated the kind of code used by people according to their social status, through the analysis of the family communication.

In addition, we considered a very important aspect of Bernstein's theory: the role of the school as an organization of official knowledge that nurtures trust in expert knowledge. It aims to transmit the elaborated code – in a form partially different from that conveyed by the upper and middle classes through mere family socialization – in order to develop the internalization of theoretical knowledge that fosters critical thinking (McLean et al. 2013). According to this perspective, the school takes on an ambivalent role: on the one hand, schools – if characterized by teachers committed to addressing cultural differences due to social origin (Giroux 2003; Parziale 2016) – can allow students from all social origins to participate in the higher levels of education, who can thus internalize the theoretical knowledge useful for developing the elaborated code. In this sense, the construction of a solid school career would favor the progressive acquisition of theoretical knowledge that requires and develops the capacity for abstraction and generalization that is typical of scientific discourse (Young and Muller 2013). On the other hand, the school can reward those students who are socially better able to handle the official culture, which is learned in the family, and offers working-class students, socialized with the restricted code, only participation in those levels of basic education, founded on the transmission of more anecdotal knowledge and close to common sense and ordinary knowledge (Bernstein 1971).

To re-state the theoretical strands that have guided our study, the perspective we have adopted suggests considering, on the one side, the broader dimensions connected to family and school socialization; and on the other, the role that the degree of social insecurity plays with regard to the way in which the various social groups orient themselves in relation to the modern institutional order, characterized by the progressive affirmation of rationality (Weber 1919).

In line with the theoretical aspects presented above, in this contribute we ask whether vaccination hesitation is one of the various ways in which the lower classes, characterized by conditions of social insecurity, express their unease against an institutional system they distrust.

Drawing inspiration from the theoretical perspective presented here, we have formulated the following hypotheses:

1 The propensity to be averse to COVID-19 vaccines is higher among members of the most disadvantaged classes, characterized by a greater social insecurity.
2 The aforementioned relationship is mediated by the type of family communication, understood as an indicator of the expressive code employed.
3 The above relationship is mediated by the level of schooling.

Considering hypothesis 1, we tried to understand whether the social origin of vaccination hesitancy can be traced back to the condition of social insecurity experienced by the disadvantaged classes. With hypothesis 2, we asked whether the possible association between social insecurity and opposition to vaccines is related to the lower likelihood for the lower classes to have a lower degree of family discussion on issues of public relevance, an indicator used to detect the level of elaborated code employed. Finally, hypothesis 3 allowed us to gain a better understanding of the link between the degree of social insecurity and of vaccination hesitancy – in particular, to examine whether vaccination hesitancy can be associated with the difficulties of the most disadvantaged groups in decoding social complexity due to low schooling.

Methodology

To answer our research question and corroborate the three hypotheses above, we administered an online survey in 2021 to a sample of 5,699 Italian students attending the fifth years of upper-secondary school in provincial capital municipalities in Italy. We adopted a probabilistic sample, stratified by geographic area and type of school track. The corroboration of the hypotheses was carried out by means of bivariate descriptive analyses (hypothesis 1) and further investigated in detail by a series of four multiple hierarchical regression models (hypotheses 1, 2 and 3).

The bivariate analyses allowed us to explore the association between the social origin of students and the degree of aversion towards COVID-19 vaccines:

- The variable related to the social origin was reconstructed from the overall most socioeconomically advantageous employment position of the mother and father of each student. The "Upper class" includes the children of professionals, managers and entrepreneurs; the "Middle class", those of clerks, technicians and teachers; the third class is represented by the sons and daughters of the self-employed. The fourth class corresponds to the "'Central' working class", formed by sons and daughters of manual workers with fixed contracts. The fifth category, the "'Peripheral working class", consists of students characterized by a marginal social background, since their parents are manual workers on temporary contracts.
- The variable related to the degree of aversion towards COVID-19 vaccines comes from a Cantril scale 1–10, and then was recoded into an ordinal scale with four response categories: not at all averse (1–3), a little averse (4–5), fairly averse (6–7), very averse (8–10).

With regard to the multiple regression models, the *dependent* variable is represented by the degree of aversion towards COVID-19 vaccines (expressed through a Cantril scale 1–10). The *independent* variable, common to all the models, concerns the social origin of the students, above described.

In the first model, built to corroborate **hypothesis 1**, the influence of social origin on the degree of aversion to the vaccine was considered by controlling for other variables conceivable as *concomitant*, such as the geographical area (North-west, North-east, Center, South of Italy), age, gender and family cultural capital. With regard to the last variable, a dichotomous variable was calculated, which distinguishes the family cultural capital into "low-medium" (the highest educational qualification held by the parents is at most a high school diploma) and "high" (at least one of both parents has a university degree).

Next, in the other three models, some intervening variables were added to the first model, since it was hypothesized that these are influenced by social background and in turn are capable of varying attitudes towards the COVID-19 vaccine. In particular, with the exception of the type of school track (high school, technical and vocational school), the *intervening* variables were summarized in numerical indices, obtained through two-stage principal component analysis (Marradi and Di Franco 2013).

To prove **hypothesis 2**, two variables were added to the previous model in order to detect the type of family communication: "communication open to issues of public relevance" ("Public family communication") and "communication directed towards issues of the private sphere" ("Private family communication"). In particular,

- The index of "communication open to issues of public relevance" reproduces 55.6 percent of the variance of three variables, concerning the frequency (measured on a 0–5 scale) with which students state that they discuss topics related to culture and entertainment (+.480), current affairs and politics (+.470), and religion (+.385) with family members.[1]
- The index of "communication directed towards issues of the private sphere" reproduces 51.6 percent of the variance concerning the frequency (measured on a scale of 0–5) of family discussion around topics such as the economic and working conditions of family members and friends (+.500), the health conditions of these actors (+.519) and the sentimental problems of the respondents (+.352).

These variables were used to detect some aspects of the family socialization according to the code theoretic perspective proposed by Bernstein. In line with what was described in the previous section, we point out that families belonging to the socially marginal social classes tend to develop communication more focused on their private matters rather than on issues of public relevance, an indicator of the use of the restricted code employed. In contrast, families belonging to the more advantaged social classes are more inclined to develop communication focusing on issues of public importance, an indicator of the elaborate code employed.

- Moreover, this model also includes a variable used to detect the level of family climate: this index synthesizes six variables and reproduces 48.5 percent of the overall variance. More specifically, respondents were asked to indicate the degree to which relations in the family were, respectively, attentive to the needs of all family members (+.238), open to dialogue (+.261), serene (+.263), rigid (–.175), cold (–.261) and hostile (–.225).

To corroborate **hypothesis 3**, in addition to the three indices above described, two more intervening variables were added to the second regression model:

- A schooling index, which reproduces 44 percent of the overall variance and relates to the degree of adherence to the education system: the most schooled students are those who obtained a better grade (average school performance in the previous year: +.585), tend to show a strong motivation to continue their studies at university (+.574) and have confidence in teachers (level of confidence in teachers: +.306).
- The type of school track chosen: this variable includes three categories of answers referring to high school, technical and vocational school.

Finally, we further investigated the relationship between social origin and vaccine aversion by building a fourth regression model, characterized by two more indices:

- The level of trust in science and expert knowledge. This index reproduces 53.7 percent of the variance and synthesizes the degree of trust in scientists (+.512), doctors (+.512) and journalists (+310).
- A conspiracy index, reproducing 36 percent of the variance of five variables. In particular, four variables indicate the degree of agreement with a number of statements related to fake news, such as the role of the 5G network in the spread of the coronavirus (+.286), the artificial creation of the coronavirus in a laboratory (+.332), the idea that the pandemic was caused by Bill Gates (+.362) and the virus was spread to convince people to be vaccinated (+.386). The last variable refers to the degree of agreement with the assertion that television and newspapers tell the truth about the coronavirus; this variable expresses significant aversion with the other four variables, showing a negative componential weight (–.286) on the conspiracy orientation index.

Results

To corroborate hypothesis 1, we carried out a bivariate analysis between social origin and level of aversion to COVID-19 vaccine. According to the results, shown in Table 15.1, it is possible to identify a relationship among the two variables: 17.9 percent of the sample stated that they were very or fairly averse to the vaccine, but this propensity increases for students from the central

TABLE 15.1 Level of Aversion to COVID-19 Vaccine by Social Condition

Social Origin	*Not at all averse (%)*	*A little averse (%)*	*Fairly averse (%)*	*Very averse (%)*	*Total (%) (n)*
Upper class	**52.7**	36.1	9.0	2.2	100 (875)
Middle class	**46.8**	39.7	**10.2**	**3.3**	100 (1,367)
Self-employed	41.4	39.1	13.3	6.3	100 (1,047)
"Central" working class	**38.4**	40.9	**15.4**	5.3	100 (1,858)
"Peripheral" working class	**28.8**	43.5	**16.9**	**10.8**	100 (552)
Total	42.2	39.8	12.9	5.0	100 (5,699)

Note: Mean values according to the social origin of the respondents.

working class (20.7 percent) and those from the marginal/peripheral working class (27.7 percent). In contrast, this value is just over 11 percent among students from upper class. Among the latter, 52.7 percent stated that they were not averse to the vaccine, whereas this figure was considerably lower in the case of students from a more disadvantaged social class: only 28.8 percent were not contrary to the vaccine.

To understand how this association reflects the existence of a connection between social origin and cognitive style, as indicated by the theoretical frame of reference outlined above, it was useful to compare the average scores on the indices calculated according to the students' social origin.

As Table 15.2 shows, in the transition from the more socially advantaged to those in a condition of greater social insecurity, there is a significant drop in the degree of schooling and trust in science and expert knowledge, alongside an increase in the score on the conspiracy orientation index. Furthermore, family communication is more focused on public issues – an indicator, according to

TABLE 15.2 Average Values of Indices by Social Origin

	Family climate	*Public family communication*	*Private family communication*	*Schooling*	*Trust in science and expert knowledge*	*Conspiracy orientation*
Upper class (875)	0.032	**0.152**	**–0.116**	**0.342**	**0.204**	**–0.202**
Middle class (1,367)	**0.063**	**0.083**	–0.025	**0.160**	0.099	**–0.146**
Self-employed (1,047)	**0.100**	–0.014	0.007	–0.049	–0.030	**0.091**
"Central" working class (1,858)	**–0.059**	**–0.095**	0.029	**–0.150**	**–0.085**	**0.072**
"Peripheral" working class (552)	**–0.196**	**–0.098**	**0.135**	**–0.338**	**–0.222**	**0.267**

Note: Mean values according to the social origin of the repsondents.

Bernstein's perspective, of the elaborate code used – among respondents from the upper and middle classes, and more based on the discussion of private issues – indicator of the restricted code employed – among students from the marginal working class, who also tend to have a worse family climate. These results suggest us that the association between disadvantaged social status and opposition to vaccines can depend on the low likelihood for marginalized groups to become familiar with the conceptual categories of scientific discourse. In other words, according to these first results, vaccination hesitancy could be related to the use of the restricted code resulting from the anxiety generated by material deprivation.

The relationship between these variables is also deepened with the use of four multiple regressions models.

In particular, the first model (Table 15.3), which reproduces the 3.6 percent variance of the dependent variable, shows that attitudes towards the COVID-19 vaccine is influenced by social origin: students belonging to the most disadvantaged classes characterized by greater social insecurity show a greater aversion to the vaccine, while upper-class students tend to have less propensity to be against the vaccine.

By also adding the intervening variables in the second model (Table 15.4), which reproduces the 5.9 percent variance of the dependent variable, it was possible to corroborate hypothesis 2: it turns out that the degree of aversion to

TABLE 15.3 First Multiple Linear Regression Model on COVID-19 Vaccine Aversion Level

	Non-standardized coefficients		*Standardized coefficients*			*Collinearity statistics*	
	B	Standard error	Beta	t	Sign	Toler-ance	VIF
Constant	–2.288	0.161		–14.238	0.000		
Middle class	0.067	0.034	0.034	1.975	0.048	0.493	2.028
Self-employed	0.194	0.038	0.089	5.163	0.000	0.492	2.032
"Central" working class	**0.225**	0.034	0.125	6.642	0.000	0.412	2.426
"Peripheral" working class	**0.465**	0.043	0.162	10.749	0.000	0.636	1.573
Female	–0.053	0.021	–0.032	–2.596	0.009	0.980	1.021
Age	–0.050	0.009	–0.072	–5.902	0.000	0.987	1.013
North-east	0.039	0.032	0.018	1.224	0.221	0.707	1.414
Center	0.045	0.029	0.023	1.532	0.126	0.668	1.498
South of Italy	–0.045	0.027	-0.025	–1.662	0.097	0.630	1.588
High family cultural capital	–0.098	0.023	–0.056	–4.252	0.000	0.830	1.205

Note: the highest values are highlighted in black.

TABLE 15.4 Second Multiple Linear Regression Model on COVID-19 Vaccine Aversion Level

	Non-standardized coefficients		*Standardized coefficients*			*Collinearity statistics*	
	B	Standard error	Beta	t	Sign	Toler-ance	VIF
Constant	–2.409	0.160		–15.075	0.000		
Middle class	0.060	0.034	0.030	1.786	0.074	0.493	2.030
Self-employed	0.180	0.037	0.082	4.832	0.000	0.491	2.036
"Central" working class	**0.196**	0.034	0.109	5.846	0.000	0.410	2.440
"Peripheral" working class	**0.424**	0.043	0.148	9.855	0.000	0.630	1.587
Female	–0.041	0.020	–0.024	–2.015	0.044	0.976	1.024
Age	–0.047	0.008	–0.066	–5.488	0.000	0.976	1.025
North-east	0.042	0.032	0.019	1.313	0.189	0.707	1.415
Center	0.053	0.029	0.026	1.801	0.072	0.666	1.502
South of Italy	–0.024	0.027	–0.014	–0.905	0.366	0.626	1.597
High family cultural capital	–0.078	0.023	-0.045	–3.413	0.001	0.822	1.217
Family climate	0.052	0.021	0.030	2.457	0.014	0.971	1.030
Public family communication	**–0.120**	0.011	–0.142	–11.061	0.000	0.862	1.160
Private family communication	0.042	0.011	0.049	3.890	0.000	0.880	1.136

Note: the highest values are highlighted in black.

the COVID-19 vaccine is influenced by the "Public family communication", i.e. the level of family discussion and of the communication centered on issues of collective importance. In other words, the degree of opposition to the vaccine depends in part on the expressive code employed in the family. Considering the negative sign this variable takes on, it emerges that a lower level of family communication open to issues in the public sphere corresponds to a higher degree of aversion to the vaccine on the part of the students.

To summarize, these two models allowed us to corroborate the first two hypotheses: indeed, even bearing mind the other conditions considered in the first model, the level of aversion to the vaccine varies according to the degree of social insecurity, with the most disadvantaged students showing a greater aversion. In turn, this relationship is in part mediated by "Public family communication", showing, therefore, the close relationship between low social status and this mode of expression, which, from the Bernsteinian analytical perspective, is an indicator of the code employed in the family – an aspect that is also explored in the following models.

By introducing the other variables, such as schooling and type of school track, into the third model (Table 15.5), which reproduces the 9.9 percent variance of the dependent variable, social status continues to exert an influence on vaccine aversion. In particular, the value of the "'peripheral' working class" decreases by a third, due to the mediated effect of schooling and type of school. This means that the positive view of vaccines grows as a function of schooling and attendance at high school, both of which are influenced by social status. In other words, those in the upper and middle classes tend to go to high school and have a good schooling, and these two factors lead to a greater propensity to accept vaccines. In contrast, students belonging to the lower class tend to be less favorable to the vaccine, because they have less schooling and have attended vocational schools, i.e. schools that generally gather people from more disadvantaged social backgrounds.

Moreover, the value of "Public family communication" – which is almost halved compared to the previous model – exerts an indirect effect on the degree

TABLE 15.5 Third Multiple Linear Regression Model on COVID-19 Vaccine Aversion Level

	Non-standardized coefficients		*Standardized coefficients*			*Collinearity statistics*	
	B	Standard error	Beta	t	Sign	Tolerance	VIF
Constant	−2.557	0.157		−16.262	0.000		
Middle class	0.021	0.033	0.011	0.638	0.524	0.490	2.041
Self-employed	0.115	0.037	0.052	3.133	0.002	0.486	2.058
"Central" working class	0.095	0.033	0.053	2.844	0.004	0.397	2.522
"Peripheral" working class	**0.282**	0.043	0.098	6.583	0.000	0.607	1.647
Female	0.044	0.021	0.026	2.078	0.038	0.877	1.140
Age	−0.053	0.008	−0.075	−6.373	0.000	0.973	1.028
North-east	0.019	0.031	0.009	0.616	0.538	0.695	1.438
Center	0.083	0.029	0.041	2.864	0.004	0.655	1.528
South of Italy	0.004	0.026	0.002	0.161	0.872	0.622	1.608
High family cultural capital	−0.018	0.023	−0.011	−0.806	0.420	0.799	1.251
Family climate	0.013	0.021	0.007	0.605	0.545	0.948	1.055
Public family communication	**−0.080**	0.011	−0.095	−7.357	0.000	0.822	1.216
Private family communication	0.035	0.011	0.041	3.300	0.001	0.879	1.138
Schooling	**−0.119**	0.011	−0.141	-10.750	0.000	0.786	1.272
Technical school	0.187	0.025	0.106	7.607	0.000	0.706	1.417
Vocational school	**0.323**	0.031	0.137	10.342	0.000	0.779	1.284

of opposition to the vaccine, especially through schooling.[2] In this sense, students who live in families characterized by greater communication on public issues are more adherent to the school system and in this sense less vaccine-averse.

This third model corroborates hypothesis 3 by allowing a greater understanding of the link between the degree of social marginalization of the disadvantaged classes and hostility to vaccines, through the role played by schooling and type of school track. Hence, according to these results, vaccination hesitancy can be attributed to the difficulty of the most disadvantaged groups in decoding social complexity, due to low schooling.

At the same time, the results confirm another important aspect: the persistence of the value of the peripheral working class, all other variables being equal, which suggests that vaccination hesitation can be one of several ways in which the disadvantaged classes express their unease against an institutional system. To investigate this relationship, a fourth model was also constructed. It explains 22.2 percent of the variance and is characterized by the addition of two important variables: trust in science and expert knowledge, and conspiracy orientation (Table 15.6). First, the values of the two new variables show that a higher conspiracy orientation leads to a greater propensity on the part of respondents to be vaccine-averse, and less trust in science is related to the greater propensity to be vaccine hostile. However, even when compared with other variables such as trust in science, schooling, family debate, school address (i.e. all factors that in some way affect the level of opposition to the vaccine), the effect of social status decreases, but not to a great extent.

In other words, observing the very low decrease in the value attributed to the lowest class between the third and fourth models, it is possible to state that social marginality has a significant direct effect on vaccine hesitancy: half of the total effect is not mediated by the other variables, including the schooling rate.

This result thus indicates the persistence of the direct effect of social status, even with the same level of trust in science, suggesting a higher likelihood of distrust of COVID-19 vaccines on the part of those in a condition of social insecurity. In other words, the reason that aversion to the vaccine is higher among the disadvantaged, even considering all the variables considered in the model, can probably be due to the condition of social insecurity in which they find themselves, which leads to a sense of fear and distrust in the institutional order.

In summary, the results of the multivariate analysis seem to support the theoretical framework of reference and corroborate the hypotheses developed through this. From a joint reading of the results obtained, it emerges that students from the "marginal" working class are more inclined to distrust, or even be openly hostile towards, COVID-19 vaccines (hypothesis 1). On the one hand, this relationship depends on the communicative code employed in the family (hypothesis 2), and, according to our findings, less discussion of issues of public importance in family leads to less acceptance of vaccines among students. On the other hand, it also depends on level of schooling and type of school (hypothesis 3), which affect the ability to decode scientific discourse, and

TABLE 15.6 Fourth Multiple Linear Regression Model on COVID-19 Vaccine Aversion Level

	Non-standardized coefficients		*Standardized coefficients*			*Collinearity statistics*	
	B	Standard error	Beta	t	Sign	Toler-ance	VIF
Constant	–2.501	0.146		-17.118	0.000		
Middle class	0.027	0.031	0.014	0.885	0.376	0.490	2.041
Self-employed	0.070	0.034	0.032	2.061	0.039	0.485	2.061
"Central" working class	0.071	0.031	0.040	2.301	0.021	0.396	2.523
"Peripheral" working class	**0.216**	0.040	0.076	5.432	0.000	0.606	1.651
Female	–0.024	0.020	-0.014	–1.244	0.214	0.867	1.153
Age	–0.045	0.008	-0.064	–5.802	0.000	0.971	1.030
North-east	0.017	0.029	0.008	0.588	0.557	0.695	1.439
Center	0.051	0.027	0.026	1.911	0.056	0.654	1.530
South of Italy	–0.023	0.025	–0.013	–0.947	0.343	0.621	1.610
High family cultural capital	–0.014	0.021	–0.008	–0.662	0.508	0.799	1.252
Family climate	–0.003	0.019	–0.002	–0.166	0.868	0.946	1.057
Public family communication	–0.057	0.010	–0.068	–5.626	0.000	0.814	1.229
Private family communication	0.025	0.010	0.029	2.527	0.012	0.878	1.139
Schooling	–0.055	0.011	–0.065	–5.195	0.000	0.749	1.334
Technical school	0.106	0.023	0.060	4.620	0.000	0.697	1.435
Vocational school	**0.159**	0.029	0.067	5.405	0.000	0.756	1.323
Trust in science and expert knowledge	**–0.137**	0.010	–0.162	-13.584	0.000	0.827	1.210
Conspiracy orientation	**0.247**	0.010	0.293	24.895	0.000	0.848	1.179

Note: the highest values are highlighted in black.

consequently the level of trust in vaccines. However, the persistence of social class and its impact on COVID-19 vaccine hostility points to the idea that the use of irrational belief systems is partly the result of material insecurity in the most disadvantaged groups.

Discussion and Concluding Remarks

This research aimed to provide an analysis of the social roots of vaccine hesitancy (in particular, the attitude of opposition to vaccines), focusing on the Italian context. Through the theoretical and analytical pathway developed, the association between social marginality and aversion to vaccines emerges. This relationship can be linked to a plurality of aspects that refer to an intricate relationship between family socialization and school socialization, both of which can more easily facilitate the understanding of social origin. In particular, the higher propensity of the most disadvantaged individuals to hold irrational beliefs is in part related to the lack of familiarity in the use of the elaborated code, due to a low level of schooling (Bernstein 1971, 1975). In fact, if we consider the degree of discussion in the family on topics of public relevance to be an indicator of the use of the elaborated code, it emerged that students who discuss these topics less often in the family are more hostile to vaccines.

Furthermore, the results showed greater vaccination hesitancy on the part of vocational students, even with the same level of schooling; this may in part depend on the role played by theoretical knowledge, which is generally less characteristic of this educational pathway. At the same time, the vocational path often represents a type of school generally aimed at young people from the lower classes (Pitzalis 2017), after they have been considered inadequate according to the criteria of the dominant culture (Bourdieu 1991, 1996). Adopting this perspective, the mistrust of COVID-19 vaccines on the part of the less educated might also depend on a lack of social recognition in its capacity to aspire, to use Appadurai's (2013) words.

Consequently, those who are socially disadvantaged tend to distance themselves from the official cultural world, also making use of other forms of knowledge dissemination and production, the highest expression of which is the infodemy of the internet. In this regard, according to our previous research, peripheral groups are more inclined than other groups to find and trust information on social media, as this form of information responds to the horizontal mode of communication that is more consistent with the restricted code they possess (Catone and Parziale 2022). In this perspective, the relationship between trust in science and the use of social media (van Dijck and Alinejad 2020) can make it possible to identify a consonance between the need to resort to social capital bonding, the focus of family communication on private issues (connected to use of the restricted code) and low institutional trust (Catone and Parziale 2022). Moreover, according to several studies, the use of certain media and information channels was an important determinant of the vaccination decision. In particular, some investigations have indicated that often misinformation produced by social media is negatively associated with the intention to vaccinate (Gehrau et al. 2021), and, at the same time, misinformation mainly characterizes contexts in which there is a lack of trust in government, politics and institutions (Jennings et al. 2021).

In light of the results obtained in our research, another key aspect emerges: social insecurity does not only influence cognitive style indirectly through mediating the level of family communication on issues of public relevance, schooling and trust in expert knowledge, but also does so directly. In fact, insecurity is linked not only to the degree of critical theoretical knowledge and the decoding of complexity, but also to the way in which one person constructs a relationship with an other, thus also influencing the determination of trust mechanisms, including institutional ones. In other words, vaccination hesitation can be read as the typical outcome of the trajectory of subjects from the disadvantaged classes, who find themselves feeling a mixture of fear and distance towards the institutions of official culture.

Therefore, it emerges that the more general vaccine hesitancy can be traced not only to forms of reaction to the vaccine, but to the global institutional apparatus, a source of social insecurity.

In this respect, in future developments of this research as well, it might be useful to trace back (at least partially) the attitude of aversion towards vaccines to an aspect of the broader social change of recent decades, i.e., to a reshaping of the traditional class conflict (based on an ideological clash founded on trust in science) towards a more cultural type of conflict characterized by the presence of groups with different value orientations. On this point, Mannheim (1929) was perhaps the first scholar to point out how social conflict, including that based on the traditional class conflicts in modern society, also concerns interpretations of the world. From this point of view, social conflict in its various forms can be traced back to a predominantly cultural dimension based on the opposition between those who have the social resources to better decode the complexity of late modernity and look forward, and those who are deprived of them.

The contrast between those who have confidence in expert knowledge and those who are more sceptical, as well as the distinction between those who are more predisposed to institutional and scientific indications and those who are more reluctant, starting with the so-called "No Vax" population, can also be placed in this long-term shift in social conflict.

Notes

1 The values in brackets are componential coefficients, i.e. values used to estimate the net contribution of each variable to the overall index.
2 The mediated effect of public family communication on vaccine aversion, which is mainly due to the mediated effect of schooling, was detected by controlling the statistical analyses performed.

References

Appadurai, Arjun. 2013. *The Future as Cultural Fact: Essays on the Global Condition*. London: Verso.

Appadurai, Arjun. 2017. "The democracy fatigue". In *The Great Regression*, edited by Heinrich Geiselberger, 1–12. Cambridge: Polity Press.

Aw, Junjie, Jun Jie Benjamin Seng, and Low Lian Leng. 2021. "COVID-19 vaccine hesitancy – a scoping review of literature in high-income countries". *Vaccines* 9, 8: 900.

Beck, Ulrich. 1986. *Risikogesellschaft: Auf dem Weg in eine andere Moderne*. Suhrkamp Verlag.

Bernstein, Basil. 1964. "Elaborated and restricted codes: their social origins and some consequences". *American Anthropologist* 66, 6: 55–69.
Bernstein, Basil. 1971. *Class, Codes and Control: Theoretical Studies towards a Sociology of Language*. London: Routledge & Kegan Paul.
Bernstein, Basil. 1975. *Class, Codes and Control: Towards a Theory of Educational Transmissions*, Vol. 3. London: Routledge & Kegan Paul.
Bourdieu, Pierre. 1991. *Language and Symbolic Power*. Cambridge: Harvard University Press.
Bourdieu, Pierre. 1996. *State Nobility: Elite Schools in the Field of Power*. Cambridge: Polity Press.
Catone, Maria Carmela, and Fiorenzo Parziale. 2022. "Digital practices, communicative codes and social inequalities: a case study during the pandemic in Italy". *Italian Journal of Sociology of Education*, 14, 3: 173–200.
Fraser, Nancy. 2017. "Progressive neoliberalism versus reactionary populism: a Hobson's choice". In *The Great Regression*, edited by Heinrich Geiselberger, 54–60. Cambridge: Polity Press.
Gehrau, Volker, Sam Fujarski, Hannah Lorenz, Carla Schieb, and Bernd Blöbaum. 2021. "The impact of health information exposure and source credibility on COVID-19 vaccination intention in Germany". *International Journal of Environmental Research and Public Health*, 18, 9: 4678.
Giddens, Anthony. 1990. *The Consequences of Modernity*. Cambridge: Polity Press.
Giroux, Henry. 2003. "Public pedagogy and the politics of resistance: notes on a critical theory of educational struggle". *Educational Philosophy and Theory*, 35, 1: 5–15.
Gobo, Giampietro, and Barbara Sena. 2019. "Oltre la polarizzazione pro-vax versus no-vax: atteggiamenti e motivazioni nel dibattito italiano sulle vaccinazioni". *Salute e società*, 2: 176–190.
Jennings, Will, Gerry Stoker, Hannah Bunting, Viktor Orri Valgarðsson, Jennifer Gaskell, Daniel Devine, Lawrence McKay, and Melinda C. Mills. 2021. "Lack of trust, conspiracy beliefs, and social media use predict COVID-19 vaccine hesitancy". *Vaccines*, 9, 6: 593.
Kerr, John R., Claudia Schneider, Gabriel Recchia, Sarah Dryhurst, Ullrika Sahlin, Carole Dufouil, Pierre Arwidson, Alexandra L.J. Freeman, and Sander van der Linden. 2021. "Correlates of intended COVID-19 vaccine acceptance across time and countries: results from a series of cross-sectional surveys". *BMJ Open*, 11, 8, e048025: 1–11.
Kessels, Roselinde, Jeroen Luyten, and Sandy Tubeuf. 2021. "Willingness to get vaccinated against Covid-19 and attitudes toward vaccination in general". *Vaccine*, 39, 33: 4716–4722.
Lin, Cheryl, Pikuei Tu, and Leslie M. Beitsch. 2020. "Confidence and receptivity for COVID-19 vaccines: a rapid systematic review". *Vaccines*, 9, 1: 15.
Mannheim, Karl. 1929. *Ideologie und Utopie*. Frankfurt am Main: Vittorio Klostermann.
Mannheim, Karl (1952). *Essays in the Sociology of Knowledge*. London: Routledge and Kegan Paul.
Marradi, Alberto, and Giovanni Di Franco. 2013. *Factor Analysis and Principal Component analysis*. Milano: Franco Angeli.
McLean, Monica, Andrea Abbas, and Paul Ashwin. 2013. "The use and value of Bernstein's work in studying (in)equalities in undergraduate social science education". *British Journal of Sociology of Education*, 34 , 2: 262–280.
Morales, Danielle Xiaodan, Tylor Fox Beltran, and Stephanie Alexandra Morales. 2022. "Gender, socioeconomic status, and COVID-19 vaccine hesitancy in the US: an intersectionality approach". *Sociology of Health & Illness*, 44: 953–971.

Parziale, Fiorenzo. 2016. *Eretici e respinti: Classi sociali e istruzione superiore in Italia.* Milano: Franco Angeli.

Pellizzoni, Luigi. 2020. "Pseudoscienza, post-verità, governo del disordine. L'esitazione vaccinale nel XXI secolo". In *Scienza in discussione? Dalla controversia sui vaccini all'emergenza Covid-19*, edited by Luigi Pellizzoni and Rita Biancheri, 31–51. Milano: Franco Angeli.

Pitzalis, Marco. 2017. Ritorno sulla riproduzione sociale. Famiglia, capitale culturale e campo scolastica. In *Il mondo dell'uomo, i campi del sapere*, edited by Emanuela Susca, 159–179. Nocera Inferiore (SA): Ortothes.

Reno, Chiara, Elisa Maietti, Maria Pia Fantini, Elena Savoia, Lamberto Manzoli, Marco Montalti, and Davide Gori. 2021. "Enhancing COVID-19 vaccines acceptance: results from a survey on vaccine hesitancy in Northern Italy". *Vaccines*, 9, 4: 378.

Soares, Patricia, João Victor Rocha, Marta Moniz, Ana Gama, Pedro Almeida Laires, Ana Rita Pedro, Sónia Dias, Andreia Leite, and Carla Nunes. 2021. "Factors associated with COVID-19 vaccine hesitancy". *Vaccines*, 9, 3: 300.

Van Dijck, José, and Donya Alinejad. 2020. "Social media and trust in scientific expertise: debating the Covid-19 pandemic in the Netherlands". *Social Media+ Society*, 6, 4: 1–11.

Vinck, Patrick, Phuong N. Pham, Kenedy Bindu, Juliet Bedford, and Eric J. Nilles. 2019. "Institutional trust and misinformation in the response to the 2018–19 Ebola outbreak in North Kivu, DR Congo: a population-based survey". *Lancet Infectious Diseases*, 19, 5: 529–536.

Vulpe, Simona Nicoleta, and Cosima Rughiniş. 2021. "Social amplification of risk and 'probable vaccine damage': a typology of vaccination beliefs in 28 European countries". *Vaccine*, 39, 10: 1508–1515.

Weber, Max. 1919. Wissenschaft als Beruf. [Science as a Vocation]. München and Leipzig: Duncker and Humblot.

Young, Michael, and Johan Muller. 2013. "On the powers of powerful knowledge". *Review of Education*, 1, 3: 229–250.

16

"FEMINISM IS THE REAL PLAGUE"

The Spanish Radical Right Antifeminism during the COVID-19 Pandemic

Antonio Álvarez-Benavides and Francisco Jiménez Aguilar

Introduction: Why Did the Spanish Radical Right Go Against Feminism during the COVID-19 Pandemic?

On March 14, 2020, Pedro Sánchez, the Spanish prime minister, announced a nationwide lockdown. Bars, restaurants, and any non-essential businesses were instructed to remain closed. People were required to stay home and only allowed to leave in order to do grocery shopping and walk their pets. The COVID-19 crisis had broken out, provoking an unseen social and political situation for most citizens. Seven days before the first confinement, on March 8 (8M), the annual women's rights demonstration took place in several cities in Spain. Thousands of religious and sporting events were held, including a far-right counterdemonstration organized by the populist radical party Vox, bringing together 9,000 to 15,000 attendees in Madrid. This rally, called Vista-legre III, was a massive party aimed at reelecting Santiago Abascal as their national leader for the following four years (Vox Spain 2020d). Some hours after that, Javier Ortega Smith, one of the most prominent responsible for the party that actively participated in the celebration, announced he was infected. Nonetheless, the 8M feminist demonstration was considered by Vox– as well as the conservative Popular Party (PP) and other moderated political forces– the primary source of infections in Spain.

Since 2020, the 8M demonstration has received furious attacks by the center and radical right. The main reason, as we will show, is not that this mass gathering was deemed a health liability but that it was a feminist demonstration. The progress of feminism in Spain has achieved unprecedented levels in recent years. In the last two decades, Spanish institutions have approved some of the most ambitious worldwide laws and politics against gender violence and for the recognition of women and LGTBIQ+ rights. The 8M mobilizations in

DOI: 10.4324/9781003459682-19

Spain since 2018 are some of the largest feminist strikes in history (Campillo 2019; Idoiaga Mongragon et al. 2022). However, feminism still faces resistance by important sectors of civil society, particularly since the creation of the coalition government of the Spanish Socialist Workers' Party (PSOE) and Unidas Podemos (UP) –an agreement between Podemos, communist, ecologist, and leftist political and social collectives.

According to antifeminists, the onslaughts against feminism do not aim to deny gender equality, but to fight against an ideological artifact that has made possible a dramatic and profound transformation of Spanish and global society. Feminist politics are, for these collective actors, the key element of a cultural, economic, and political decadence that goes beyond some specific rights or conditions. The nature of the movement is associated with ideologies such as anarchism, communism, socialism, ecologism, or pacifism. Hence, and paradoxically, the transversal, intersectional, translocal, and transformative character that feminism has always reclaimed for itself (Cabezas González 2021) is recognized by those who repudiate it.

Various political parties have articulated multiple forms of sexism and LGTBIQphobia. Recently, though, some have openly and clearly identified themselves as antifeminist and antigender (Graff and Korlczuk 2022). This is the case of the Spanish radical right party Vox, a PP spinoff founded on December 17, 2013. Beyond claims formulated by the conservative party against abortion rights and homosexual marriage, no other right-wing party had explicitly rejected all forms of equality policy and feminism. Vox embodies a "party antifeminism" that threatens implementing a complete "state antifeminism" (Dupuis-Déri 2016). Sexism has thus become a primary discursive node for this new far-right group since its emergence and participation in national institutions (Alonso and Espinosa-Fajardo 2021; Álvarez-Benavides and Jiménez Aguilar 2021; Cabezas 2022).

The COVID-19 crisis is an excellent example of how antifeminism/antigenderism has become an essential agent of change to structure the far-right political and cultural response to the ideas and people that feminism represents. The Spanish radical right has identified the pandemic as a multidimensional crisis, a broad process, which is not limited to its epidemiological consequences. The critics of the "communist-feminist" government are supported by the lack of a "strong government", due to the displacement of masculinity as a central figure and the progressive disappearance of conservative conceptions of femininity and family. The existence of a progressive and feminist government is, per se, the consequence of a historical and cultural process that has spread weak ideas, politics, and agents but paradoxically also defined as totalitarian. Their health crisis management is one of the costs of a long-term crisis provoked by the "Trojan horse of equality". All these complex and contradictory stances led to a complete rejection of feminism.

In this chapter, we will explain why Vox has interpreted the COVID-19 crisis in antifeminist terms. To do so –through Vox's public statements, political speeches, interviews, official party webpage and social media posts, and parliamentary interventions between 2020 and 2022– we will analyze how this radical right party has evaluated the health crisis and its political consequences in Spain, what measures they have proposed to solve it, and the responses they have given. The cross-sectional study of its organization, performance, and agenda-setting will permit us to point out that feminism, among other agents, is, in their view, an explicative element of the origins of the pandemic crisis. In this sense, any feminist idea or measure has delayed or hampered the recovery of normality, even in the survival of democracy. For that reason, national policy must directly end state and social feminism. To address it, in the following sections we will focus on the different forms of sexism and antifeminism displayed by Vox when facing a health crisis with substantial political, economic, and cultural consequences.

More Than Benevolent Sexism: Nativist and Antifeminist Femininities for a "New Normal"

Recent far-right studies distinguish between benevolent sexism and hostile sexism in order to talk about ways of imagining normative sexual difference and their counterparts (Mudde 2019). As we will show in this section, rather than being two distinct elements, they are complementary. Vox's gender discourse and practices during the pandemic show ambiguous signs of a benevolent sexism. The party claims the need for recovering traditional female roles based on Christian and neoliberal models of femininity, further denigrated by the social precariousness derived from the economic crises rooted in both the Great Recession as well as the recent health emergency. It resorts to the traditional sources of Catholicism to idealize Spanish women as wives and mothers. The Virgin Mary symbolizes the ultimate female representation. Using the hashtag #TheBestWoman (*#LaMejorMujer*), they define her as "devoted, attentive, sweet, generous, strong, helpful, modest, faithful, prayerful, guide, companion, wife, mother, queen", in a campaign with billboards in multiple Spanish cities, on March 8, 2021 (Toscano, March 8, 2021c). This femininity is based on a biologically and culturally differentiated conception of women and men. It does not question the roots of family and maternal issues that have risen from different patterns and forms of inequality, not even in the context of the COVID-19 care crisis. It seeks to preserve this model. They stand for "a woman who wants to fulfill herself in the private sphere and form a home" (Vox Spain, May 11, 2022i).

Due to the secularization processes in Spain, Vox also incorporates other new profiles of women that justify their ideology. These profiles became especially significant in addressing the care and security demands during the periods of confinement. They accept and promote a model of working women when it legitimizes their national, military, and neoliberal collective imaginary. For example, María Bernardo de Quirós (1898–1983), the first Spanish airplane pilot, is presented as a "woman without quotas", whose "spirit is completely different from that of current feminism, a feminism that has become a hateful ideology" (Vox Spain, March 7, 2022b). Clara Campoamor (1888–1972), one of the leading promoters for women's suffrage in Spain and a member of the center and right-wing republican parties, is defined as a "feminist against socialism" (Vox Spain, March 4, 2019a). "Traditional" male professions are acceptable as long as they do not contradict the basis of their ultranationalist ideology. In this case, these female models are well accommodated to the punitive and neoliberal dimension Vox has sheltered so far (Brown 2019, 39–46). This woman represents an empowered subject who obtains her authority by herself through work (Rottenberg 2018), which usually coincides with the nation's interests, such as civil agents, police officers, and soldiers (Vox Castellón, March 8, 2022), but also as domestic and care workers (Vox Spain, March 8, 2021b). This type of femininity, despite taking place within a more secular nature, continues to refer to a cultural Christianity, no longer based on creed but on a native worldview, customs, and traditions which are considered superior (Cornejo and Pichardo Galán 2017).

Vox female political representatives personify the femininity types demarcated by this radical party and it is indeed these women who lead and provide impetus to this antifeminist backlash. Right-wing parties such as PP or Ciudadanos, which articulate some sexist practices, accept equality policies and have members self-defined as feminists. On the other hand, most Spanish far-right feminine representatives are self-proclaimed antifeminists. Deputies such as Rocío de Meer, Lourdes Méndez, María Ruiz, Carla Toscano, Alicia V. Rubio, Rocío Monasterio, or Macarena Olona led the antifeminist discourse in the Congress of Deputies, the Senate, or the Assembly of Madrid. They are self-presented in the political institutions and media as women who resist "aversive" forms of being a woman. Most male representatives do not generate these discourses –except for some cases of misogynistic outbursts– and participate in a rather minor role as disseminators. Paradoxically, Vox's sexism and antifeminism are compatible with apparently more egalitarian forms of party structure. Many of its representatives and spokespersons are women and have employed a "zipper system" in most of the elections they have run since 2017. They have even defined themselves as "the party of women", in opposition to those who accuse Vox of being "sexist" (*machistas*) (Vox Spain, February 7, 2022a). Another question still to be studied is women's real power behind Vox closed doors.

At this point, it is necessary to emphasize that there is a clear analogy between Vox's definition of womanhood and nation. The nation must be protected because it is weakened by its enemies, even though it is in essence strong, undisputable, and sublime. Only they represent and care about it, they are the nation's sole savior. Spanish women are also weakened by the same actors who ruin the nation and dispossess it of its soul. However, from their conception of femininity and gender relations, women will have the strength to become women again. It is for this reason that they deny that feminism represents women, their campaign *#Don'tSpeakInMyName* (*#NoHabléisEnMiNombre*) being one of the most obvious examples of this notion (Vox Spain, March 8, 2022h). Given that Vox is the unique party that defends the "real woman", who sacrifice, fulfill themselves being mothers, at home or working for their fatherland, the idea of sacrifice is powerful. In this sense, they justify the suppression of equality laws arguing that women should not be protected, because they are self-sufficient, and able to maintain the same rights as men through effort, tenacity, and acceptance. Sacrifice refers to the religious aspect of life, but also the sacredness of the nation. Again, it offers an ideological articulation that combines elements of religion with other secularized axioms –such as a neoliberal individualized conception of agency (Álvarez-Benavides and Turnbough 2022, 2–5)– to construct its vision of national and gender relations. It is also evident in their worldview the analogy between a nation conceived as a mother and a woman who finds in motherhood her true *raison d'être*. Anything that questions these types of women and nation, by the simple fact of conceiving the possibility of other models, is considered an enemy.

Antifeminism and ultranationalism constitute an inseparable pairing in Vox. Their main antagonist is gender ideology. This idea was developed by the Catholic Church during the 1980s and 1990s as a religious opposition to feminism and sexual diversity. It has also been a central component of the response to many recent reforms in secular law governing the sexes, sexuality, reproduction, and the family promoted by the UN and the UE. These include laws leading to the dismantling of sex roles, the acceptance of homosexuality, the recognition of a diversity of family types and of sexual and gender expression, and access to new reproductive technologies, condoms, other contraceptives, and abortion (Case 2019, 640–641). In this view, feminism and gender ideology are the same thing, referring to an ideology that, under the guise of fighting against women's inequality, sneaks in a complete battery of progressive and relativistic cultural politics that head towards national and Western decadency. For these reasons, feminism and gender ideology are held responsible for the destruction of the family, the individual's moral deterioration, and the natality crisis.

Left-wing parties, particularly during the COVID-19 crisis, were considered the enemies of democracy. The connection between gender ideology and communism is systematic and especially powerful in Spain, first, because this radical right is self-defined as liberal or neoliberal (Ferreira 2019), and second, because it has not entirely detached from Francoism, which based its legitimation on the myth of fighting communism in Spain. This approach is an example of some far-right ideological assumptions shared by political actors and parties not considered extremists (Álvarez-Benavides 2018). For instance, the Madrilenian PP used the slogan "communism or freedom" (El País, March 15, 2021) in the 2021 regional election, claiming that the measures to contain the virus approved by the central left-wing government were unjustified, authoritarian, and attacked freedom as a communist system does.

Neither communism nor feminism is acceptable for Vox, even as political options. The starting point for recovering the glory of the Spanish nation involves the eradication of its enemies, and the pandemic has proven to be an excellent opportunity for this purpose. They have demanded the illegalization of UP and any communist party, the regional independentist parties, as well as any political organization that, in their view, jeopardizes Spain and its democracy (Vox Spain, July 23, 2021f). For them, these parties and ideas are dangerous for the nation and are using the pandemic to impose politics that erode citizens' rights. Their concept of freedom is tremendously restrictive, as is its idea of the national community. They consider the nation to be a homogeneous entity; thus any other interpretation based on ethnic, cultural, linguistic, religious, or ideological diversity is incompatible with its national being and is rejected outright. Something similar happens with its conception of femininities. Vox only recognize the agency of the women that align with their gender values and nationalism. To justify that, these free women can assume only these specific characteristics; they ignore and deny any other women. They constantly contrast the women they envisage with other women who are supposedly amoral, weak, uneducated, resentful, misandrist, and unpatriotic. These are no-women, the same way that those who do not recognize themselves in their idea of the nation are no-Spaniards. The women that do not coincide with the radical right canon are naturalized and objectivated through a patriarchal process of homogenization carried out in the traditional media, social networks, and political institutions (Alcaide Lara 2022).

Generally, Vox rejects debate because its arguments are addressed as axioms. Their main objective in the political arena is to discredit and nullify their opponents, avoiding any kind of discussion. The rejection of feminist women is articulated through an antidemocratic and antiegalitarian speech supported by the connections between anticommunism and gender ideology. When left-wing parties defend women's rights, they are stigmatized as "feminist supremacist", putting them on the same level as white nationalism (Vox Spain, December 2, 2021i). Feminism is accused of being a "Thought Police", referring to George Orwell's dystopic novel *1984* (Vox Spain, October 12, 2021g). They are also called "feminazis", a portmanteau popularized by the American conservative commentator Rush Limbaugh (Vox Spain, March 8, 2019b), or "totalitarians", as was the case for the representatives of the Basque independentist left-wing party EH-Bildu during a session of the European Parliament (Toscano, November 26, 2020d). This idea of a "lefty totalitarianism" is usually evoked by Vox Spain (February 27, 2020c), aiming to make fascism and communism morally equal, and in such a manner to invalidate any left-wing politics (Traverso 2001). Feminists are even accused of being sexist for promoting, for example, bicycle courses for women (Vox Spain, October 28, 2020f). There are also references to colonialism when they are called "feminism's slaves" (El Debate, October 24, 2021). During the pandemic, this discourse has been radicalized with the definition of feminism as a cancer or a plague which threatens the health of democracy, society, and the nation (GranCanariaTv.com, November 15, 2019). The use of such biological metaphors involves not only their moral or political delegitimization, but also their dehumanization.

In this way, for Vox, Minister of Equality Irene Montero embodies all the negative features of a leftist feminist politician. She is the antithesis of the Spanish woman. Attacks against Montero exhibit the most hostile and violent antifeminism deployed by the radical right party. The minister is not only questioned for the politics she is promoting but also herself as a woman and person. The intervention of radical right deputy Carla Toscano in the Congress of Deputies on November 23, 2022, illustrates perfectly the radical party strategy against feminism since its arrival to the political arena. She blamed the minister for imposing the "infamous gender ideology" and a "deranged and hung-up feminism", of "destroying human nature", "abandoning women and children", "criminalizing men", "promoting pedophilia", and "releasing rappers". Toscano stated that her unique merit for being a minister was "to have deeply studied Pablo Iglesias", former UP leader and her current partner. Montero is not judged for her role as a politician, but because of her sexuality, due to (according to Toscano) her "vices", "traumas", and "sexual obsession". This was not the first time a representative of the radical right party called her a "whore" (Sánchez, August 25, 2022), though this political speech includes a compendium of Vox political styles, never seen before in the parliament, as well as its animadversion to every woman that does not fit their patriarchal and ultranationalist worldview of gender relations. Toscano ended her intervention affirming that Montero as a woman, activist, and public representative is "the worst thing that has happened to Spain in the last few years" (Deputy Congress, November 23, 2022). As maternity is a central element in Vox's conception of women, Montero has also been attacked in this regard. The far right have disseminated a hoax, accusing the minister of using cabinet members as babysitters.

Therefore, the pandemic has allowed them to amplify, diversify, and radicalize their discursive frameworks and tactics. This antifeminist backlash has sometimes adopted benevolent types of sexism, aiming to propose and promote both traditional and more modern ultranationalist femininities. However, most of the time, it aggressively assumes the most radical forms of hostile sexism, even breaking the rules of the democratic system as they aim to remove their enemies.

The Antifeminist Agenda for the Crisis: Lawfare, Neoliberalism, Protest, and Mainstreaming

Vox has put this sexist outlook into practice through a series of measures, with the intention of setting the political agenda during the COVID-19 crisis. There are at least four types of strategies that the radical right party employs to attain its antifeminist goals: first, using legal means to criminalize feminism, question the legality of equality politics, and harass those considered enemies; second, arguing from a neoliberal perspective that any feminist politics involve an unnecessary expense within a context of global health crisis marked by shortage, unemployment, and uncertainty; third, stirring up citizens via the imitation of national and transnational far-right and progressive social movements' collective contention repertories; and finally, developing their antifeminist culture through slogans, celebrations, and clothes aims to create common symbols and spaces that generate a collective identification against feminism.

The celebration of Vistalegre III on May 8, 2020, is remarkable, because it confirmed Vox's antifeminism logic reinforced during the health crisis. The event was conceived as a response to the "leftist cultural agenda" after "decades of progressive politics", and at the same time as an alternative place to "leftist thought" where people can freely express ideas against the "feminist establishment" in a space of fraternity and freedom (Vox Spain, March 8, 2020a). Following the member of the European Parliament Jorge Buxadé, they faced the "inappropriate use of women with political purposes" by the "radical and violent feminism" against men and other women that dissent from their "gender ideology". He continued affirming that feminists deny admitting the sexual violence of immigrants and, at the same time, that the only worthy identity is the native one (Vox Spain, March 8, 2020i). The idea that Vox is the one who dares to give voice to what many people think without saying is a recurrent element in their speeches which generates a feeling of distinction and comradeship. Moreover, this is why there is a constant definition of what they are, true Spaniards, in opposition to all the rest: feminists, migrants, left-leaning people, etc. This rhetoric is tinged with a constant feeling of superiority, audacity, rejection, blaming others, and, consequently, ultranationalism.

Vox's recent participation in the political institutions has provoked unprecedented effects on the Spanish far right that have aimed to set in the center of the political arena debates that were minoritarian and seldom formulated previously. For this objective, one of its four strategic pillars is employing the courts of law as a political struggle mechanism. Days after Vistalegre III, when the health crisis was confirmed, and even though hundreds of people were infected there, Vox leaders blamed the 8M demonstration, the government, and especially the Minister of Equality, for the outbreak. In addition to demanding their resignation, they opened the "legal course of action". This policy has become essential for the far right in the public sphere, following the path introduced by secular associations associated with Christian values at the beginning of the 2000s. It was precisely these new ultraconservative social collectives who launched the first judicial proceedings as a systematic tactic against the socialist government of Jose Luis Rodríguez Zapatero, which approved what they considered sensitive political issues, such as same-sex marriage, abortion, or divorce (Álvarez-Benavides and Jiménez Aguilar 2021, 5–7).

The judicial proceedings against the government for allowing and promoting the 8M demonstration failed, and the court dismissed the lawsuit in June 2020, but the radical right party realized the possibilities of this avenue as a way to dictate the political agenda and to publicize their topics in public opinion. In addition to this cause, Vox has reported any individuals who have defined this political organization as extreme right or who have signaled its links with ideologies such as fascism, Nazism, and Francoism, or even those who consider its political ideas an actual risk for the social rights achieved in Spain. As an example of its targets, Vox has reported several members of the government, such as the Gender Violence Delegate (Vox Spain, July 6, 2022l), the Minister of Industry (Vox Spain, May 11, 2021d), the former Second Deputy Prime Minister and leader of UP (Vox Spain, November 5, 2022o), the Minister of Equality –including a complaint for incitement because of promoting sexual education courses for children– as well as different political leaders (Vox Spain, May 7, 2021c) and social network activists (Vox Spain, July 13, 2021e).

This judicial scheme makes sense and has become particularly useful for the radical right during the pandemic. In a scenario of uncertainty and exceptionality, a national and global emergency, the idea of accountability and assumption of responsibility has become a central claim for citizens as they seek to understand the crisis's origins and development, as well as the manner in which it has been managed. Through its decisions and interactions, the judicial institution legitimizes certain narratives about the causes of the crisis. Consequently, the instrumentalization of the judiciary allows the feminist movement and its leading voices to be singled out and tarnished in a context where many citizens "need" scapegoats.

Another strategy employed during the COVID-19 crisis against feminism involves a turn to a neoliberal (Ferreira 2019, 91) and welfare-chauvinist logic (Rama et al. 2021). Vox has employed arguments that aim to be based on economic rationality, looking to reduce or eliminate any social policies not in line with this view and to present feminism as a source of economic harm related to tax increases and non-justified expenses (Vox Spain, November 6, 2020e). Their political program "Let's Protect Spain" (*Protejamos España*), published at the end of March 2020, was dedicated to tackling the epidemiological and economic consequences. It is another example of how Vox considered the pandemic as a perfect chance to insert its political targets into the public debate. The "Ten urgent measures to safeguard the health and economy of the Spanish people" (Vox Spain, 2020b) perfectly summarize their ideological objectives: shrinking the State, centralization, and eradication of subsidies to political parties, trade unions, business organizations, and NGOs (measures 3, 7, 8, 9, and 10); militarization, securitization, and strengthening border controls (measures 2, 6, and 7); anti-Europeanism, anti-globalization, anti-environmentalism, and populism (measures 1, 2, 3, 4, 5, 6, and 10).

Consequently, the reason for eradicating institutions and politics favoring women's rights is that it is a means to eliminating unnecessary public spending, especially during a national emergency. This discourse, even with the intention of being rooted in rationality, is nevertheless formulated with aggressivity and verbal abuse. Therefore, feminist and gender equality institutions are defined as "lobbies", "shady feminist companies", or even a "mafia" (Vox Collado Mediano 2021). Feminism is considered a social actor that uses lies and intimidation to obtain political and economic benefits. For that reason, the mere existence of the Ministry of Equality is unacceptable. Vox rejects any measure coming from this department and constantly disseminates hoaxes and fake news related to its budget or the cost of different campaigns in favor of gender equality at the regional (Vox Spain, November 24, 2021h, September 20, 2022m, September 21, 2022n) and national levels (Vox Spain, March 30, 2022f, March 31, 2022g). Macarena Olona, former representative, summarized in a few words the party's view about the Ministry when she stated that "the best equality policy is to make the Ministry of Equality disappear" (Vox Spain, December 22, 2021j).

This institutional antifeminism has an international scope, promoted from outside Spain, which Vox has rapidly joined. They supported, for example, the campaign against the 2030 Agenda –The Sustainable Development Goals– formulated in 2015 by the United Nations General Assembly, and whose principles guided the European Union Recovery Instrument and the Spanish Government's Recovery, Transformation, and Resilience Plan. For the radical right organization, these blueprints are a manifestation of globalist agents conniving with the feminist struggle that consists of destroying the nation and the natural order. Vox representative Carla Toscano explained this theory on Instagram:

> Gender ideology is the cultural battle of our time. There are supranational powers and organizations that seek the destruction of human nature, the destruction of the family. This can only be achieved with a lot of propaganda and unjust laws, such as gender and "equality" laws, LGBT laws, abortion and euthanasia laws. It is about evil triumphing. That is why I speak of Good, Truth and Beauty, because only when we make these values prevail can we effectively combat everything that this gender ideology stands for
>
> *(Toscano, October 5, 2021g)*

A third strategy during the pandemic entailed discrediting feminism, its demands, and symbols, by emptying them of meaning or resignifying them. In 2021, they proposed to rename 8M as the "National Day for Victims of Coronavirus" to honor the dead persons due to the previous year's demonstration (LibertadDigital, March 6, 2021) and, in the process, eliminating the most important feminist celebration. Even in 2022, though they did not echo this proposal again, they refused to participate in any event in favor of equality, arguing again the unnecessary waste that feminist politics entails, particularly because of the recent war in Ukraine (Vox Spain, March 8, 2022c). In a clip entitled #NoHablesEnMiNombre, they included different images of the feminist movement in between references to the increase of squatting, energy poverty, inflation, and the reduction of families' purchasing power (Vox Spain, March 8, 2022h). This imbrication of antifeminism and neoliberal rationality is also completed with an Islamophobic pattern, as they used the hashtag that went viral after several incidents against Muslim people following the terrorist attacks on Charlie Hebdo and Bataclan in Paris in 2015.

They have also tried to establish a counter-calendar of antifeminist festivities. For example, they attempt to redefine the International Day for the Elimination of

Violence against Women, celebrated on November 25. In 2020, Vox representative Patricia Rueda read a statement and asked people to observe a minute's silence in "defense of all victims of violence, no matter their sex, nationality or any other characteristics" (Vox Spain, November 24, 2020g, November 25, 2020h). Thus, she wanted to deny the gender violence frame, speaking about "intrafamilial violence" to justify the abolition of the law to prevent male violence against women. She proposed a new law that does not "criminalize men" but punishes convicted felons with tougher sentences (Toscano, May 25, 2021d; Vox Spain, June 8, 2022k). Vox also joined other transnational antifeminist celebrations as the "Falsely Accused Day" on September 9, 2022. This initiative, born in the United Kingdom in 2021, and which has expanded to America the following year, was popularized thanks to Carla Toscano, aiming to justify the abolition of any kind of gender violence law due to the injustices and false accusations that thousands of men supposedly suffer (Toscano, June 8, 2021e, March 19, 2022a; Vox Spain, May 26, 2022j).

Vox is supported by a growing antifeminist culture and, at the same time, wants to be a central national and international social actor in the production and reproduction of this culture. Hence, in its everyday ultranationalism (Fox and Miller-Idris 2008), the political party is developing a type of far-right activism where antifeminism also plays a central role. In addition to the constant presence of the Spanish flag in rallies, demonstrations, and as an outfit element –used to distinguish the real and the non-Spaniards– they have created a whole structure of artifacts and practices to distribute systematically different antifeminist mottos, slogans, and chants, combined with other ideological mantras tied to ultranationalism, anti-multiculturalism, or islamophobia.

It is precisely in daily life where its antifeminism has become a potent discursive and practical element, beyond its opposition to equality politics, new plural gender roles, and public feminist institutions. Vox conceive their antifeminism as a symbolic component of collective identity that provides them with a sense of pride, develops a feeling of belonging and of being different. This new political field, which it has explored intensely during the pandemic, has involved different shapes and tactics. In addition to the resignification or appropriation of common feminist symbols, they have also used performances, humor, and parodies, especially through social network sites, and aimed to connect with a wider and more plural audience to enhance their institutional antifeminist backlash with an everyday and more social outlook.

In the same way that the market has coopted feminism through merchandising, such as mugs, films, or music (Zeisler 2016), it has also started to offer new products for the antifeminist public. Politicians such as Macarena Olona and Carla Toscano usually dress in clothes with antifeminist slogans. These outfits resemble sports and music merchandising, with the goal of providing a fresher, more youthful image, and generating a kind of brand identity (Miller-Idriss 2017, 51–81). The slogans refer to well-known right-wing mottos, such as "Make Men Great Again" –Trumpism– or "Stop This Feminist Agenda" – Identitarianism – or national and international feminist, housing, or antiracist movements, such as: "Non feminist" (Toscano, September 24, 2022d); "Stop false accusations" (Toscano, September 13, 2022c); "This is what an anti-feminist looks like" (Toscano, September 7, 2022b); "*#NotMeToo*" (Toscano, October 23, 2021h); or "Unborn Lives Matters" (Toscano, January 26, 2021a). They also introduce souvenirs with common quotes like "I love patriarchy" (Toscano, October 14, 2022e) or "Keep Calm and Ignore Feminazis" (Toscano, September 24, 2021f). They mostly use English in this propaganda, primarily when they create their own sexist and antifeminist slogans, as a mark of distinction and to connect with a younger audience that constantly shares them on the manosphere. Some of them are: "Feminist Tears" (Toscano, February 13, 2021b), "Biology is real" (Toscano, November 19, 2020c), "Anti-Feminist" (Toscano, November 11, 2020b), and "You are not oppressed" (Toscano, September 25, 2020a). Finally, in addition to Vox's discursive violence and the common use of a language that combines yelling, axioms, and insults, some representatives have tried to innovate, making their speeches fashionable. Olona, in a public intervention in the Congress of Deputies, pronounced: "A man does not rape, a rapist does/ A man does not murder, a murderer does/ A man does not mistreat. An abuser mistreats. And a man does not humiliate. Humiliates the coward" (Olona, April 24, 2021). In short, we can identify different ways of combining tradition and modernity, which Vox explores, aspiring to articulate a more conscious antifeminism.

Conclusion

Vox has viewed the latest crisis provoked by the COVID-19 as an incredible opportunity to deploy all its antifeminist discourse and contention repertoires from a diversity of scopes. The far-right party's discourse against feminism was employed as the explanation for the vast majority of the pandemic issues, from the very beginning to the end. They affirmed that the explosion of infections in Spain occurred during the 8M feminist demonstrations, celebrated one week before the lockdown. During the next two years, they accused the Spanish government of being weak and authoritarian at the same time, because of supporting feminism. Over this period, Vox antifeminism has appeared in diverse places, with a range of intensity levels. Like other radical right parties, it manages several forms of sexism and misogyny, as well as various femininities. They propose different types that concur with its ultranationalist, neoliberal, familistic, antifeminist, and xenophobic worldview, both at the national and global level, while rejecting and denying any other type of woman outside the limits of their interpretive framework.

The COVID-19 crisis has permitted Vox to explore and develop its gender relations worldview in depth and to deploy its antifeminism in the institutions, streets, and everyday life. Among its strategies to fight feminism, they have emphasized the litigation culture started two decades ago by recently created secular associations loosely inspired by Christian values. They brought actions against the entire government, different ministers, political opponents, and activists, and have filed complaints against every law approved by the Ministry of Equality. At the same time, they have adopted an openly neoliberal position, consisting of questioning and rejecting every feminist institution or policy, using the economic situation brought about by the crises as an excuse. The party augments this discourse with a populist logic blaming every feminist actor, politician, institution, or policy for corruption. They assert that the true motivation of these agents is not equality, but personal gain.

Nevertheless, their symbolic and everyday strategies are probably the element which has gained the greatest relevance during the pandemic. Vox presents itself as the only party that proposes to reply and fight feminism on all the frontlines. For that, they try to empty of significance or resignify institutionalized feminist symbols and celebrations, and, simultaneously, to create an openly antifeminist culture. The radical right party proposed to rename the 8M as the "National Day for the Victims of Coronavirus". They refuse to participate in any institutional minute of silence for women victims of gender violence. They have also joined international antifeminist festivities, such as Falsely Accused Day. On the other hand, they have developed a complete marketing display consisting of antifeminist messages, hashtags, and slogans shared on social networks and printed on T-shirts and mugs. This everyday antifeminism is conceived as a civic act of rebellion, versus the "leftist dictatorship" and the "totalitarian feminism", as a response to the establishment that only they dare to formulate.

Antifeminism is a global upward tendency, and the pandemic has become an ideal scenario for normalizing this political trend. In this regard, Spain is not an exception, and the far right has focused on trying to set their antifeminist agenda at the center of public debate. Like feminism, antifeminism is transverse, and is the reason why denying sexism and gender inequality also involves rejecting most of the different forms of sexual, ethnic, racial, and religious diversity. We must insist on the growing importance of these "normalized" radical right parties such as Vox, which consciously articulates ultranationalist, antifeminist, and xenophobic discourses and practices. Like a virus, the populist radical right infects and transforms civil society and its institutions, and represents an increasingly real threat to equality and, ultimately, to democracy.

References

Alcaide Lara, Esperanza R. 2022. "La imagen de la mujer en VOX: el discurso antifeminista de la 'derecha radical' en España". *Discurso & Sociedad* 16, 2: 275–302.

Alonso, Alba, and Julia Espinosa-Fajardo. 2021. "*Blitzkrieg* against democracy: gender equality and the rise of the populist radical right in Spain". *Social Politics: International Studies in Gender, State & Society* 28, 3: 656–681. https://doi.org/10.1093/sp/jxab026.

Álvarez-Benavides, Antonio. 2018. "Fascism 2.0: the Spanish case". *Digitcult Sientific Journal on Digital Cultures* 3, 3: 61–74. https://doi.org/10.4399/97888255208976.

Álvarez-Benavides, Antonio, and Francisco Jiménez Aguilar. 2021. "La contra-programación cultural de Vox: secularización, género y antifeminismo". *Política y Sociedad* 58, 2. https://doi.org/10.5209/poso.74486.

Álvarez-Benavides, Antonio, and Matthew L. Turnbough. 2022. "Supporting oneself: the tensions of navigating a prolonged crisis among Spanish youth". *Current Sociology*. https://doi.org/10.1177/00113921221093094.

Brown, Wendy. 2019. *In the Ruins of Neoliberalism: The Rise of Antidemocratic Politics in the West*. New York: Columbia University Press.

Cabezas, Marta. 2022. "Silencing feminism? Gender and the rise of the nationalist far right in Spain". *Signs: Journal of Women in Culture and Society* 47, 2: 319–345. https://doi.org/10.1086/716858.

Cabezas González, Almudena. 2021. "Los Feminismos Ante La Nueva Extrema Derecha: Prácticas De Acuerpe Y Sororidades estratégicas Para La construcción De Un Horizonte De Equidad E Igualdad". *Encrucijadas. Revista Crítica De Ciencias Sociales* 21, 2.

Campillo, Inés. 2019. "'If we stop, the world stops': the 2018 feminist strike in Spain". *Social Movement Studies*, 18, 2: 252–258. https://doi.org/10.1080/14742837.2018.1556092.

Case, Mary Anne. 2019. "Trans formations in the Vatican's war on 'gender ideology'". *Signs: Journal of Women in Culture and Society* 44, 3: 639–664. https://doi.org/10.1086/701498.

Cornejo, Mónica, and José Ignacio Pichardo Galán. 2017. "From the pulpit to the streets: religious activism against gender issues in Spain". In *Anti-Gender Campaigns in Europe: Mobilizing against Equality*, edited by Roman Kuhar and David Paternotte, 152–165. Rowman & Littlefield.

El Debate. 2021. *Carla Toscano (Vox):* "Las mujeres ahora somos esclavas del feminismo". Filmed October 24, at YouTube. Video, 5:24. www.youtube.com/watch?v=IGngyhq1NxA.

Deputy Congress. 2022. "Sesión Plenaria" (23/11/2022)". Filmed November 23, 2021, at YouTube. Video, 11:54:58. www.youtube.com/watch?v=aB_NuDKa71g&t=35568s.

Dupuis-Déri, Francis. 2016. "State antifeminism". *International Journal for Crime, Justice and Social Democracy* 5, 2: 21–35. https://doi.org/10.5204/ijcjsd.v5i2.315.

Ferreira, Carles. 2019. "Vox como representante de la derecha radical en España: un estudio sobre su ideología". *Revista Española de Ciencia Política* 51: 73–98. https://doi.org/10.21308/recp.51.03.

Fox, Jon E., and Cynthia Miller-Idriss. 2008. "Everyday nationhood". *Ethnicities* 8, 4: 536–576. https://doi.org/10.1177/1468796808088925.

Graff, Agnieszka, and Elżbieta Korlczuk. 2022. *Anti-Gender Politics in the Populist Moment*. New York: Routledge.

GranCanariaTv.com. 2019. "'Costura en vez de feminismo, que es cancer' Alicia Rubio (Vox)". Filmed November 15, at YouTube. Video, 2:09. https://www.youtube.com/watch?v=9ADq8NgLcNA.

Idoiaga Mondragon, Nahia, Naiara Berasategi Sancho, Nekane Beloki Arizti, and Maite Belasko Txertudi. 2022. "#8M women's strikes in Spain: following the unprecedented social mobilization through Twitter". *Journal of Gender Studies* 31, 5: 639–653. https://doi.org/10.1080/09589236.2021.1881461.

LibertadDigital. 2021. "Entrevista a Carla Toscano: 'Vox es el partido que más protege a la mujer'". Filmed March 6, 2021, at YouTube. Video, 5:52. https://www.youtube.com/watch?v=Xz_GZci01qU.

Miller-Idriss, Cynthia. 2017. *The Extreme Gone Mainstream: Commercialization and Far Right Youth Culture in Germany*, Princeton and Oxford: Princeton University Press.

Mudde, Cas. 2019. *The Far Right Today*. Cambridge and Malden: Polity Press.

Olona, Macarena (@macarenaolona). 2021. "El hombre no viola, viola un violador". Instagram photo, April 24. www.instagram.com/p/COCswKRhvXL/.
El País. 2021. *Ayuso, sobre Iglesias:* "Voy a cambiar el lema: Comunismo o Libertad". Filmed March 15, at YouTube. Video, 1:55. www.youtube.com/watch?v=JFAvF7sMjdg.
Rama, José, Lisa Zanotti, Stuart J. Turnbull-Dugarte, and Andrés Santana. 2021. *Vox: The Rise of the Spanish Populist Radical Right*, London and New York: Routledge.
Rottenberg, Catherine. 2018. *The Rise of Neoliberal Feminism.* New York: Oxford University Press.
Sánchez, Rubén. 2022. "Carlos Corvalán es concejal de Vox en Mazarrón. Ha llamado 'puta' a la ministra Irene Montero. Ningún dirigente de su partido lo ha desautorizado todavía por ello: ni @Santi_ABASCAL, ni @ivanedlm, ni @monasterioR…" Twitter post, August 25. https://twitter.com/rubensancheztw/status/1562789290190393345?lang=es.
Toscano, Carla (@carla_eledh). 2020a. "Con mi queridísima Mazaly Aguilar en @restaurantedelariva. Como en casa. ¡Viva España!" Instagram photo, September 25. www.instagram.com/p/CFkTIYfJTtQ/.
Toscano, Carla (@carla_eledh). 2020b. "Las mujeres en España tenemos los mismos derechos que los hombres". Instagram photo, November 11. www.instagram.com/p/CHdHnFMq8Ic/.
Toscano, Carla (@carla_eledh). 2020c. "Señores del Partido Popular: la izquierda no les va a votar". Instagram photo, November 19. www.instagram.com/p/CHw3uTzKtWG/.
Toscano, Carla (@carla_eledh). 2020d. "Hoy con @crisesteb en el Parlamento vasco acompañando a nuestra valiente Amaia Martínez. Un honor escucharle oponerse a las propuestas feministas y totalitarias de Bildu. ¡Orgullosa de ti, Amaia!" Instagram photo, November 26. www.instagram.com/p/CIDvlzVpZHM/.
Toscano, Carla (@carla_eledh). 2021a. "Pendiente de ratificar y con fuertes presiones internacionales que promueven el crimen del aborto, hay que felicitar a los diputados hondureños por su valentía en defender el derecho a la vida de los más vulnerables". Instagram photo, January 26. www.instagram.com/p/CKgGmJ9KHNk/.
Toscano, Carla (@carla_eledh). 2021b. "Hoy quiero felicitar por su cumpleaños a nuestra inefable Irene Montero, comisaria de desigualdad del reino de España". Instagram photo, February 6. www.instagram.com/p/CLO_1QiBPXf/.
Toscano, Carla (@carla_eledh). 2021c. "En el #8M, la mejor referencia, la mejor madre". Instagram photo, March 8, 2021. www.instagram.com/p/CMKGKu2qnBu/.
Toscano, Carla (@carla_eledh). 2021d. "#LaViolenciaNoTieneSexo". Instagram photo, May 25, 2021. www.instagram.com/p/CPTx8Cqt64H/.
Toscano, Carla (@carla_eledh). 2021e. "Siempre con los padres inocentes víctimas del feminismo". Instagram photo, June 8. www.instagram.com/p/CP3ybxUNbSk/.
Toscano, Carla (@carla_eledh). 2021f. "Conspirando contra las feminazis con mi querido @pedromorenogmz. Por la igualdad de derechos de todos". Instagram photo, September 24, 2021. www.instagram.com/p/CUNJbIHtayu/.
Toscano, Carla (@carla_eledh). 2021g. "Gender ideology is the cultural battle of our time". Instagram photo, October 5. www.instagram.com/p/CUppWSWNGOg/.
Toscano, Carla (@carla_eledh). 2021h. "Las feministas no pueden negar la verdad: que en el fondo las mujeres les importan un bledo". Instagram photo, October 21. www.instagram.com/p/CVXsyIrAAI4/.
Toscano, Carla (@carla_eledh). 2021i. "EA". Instagram photo, October 24. www.instagram.com/p/CVa4xerNiUk/.
Toscano, Carla (@carla_eledh). 2022a. "#SanJosé #DíaDelPadre". Instagram photo, March 19. www.instagram.com/p/CbSHHyCtlP5/.

Toscano, Carla (@carla_eledh). 2022b. "El 9 de septiembre es el #DíaContraLasDenunciasFalsas". Instagram photo, September 7. www.instagram.com/p/CiOHQ8OMStz/.

Toscano, Carla (@carla_eledh). 2022c. "Hemos presentado una PNL de Custodia Compartida". Instagram photo, September 13. www.instagram.com/p/CickmPIuzH4/.

Toscano, Carla (@carla_eledh). 2022d. "Viva Chamartín". Instagram photo, September 24. www.instagram.com/p/Ci474b7NYr2/.

Toscano, Carla (@carla_eledh). 2022e. "Las dos camisetas más molonas que vais a ver hoy". Instagram photo, October 14. www.instagram.com/p/CjsVvGatNoM/.

Traverso, Enzo. 2001. *El totalitarismo. Historia de un debate.* Buenos Aires: Eudeba.

Vox Castellón (@CastellonVox). 2022. "Manifestación #8M en #Castellón". Twitter post, March 8. https://twitter.com/CastellonVox/status/1501271024087666691.

Vox Collado Mediano. 2021. "No hables en mi nombre". Facebook, March 9. www.facebook.com/watch/?v=263864091901628.

Vox Spain (@vox_es). 2019a. "Las mujeres de VOX rompen con la huelga feminista del 8M". Filmed March 4, at YouTube. Video, 2:59. www.youtube.com/watch?v=xmzYJxOwHuE.

Vox Spain (@vox_es). 2019b. "Así visitan las feminazis la sede de Vox… #8M". Filmed March 8, at YouTube. Video, 1:41. www.youtube.com/watch?v=ZNsFc5Ne9CQ.

Vox Spain (@vox_es). 2020a. "DIRECTO | VISTALEGRE III - LA ALTERNATIVA". Filmed March 8, at YouTube. Video, 1:59:28. www.youtube.com/watch?v=4jKQ7vtfETQ.

Vox Spain (@vox_es). 2020b. "Programa Protejamos España". Accessed July 2, 2023. www.voxespana.es/programa-protejamos-espana.

Vox Spain (@vox_es). 2020c. "Buxadé: 'En Vox ejercemos el derecho a disentir frente al totalitarismo progre'". Accessed July 2, 2023. www.voxespana.es/actualidad/buxade-en-vox-ejercemos-el-derecho-a-disentir-frente-al-totalitarismo-progre-20200227.

Vox Spain (@vox_es). 2020d. "Una alternativa para España". Accessed July 2, 2023. www.voxespana.es/vox-opinion/una-alternativa-para-espana-20200309.

Vox Spain (@vox_es). 2020e. "'En defensa de la dignidad de los españoles', enmienda a la totalidad". Accessed July 2. www.voxespana.es/grupo_parlamentario/actividad-parlamentaria/en-defensa-de-la-dignidad-de-los-espanoles-enmienda-a-la-totalidad-20201106.

Vox Spain (@vox_es). 2020f. "Vox califica de machista los cursos municipales para que las mujeres aprendan a conducir bicicletas". Accessed July 2, 2023. www.voxespana.es/noticias/vox-califica-de-machista-los-cursos-municipales-para-que-las-mujeres-aprendan-a-conducir-bicicletas-20201028?provincia=sevilla.

Vox Spain (@vox_es). 2020g. "Vox presenta una Declaración Institucional con motivo del Día Contra la Violencia Hacia la Mujer". Accessed July 2, 2023. www.voxespana.es/noticias/vox-presenta-una-declaracion-institucional-con-motivo-del-dia-contra-la-violencia-hacia-la-mujer-20201124?provincia=castellon.

Vox Spain (@vox_es). 2020h. "Vox guarda un minuto de silencio por todas las personas víctimas de violencia". Accessed July 2, 2023. www.voxespana.es/actualidad/vox-guarda-un-minuto-de-silencio-por-todas-las-personas-victimas-de-violencia-20201125.

Vox Spain (@vox_es). 2020i. "Vox ante el #8M". Filmed March 8, at YouTube. Video, 7:24. www.youtube.com/watch?v=BG_gQnpnx-M.

Vox Spain (@vox_es). 2021b. "El feminismo radical no entiende ni atiende a las necesidades reales de las mujeres que limpian sus porquerías". Twitter post, March 8. https://twitter.com/vox_es/status/1368998589037481984.

Vox Spain (@vox_es). 2021c. "Vox se querella contra Ione Belarra por delito de odio al identificar a la formación con el nazismo". Accessed July 2, 2023. www.voxespana.

es/actualidad/vox-se-querella-contra-ione-belarra-por-delito-de-odio-al-identificar-a-la-formacion-con-el-nazismo-20210507.

Vox Spain (@vox_es). 2021d. "Vox se querella contra Reyes Maroto por injurias, calumnias y delito de odio tras acusar a la formación de amenazar de muerte a los demócratas". Accessed July 2, 2023. www.voxespana.es/actualidad/vox-se-querella-reyes-maroto-injurias-calumnias-delito-odio-acusar-formacion-amenazar-muerte-democratas-20210511.

Vox Spain (@vox_es). 2021e. "Vox se querella contra la tuitera Martu Garrote por acusar a este partido de estar detrás de la muerte de Samuel Luiz". Accessed July 2, 2023. www.voxespana.es/noticias/vox-querella-la-tuitera-martu-garrote-acusar-este-partido-estar-detras-la-muerte-samuel-luiz-20210713.

Vox Spain (@vox_es). 2021f. "@Macarena_Olona sobre la ilegalización de Podemos y partidos separatistas". Twitter post, July 23. https://twitter.com/vox_es/status/1418622431716155395.

Vox Spain (@vox_es). 2021g. "Rubén Manso reivindica el orgullo de pertenencia a la familia, a España y a la Hispanidad". Accessed July 2, 2023. www.voxespana.es/noticias/ruben-manso-reivindica-el-orgullo-de-pertenencia-a-la-familia-a-espana-y-a-la-hispanidad-20211012?provincia=malaga.

Vox Spain (@vox_es). 2021h. "Ana Gil desmonta al feminismo más radical: 'Las leyes de género no sirven'". Accessed July 2, 2023. www.voxespana.es/noticias/ana-gil-desmonta-al-feminismo-mas-radical-las-leyes-de-genero-no-sirven-20211124.

Vox Spain (@vox_es). 2021i. "Vox exige acabar con el 'supremacismo feminista' y con la politización de la ideología de género". Accessed July 2, 2023. www.voxespana.es/vox-en-el-parlamento-de-cataluna/vox-exige-acabar-con-el-supremacismo-feminista-y-con-la-politizacion-de-la-ideologia-de-genero-20211202?provincia=barcelona-lerida-tarragona.

Vox Spain (@vox_es). 2021j. "Olona: 'La mejor política de igualdad es que desaparezca el Ministerio de Igualdad '". Accessed July 2, 2023. www.voxespana.es/grupo_parlamentario/actividad-parlamentaria/olona-la-mejor-politica-de-igualdad-es-que-desaparezca-el-ministerio-de-igualdad-20211222.

Vox Spain (@vox_es). 2022a. "¡Conoce a las valientes mujeres de VOX!" Filmed February 7, at YouTube. Video, 7:11. www.youtube.com/watch?v=kgdnCtiIbi0.

Vox Spain (@vox_es). 2022b. "Vox homenajea a la primera mujer piloto, una 'mujer sin cuota' que 'apostó por la igualdad de oportunidades'". Accessed July 2, 2023. www.voxespana.es/grupo_parlamentario/actividad-parlamentaria/vox-homenajea-a-la-primera-mujer-piloto-una-mujer-sin-cuota-que-aposto-por-la-igualdad-de-oportunidades-20220307.

Vox Spain (@vox_es). 2022c. "Espinosa: 'La luz al alza y más de 20.000 millones para políticas feministas ... es un insulto'". Accessed July 2, 2023. www.voxespana.es/grupo_parlamentario/espinosa-la-luz-al-alza-y-mas-de-20-000-millones-para-politicas-feministas-es-un-insulto-20220308.

Vox Spain (@vox_es). 2022d. "Ángela Mulas confirma que VOX no participará en la 'farsa feminista del 8M' que busca 'colectivizar e instrumentalizar a las mujeres'". Accessed July 2, 2023. www.voxespana.es/noticias/angela-mulas-confirma-que-vox-no-participara-en-la-farsa-feminista-del-8m-que-busca-colectivizar-e-instrumentalizar-a-las-mujeres-20220308.

Vox Spain (@vox_es). 2022e. "Vox no se adhiere a los manifiestos ni del 8M ni del Consejo Local de la Mujer". Accessed July 2, 2023. www.voxespana.es/noticias/vox-no-se-adhiere-manifiestos-8m-consejo-local-mujer-20220308?provincia=toledo.

Vox Spain (@vox_es). 2022f. "De Meer, a Montero: 'Se va a gastar cuatro veces el presupuesto del ministerio de Sanidad en un plan ideológico'". Accessed July 2, 2023. www.voxespana.es/grupo_parlamentario/actividad-parlamentaria/de-meer-a-montero-se-va-a-gastar-cuatro-veces-el-presupuesto-del-ministerio-de-sanidad-en-un-plan-ideologico-20220330.

Vox Spain (@vox_es). 2022g. "Vox exige a Ruiz que deje de gastar dinero en políticas de género 'que no llevan a defender a la mujer' tras conocer que la publicidad del 8M costó más de 123.000 €". Accessed July 2, 2023. www.voxespana.es/noticias/vox-demanda-a-ruiz-que-deje-de-gastar-dinero-en-politicas-de-genero-que-no-llevan-a-defender-a-la-mujer-y-se-centre-en-politicas-de-conciliacion-de-la-familia-20220331.

Vox Spain (@vox_es). 2022h. "#NoHablesEnMiNombre | Stop feminismo". Filmed March 8, at YouTube. Video, 1:41. www.youtube.com/watch?v=RIeR1qvuztk.

Vox Spain (@vox_es). 2022i. "Macarena Olona a Irene Montero: 'Quiero romper las cadenas que nos ha impuesto el feminismo'". Filmed May 11, at YouTube. Video, 2:34. www.youtube.com/watch?v=eO8BwVDzC28.

Vox Spain (@vox_es). 2022j. "'Ley solo sí es sí: Toscano rechaza al 'Gobierno que indulta a secuestradoras; de sus manos contaminadas no puede salir una ley justa'". Accessed July 2, 2023. www.voxespana.es/grupo_parlamentario/actividad-parlamentaria/ley-solo-si-es-si-toscano-rechaza-al-gobierno-que-indulta-a-secuestradoras-de-sus-manos-contaminadas-no-puede-salir-una-ley-justa-20220526.

Vox Spain (@vox_es). 2022k. "La contundente respuesta de Olona frente al feminismo: 'hombres y mujeres somos complementarios'". Filmed June 8, at YouTube. Video, 2:43. www.youtube.com/watch?v=Q17aWaMXyvs.

Vox Spain (@vox_es). 2022l. "Vox se querella contra la delegada del Gobierno de Violencia de Género tras afirmar en TVE que la formación 'es un riesgo' para las menores". Accessed July 2, 2023. www.voxespana.es/actualidad/vox-querella-delegada-gobierno-violencia-genero-afirmar-tve-formacion-riesgo-menores-20220706.

Vox Spain (@vox_es). 2022m. "'El camino del arcoíris', lenguaje no sexista … los 500.000 euros de Igualdad a examen: Vox pregunta por el despilfarro en el ministerio de Irene Montero". Accessed July 2, 2023. www.voxespana.es/grupo_parlamentario/actividad-parlamentaria/el-camino-del-arcoiris-lenguaje-no-sexista-los-500-000-euros-de-igualdad-a-examen-vox-pregunta-por-el-despilfarro-en-el-ministerio-de-irene-montero-20220920.

Vox Spain (@vox_es). 2022n. "Vox critica las nuevas ayudas de Igualdad de la Xunta de Galicia porque "promueven la desigualdad entre hombres y mujeres". Accessed July 2, 2023. www.voxespana.es/noticias/vox-critica-las-nuevas-ayudas-de-igualdad-de-la-xunta-de-galicia-porque-promueven-la-desigualdad-entre-hombres-y-mujeres-20220921?provincia=la-coruna-lugo-ourense-pontevedra.

Vox Spain (@vox_es). 2022o. "'Tarjeta SIM': VOX quiere llegar hasta el final y se querella contra Dina por simulación de delito, estafa procesal y falso testimonio". Accessed July 2, 2023. www.voxespana.es/noticias/tarjeta-sim-vox-quiere-llegar-hasta-el-final-y-se-querella-contra-dina-por-simulacion-de-delito-estafa-procesal-y-falso-testimonio-20221105.

Zeisler, Andi. 2016. *We Were Feminists Once: From Riot Grrrl to CoverGirl®, the Buying and Selling of a Political Movement*. New York: Public Affairs.

INDEX